Managing the Side Effects of Psychotropic Medications

Second Edition

Managing the Side Effects of Psychotropic Medications

Second Edition

Joseph F. Goldberg, M.D., M.S.

Clinical Professor of Psychiatry
Icahn School of Medicine at Mount Sinai
New York, New York

Carrie L. Ernst, M.D.

Associate Professor of Psychiatry and Medical Education
Icahn School of Medicine at Mount Sinai
New York, New York

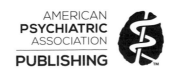

AMERICAN
PSYCHIATRIC
ASSOCIATION
PUBLISHING

Copyright © 2019 American Psychiatric Association
ALL RIGHTS RESERVED

Manufactured in the United States of America on acid-free paper
26 25 24 23   9 8 7 6
Second Edition

Typeset in The Mix and Book Antiqua.

American Psychiatric Association
800 Maine Ave., SW
Suite 900
Washington, DC 20024-2812
www.appi.org

Library of Congress Cataloging-in-Publication Data
Names: Goldberg, Joseph F., author. | Ernst, Carrie L., author.
Title: Managing the side effects of psychotropic medications / Joseph F. Goldberg, Carrie L. Ernst.
Description: Second edition. | Washington, D.C. : American Psychiatric Association Publishing, [2019] | Includes bibliographical references and index.
Identifiers: LCCN 2018023606 (print) | LCCN 2018024418 (ebook) | ISBN 9781615372034 (ebook) | ISBN 9781585624881 (pbk. : alk. paper)
Subjects: | MESH: Psychotropic Drugs—adverse effects
Classification: LCC RM315 (ebook) | LCC RM315 (print) | NLM QV 77.2 | DDC 615.7/88—dc23
LC record available at https://lccn.loc.gov/2018023606

British Library Cataloguing in Publication Data
A CIP record is available from the British Library.

To our children, Joshua, Brian, Hannah, and Jonah,
for their patience, encouragement, and love;
and to our parents, Arline and Robert Zinaman,
Ethel Goldberg, and to the memory of Daniel Goldberg,
for their commitment and omnipresence;

and to each other,
for everything in between

Contents

PART I

General Considerations

PART III

Summary Recommendations

Foreword to the Second Edition

This second edition of *Managing the Side Effects of Psychotropic Medications* by Drs. Goldberg and Ernst builds powerfully on the first edition, providing updated information that is otherwise unavailable in psychopharmacology textbooks. The book is a thoughtful yet practical compendium of why psychotropic drugs cause side effects and what to do about them. We practitioners are inundated with clinical trial data that generally emphasize efficacy over tolerability. If results from randomized controlled trials generate efficacy information that is sometimes difficult to figure out how to apply in a clinical practice setting, translating tolerability data from these trials into what to expect in terms of side effects in a real-world setting can be even more difficult. Often, relevant information on tolerability is simply lacking because of the way that these data are collected and presented for regulatory purposes. Furthermore, the data on side effects usually end up in a blizzard of unreadable small-font package inserts from the U.S. Food and Drug Administration (FDA) or buried in clinical trial reports on sometimes obscure Web sites. We consult these sources to learn about side effects, but frequently we find such sources of information not very useful because these data really are presented as rules for what pharmaceutical sales personnel can say and not guidelines for how to practice psychiatry. It takes the approach adopted here by Drs. Goldberg and Ernst to help us know the straight story on what really to expect and what to do when we see the unexpected.

How do these authors do it? They combine comprehensive and scholarly coverage of just about everything that can happen after taking a psychotropic drug, with pragmatic, old-fashioned "bedside" tips and pearls about how to manage these problems, explaining the rationale and not merely giving empirical instructions. Their advice makes sense, and thus readers are likely to use this information. I found myself learning a number of things I did not know, remembering numerous facts I had long forgotten, and comprehending a number of points that I knew empirically but did not really understand. For example, I particularly enjoyed the section helping me to become an amateur dermatologist and the tables on sexual dysfunction and weight gain. Rashes freak out most psychiatrists, and sexual dysfunction and weight gain are the kiss of death for adherence by most patients, and I very much appreciated the advice of the authors. There are many other examples of particularly helpful areas, ranging from what is the most common to what is the most dangerous. Every reader will have his or her own response to the various sections, but probably no reader knows all of the information presented here, and thus every clinician is likely to benefit from this text in a very unique and personalized manner.

The fingerprints of wise clinician-authors are all over this text, as exemplified by the way they set a context, weigh the strength of the evidence honestly, and discuss broad as well as niche issues. For example, their discussion in Chapter 1, "The Psychiatrist as Physician," on the nocebo phenomenon (a particularly frustrating bugaboo for me in clinical practice) gently reminded me that some patients, for their own psychodynamic reasons, try to frustrate our helping efforts rather than align with them. Where do readers ever see that topic discussed in a textbook of psychopharmacology or a manufacturer's package insert?

The authors also deconstruct complex situations into understandable component parts, ranging from the pharmacokinetic, with useful resurrection of often-neglected use of judicious and targeted therapeutic drug monitoring, to the pharmacodynamic, explicating one drug and one mechanism at a time in a specialty filled with combination treatments. The authors grab the bull by the horns to grapple with the question of what does a clinician do when certain side effects cannot be avoided — resolving this quandary by providing thoughtful approaches on how to weigh risks with benefits — and reminding us that sometimes greater benefits come with justifiable but necessarily greater risks. This is an example of how these authors handle numerous and quite sophisticated clinical issues. That is, not only do the authors tell readers a lot, because the authors clearly know a lot, but they also present information in a way that reminds us that it is not enough to know it all. In fact, it is only realistic to have all the information available in a reference source such as this and not complete in our memory. However, the authors leave us with something else: they impart a bit of wisdom, which is what we learn *after* we know it all.

Welcome to a valuable and unique work of practical scholarship to help readers on their voyage through the entire field of psychopharmacology.

Stephen M. Stahl, M.D., Ph.D.
Adjunct Professor of Psychiatry, University of California, San Diego

Preface

In developing the second edition of this text, we sought to incorporate information about new psychotropic drugs since publication of the first edition, as well as summarize advances in knowledge about identifiable risk factors for adverse effects (particularly in pharmacogenetics) and update recommendations on viable "antidote" management strategies. The latter strategies include recognizing emerging novel pharmacotherapies for tardive dyskinesia, newer agents for weight loss, and newer meta-analytic data on comparative risks for cardiovascular and metabolic adverse effects from second-generation antipsychotics and other psychotropic agents. We are grateful for the enthusiastic positive feedback we have received from many readers of the first edition and have attempted to incorporate many useful points and ideas brought to our attention.

As we noted in the first edition, to understand the adverse effects of a medication means to fully appreciate its effects on the body. The pharmacodynamic and pharmacokinetic profile of a drug is manifested by the entirety of its actions, intended and unintended, beneficial or adverse, expected or unexpected. We undertook the writing of this book to help mental health practitioners better understand the consequences of drug therapies they may prescribe (or avoid), the range of available strategies to effectively manage adverse effects, and the scientific and practical implications of their treatment decisions.

We interchangeably use the terms *adverse effect* and *side effect* to indicate any undesirable or unintended pharmacodynamic event that is separate from the intended main effects of a medication, although the World Health Organization links "noxious" with "unintended" in defining a drug's effect as "adverse." "Side" effects, by contrast, may sometimes be capitalized on for their unintended but potentially beneficial actions — as in the case of soporific effects caused by strong histamine H_1 receptor antagonists such as quetiapine or mirtazapine, or the appetite suppressant and weight-loss effects that are associated with a drug such as topiramate.

When should a drug be stopped or avoided because of adverse effects, or when do benefits outweigh risks of continuing? Clinicians must consider the medical seriousness of an apparent side effect, its tran-sience or persistence, its impact on adherence, and the availability of alternative therapeutics. As in other areas of medicine, practitioners must gauge the severity of the ailment being treated and the uniqueness of an existing efficacious therapy.

Some readers of the first edition of this book shared with us their impressions that, while we described possible remedies for managing many adverse drug effects, a more directive or algorithmic approach of "what to do" might be preferable. We agree that a definitive management strategy should be adopted if it exists (e.g., immediate cessation of lamotrigine after a severe skin rash). However, dogmatic recommendations are often impractical and fail to take into account the unique risk–benefit circumstances that vary from patient to patient. Rather than provide a "cookbook" approach to clinical management, our hope has instead been to provide practitioners with a sufficient breadth of information necessary for them to make informed decisions on a case-by-case basis.

Strategies to best anticipate, identify, and manage drug side effects vary considerably. Sometimes, fairly extensive databases exist, comparing different types of interventions that have been empirically studied to counteract a well-known side effect, with varying levels of scientific rigor and support (e.g., antidotes for antidepressant-induced sexual dysfunction); at other times, little or no empirical data are available apart from anecdotal experience. Overreliance on anecdotal impressionism incurs the risk of forming wrong or scientifically implausible inferences about cause and effect. At the opposite extreme, when controlled trials do exist that study interventions to counteract a drug side effect, they may have limited value because they are seldom conducted with adequate statistical power to stratify or control for possible confounding factors (e.g., medications that are intended to counteract psychotropic-induced weight gain may vary in efficacy depending on which agents cause the weight gain, patients' baseline body mass index and other clinical features, concomitant therapies, and other relevant characteristics). Pharmacotherapy trials undertaken by industry sponsors are usually driven by the pursuit of product indications from the U.S. Food and Drug Administration (FDA), rather than by initiatives to counteract (and draw attention to) the adverse effects of a proprietary drug—in other words, there is a dearth of systematic research on the treatment of side effects.

Because the information that exists about options for managing side effects is often variable in volume and content, we have prefaced discussions about many clinical problems with general recommendations that synthesize research-based findings with our own clinical experience to provide "bottom-line" suggestions for clinical management. A balance always needs to be struck between scientifically grounded, empirically studied interventions (which often require extrapolation to heterogeneous patient groups) and homespun remedies that may be too idiosyncratic or untested to be considered generalizable. For situations in which little or no data are available in the literature to inform treatment recommendations specific to counteracting adverse drug effects, we have relied on clinical experience, theoretical rationales, and inferences from other areas to the extent doing so seemed appropriate. Although virtually all of the suggested pharmacological strategies to counteract adverse drug effects that are described in this volume are "off label" from FDA-approved uses, we sought to ensure that they are scientifically plausible and informed by the experience of empirical observations.

As in the first edition, we deliberated over how annotated a text of this nature should be. Our purpose was to provide a readable and accessible compendium of practical information for busy clinicians, rather than a comprehensive, scholarly review of the supportive literature for any and all possible iatrogenic drug effects. We therefore supplemented our own clinical experience with selective literature reviews when it seemed wise to do so, citing pertinent randomized trials, open trials, and case reports where useful. Where data were lacking on issues that clinical experience alone seemed insufficient to offer recommendations, we contacted pharmaceutical manufacturers to determine the availability of information on areas of clinical concern (e.g., the cross-sensitivity of anticonvulsant rashes with sulfa antibiotics). The citation of individual case reports always poses difficulties for purposes of generalizability; they provide a very limited degree of evidence that may point to an association between an intervention and an untoward outcome, and their purpose in the literature is more to prompt thinking or generate hypotheses rather than test them. On the other hand, for purposes of a book such as this, case reports afford documentation not on the incidence or generalizability of an adverse effect, but rather of the recognition and plausibility for a suspected link between a treatment and an outcome.

We have strived to provide a reasonably thorough review of common or clinically important adverse effects while at the same time offering a context that does not overstate trivial or obscure reported side effects that have little relevance to everyday practice. Sufficient detail is crucial for practitioners to feel they are well equipped to manage such bread-and-butter issues as psychotropic-induced weight gain, metabolic dysregulation, sexual dysfunction, skin rashes, sleep disturbances, cognitive complaints, and other neurological concerns. Our hope is that readers will gain a greater sense of confidence in their medical decision making and comfort level in understanding, anticipating, and managing (rather than simply avoiding) the relative risks of psychotropic agents.

The book has been divided into three main sections. Part I deals with global issues that bear on the assessment and formulation of possible adverse effects and with pertinent concepts related to basic pharmacology, physiology, and medical monitoring. The chapters in Part II present information organized by individual organ systems or specific medical circumstances rather than by drugs or drug classes. This approach seems to provide a logical and comprehensible format that allows readers to search out information as referenced by a particular side effect (and its varied potential causes) and to locate a discussion of practical management strategies. Part III focuses on summary recommendations covering all the material presented in the book and is followed by helpful appendixes on self-assessment questions and resources for practitioners. The book is meant to serve as a ready reference that simultaneously provides scientific and scholarly discussion of available treatment options and presents their scientific rationales.

Clinicians who teach medical students and psychiatry residents, who collaborate with colleagues from other medical disciplines, and who treat many patients quickly realize that skillful psychopharmacology demands a reasonable working knowledge of primary care medicine—a knowledge base that is often minimally addressed during most internships or residencies in psychiatry—and remarkably, is seldom incorporated into formal continuing medical education activities for psychiatrists. This book is intended as a tool to help bridge that educational gap.

We are deeply grateful to a number of colleagues who have kindly offered their expertise and provided us with helpful comments on sections of this book, including Ross J. Baldessarini, M.D.; Richard Balon, M.D.; Lesley Berk, M.A.; Beth Counselman Carpenter, Ph.D., L.C.S.W., M.S.W.; Anita H. Clayton, M.D.; David Colbert, M.D.; Andrew Cutler, M.D.; Howard Eison, M.D.; Marlene Freeman, M.D.; Glen O. Gabbard, M.D.; Steven Glazer, M.D.; James W. Jefferson, M.D.; Ethan Kisch, M.D.; Rajnish Mago, M.D.; Henry Nasrallah, M.D.; Sheldon Preskorn, M.D.; Stephen M. Stahl, M.D., Ph.D.; Neil J. Stone, M.D.; Holly Swartz, M.D.; Peter J. Weiden, M.D.; Kimberly Yonkers, M.D.; and Rachel Fischer, M.P.A., R.D., C.D.N.

As clinicians and educators, we could not have undertaken this task without the stimulation provided by our patients, students, and colleagues. A tremendous sense of gratification comes from being able to explain in clear and simple terms how and why an intervention causes an understandable effect—whether desirable or undesirable—and from navigating through logical strategies to maximize benefits while minimizing risks. At its best, medical decision-making hinges on thoughtful deliberation and problem solving—reflecting the capacity to integrate the clinician's own experience with an awareness of empirically validated findings and the ability to differentiate between problems caused by diseases and problems caused by their intended remedies. The sum of these skills finds its ultimate expression in the ability to balance treatment risks and benefits with logic, forethought, and wisdom.

Joseph F. Goldberg, M.D., M.S.
Carrie L. Ernst, M.D.

Disclosures of Interest

Joseph F. Goldberg, M.D., M.S.—*Speakers' bureau:* Merck and Co. Inc., Neurocrine, Otsuka Pharmaceuticals, Sunovion Pharmaceuticals, Takeda-Lundbeck; *Advisor/consultant:* Medscape, Neurocrine Continental Inc., Otsuka Pharmaceutical Development and Commercialization Inc., Sunovion Pharmaceuticals, Supernus Pharmaceuticals, WebMD; *Major stockholder:* None; *Employee:* None.

Carrie L. Ernst, M.D., is married to Joseph F. Goldberg, M.D., and has no independent competing interests to disclose.

List of Abbreviations

The following abbreviations are used frequently throughout this book without being spelled out.

ACE	angiotensin-converting enzyme
ADHD	attention-deficit/hyperactivity disorder
ALT	alanine aminotransferase
ASCVD	atherosclerotic cardiovascular disease
AST	aspartate aminotransferase
AUC	area under the curve
A-V	atrioventricular
bid	twice daily (bis in die)
BMI	body mass index
CATIE	Clinical Antipsychotic Trials of Intervention Effectiveness
CBC	complete blood count
CI	confidence interval
CK	creatine kinase
Cmax	maximal drug plasma concentration
CNS	central nervous system
Cr	creatinine
CR	controlled release
CrCl	creatinine clearance
CRP	C-reactive protein
C_{ss}	steady-state plasma concentration
CYP	cytochrome P450
DORA	dual orexin receptor antagonist
DR	delayed release
eGFR	estimated glomerular filtration rate
EPS	extrapyramidal symptoms
ER	extended release
ESRD	end-stage renal disease

FAERS	FDA Adverse Event Reporting System
FDA	U.S. Food and Drug Administration
FGA	first-generation antipsychotic
FRS	Framingham Risk Score
GABA	γ-aminobutyric acid
GAD	generalized anxiety disorder
HbA_{1C}	hemoglobin A1C
HDL	high-density lipoprotein
hERG	human ether-à-go-go–related gene
HMGCR	3-hydroxy-3-methylglutaryl-coenzyme A reductase
IgE	immunoglobulin E
IM	intramuscular
INR	international normalized ratio
IR	immediate release
K^+	potassium
LA	long acting (sustained release)
LAI	long-acting injectable
LDL	low-density lipoprotein
MAOI	monoamine oxidase inhibitor
Mg^+	magnesium
MI	myocardial infarction
MMSE	Mini-Mental State Exam
NAION	nonarteritic anterior ischemic optic neuropathy
NAS	neonatal abstinence syndrome
NDI	nephrogenic diabetes insipidus
NMS	neuroleptic malignant syndrome
NNH	number needed to harm
NNT	number needed to treat
NSAID	nonsteroidal anti-inflammatory drug
OCD	obsessive-compulsive disorder
OR	odds ratio
PCOS	polycystic ovary syndrome
PDE	phosphodiesterase
PDSS	post-injection delirium/sedation syndrome
PLLR	Pregnancy and Lactation Labeling Rule
PM	poor metabolizer
po	by mouth (per os)
PO_4	phosphorous
PPARγ	peroxisome proliferator-activated receptor gamma
PPHN	persistent pulmonary hypertension of the newborn
prn	as needed

PSM	perceived sensitivity to medicines
PUVA	psoralin plus ultraviolet A light
PVC	premature ventricular contraction
qd	once a day (quaque die)
qhs	every night at bedtime (quaque hora somni)
qid	four times daily (quarter in die)
REM	rapid eye movement
REMS	Risk Evaluation and Mitigation Strategies
SC	subcutaneous
SERM	selective estrogen receptor modulator
SGA	second-generation antipsychotic
SNP	single-nucleotide polymorphism
SNRI	serotonin-norepinephrine reuptake inhibitor
SR	sustained release
SRM	statin-related myotoxicity
SSRI	selective serotonin reuptake inhibitor
TCA	tricyclic antidepressant
TdP	torsades de pointes
tid	three times daily (ter in die)
Tmax	time until maximal drug plasma concentration
UGT	uridine 5′-diphosphate (UDP) glucuronosyltransferase
URM	ultrarapid metabolizer
V_d	volume of distribution
VLDL	very low density lipoprotein
XL	extended release
XR	extended release

List of Drugs

The following drugs mentioned or discussed in this book are listed alphabetically by drug class, with brand names in parentheses following the generic name (only generic names are used in the text). For classification of topical steroids for dermatological conditions, see Table 8–3.

Alcohol abuse or dependence treatments
Acamprosate (Campral)
Naltrexone (Revia) [opioid receptor antagonist]

Alzheimer's disease medications
Acetylcholinesterase inhibitors
　　Donepezil (Aricept)
　　Galantamine (Razadyne, Reminyl)
NMDA receptor antagonists
　　Memantine (Namenda)

Analgesics (nonnarcotic)
Acetaminophen (Tylenol)
Phenazopyridine (Pyridium) [urinary tract local analgesic]
Tramadol (Ultram) [agonist at μ-opioid receptor, serotonin-releasing agent, norepinephrine reuptake inhibitor]

Anorexiants
Lorcaserin (Belviq)
Naltrexone-bupropion (Contrave)
Phentermine–topiramate ER (Qsymia)

Antiarrhythmics
Amiodarone (Cordarone) [Class III antiarrhythmic]
Disopyramide (Norpace) [Class Ia antiarrhythmic]
Flecainide (Tambocor) [Class Ic antiarrhythmic]
Procainamide (Pronestyl) [Class Ia antiarrhythmic]
Propafenone (Rythmol) [Class Ic antiarrhythmic]
Sotalol (Betapace) [Class III antiarrhythmic and β-blocker]

Antibiotics
Azithromycin (Zithromax)
Ciprofloxacin (Cipro)
Clarithromycin (Biaxin)
Erythromycin (E-Mycin)
Gemifloxacin (Factive)
Levofloxacin (Levaquin)
Lomefloxacin (Maxaquin)
Moxifloxacin (Avelox)
Norfloxacin (Noroxin)
Ofloxacin (Floxin)
Rifampin (Rifadin, Rimactane)
Rufloxacin (Ruflox)
Trimethoprim-sulfamethoxazole (Bactrim)

Anticholinergc agents (all antimuscarinic)
Benztropine (Cogentin) [H_1 antihistamine/antiparkinsonian]
Glycopyrrolate (Robinul)
Ipratropium bromide (Atrovent spray) [inhaler]
Orphenadrine (Norflex) [H_1 antihistamine/antispasmodic
    analgesic, for muscle injuries]
Oxybutynin (Ditropan) [bladder antispasmodic; treatment for
    urinary urgency/incontinence]
Solifenacin (VESIcare) [bladder antispasmodic; treatment for
    urinary urgency]
Tolterodine (Detrol) [treatment for urinary incontinence]
Trihexyphenidyl (Artane) [antiparkinsonian]

Anticoagulants
Warfarin (Coumadin)

Anticonvulsants
Carbamazepine (Tegretol, Equetro)
Divalproex or valproic acid (Depakote, Depakene)
Eslicarbazepine (Aptiom)
Gabapentin (Neurontin)
Gabapentin enacarbil (Horizant)
Lamotrigine (Lamictal)
Levetiracetam (Keppra)
Oxcarbazepine (Trileptal)
Phenytoin (Dilantin)
Primidone (Mysoline)
Progabide (Gabrene)
Topiramate (Topamax)

Antidepressants
Amitriptyline (Elavil)
Bupropion (Wellbutrin, Zyban)
Citalopram (Celexa)
Desipramine (Norpramin)
Desvenlafaxine (Pristiq)
Doxepin (Silenor, Sinequan)
Duloxetine (Cymbalta)
Escitalopram (Lexapro)
Fluoxetine (Prozac, Sarafem)
Fluvoxamine (Luvox)
Imipramine (Tofranil)
Isocarboxazid (Marplan)
Levomilnacipran (Fetzima)
Maprotiline (Ludiomil)
Mirtazapine (Remeron)
Moclobemide (Aurorix, Manerix)
Nefazodone (Serzone)
Nortriptyline (Pamelor)
Paroxetine (Paxil)
Phenelzine (Nardil)
Sertraline (Zoloft)
Transdermal selegiline (Emsam)
Tranylcypromine (Parnate)
Trazodone (Desyrel)
Venlafaxine (Effexor)
Vilazodone (Viibryd)
Vortioxetine (Trintellix)

Antidiarrheal agents
Loperamide (Imodium) [opioid receptor agonist]

Antiemetic/antinausea agents
Metoclopramide (Reglan) [gastroprokinetic]
Ondansetron (Zofran) [$5HT_3$ receptor antagonist]
Prochlorperazine (Compazine)
Trimethobenzamide (Tigan)

Antiestrogen agents
Clomiphene (Clomid) [selective estrogen receptor modulator]
Letrozole (Femara) [aromatase inhibitor]
Tamoxifen (Nolvadex) [estrogen receptor antagonist]

Antifungal agents
Ketoconazole (Feoris, Nizoral)

Antihistamines
Cetirizine (Zyrtec)
Cyproheptadine (Periactin)
Diphenhydramine (Benadryl)
Hydroxyzine (Atarax, Vistaril)
Loratadine (Claritin)
Promethazine (Phenergan) [phenothiazine derivative]

Antihypertensive agents
ACE inhibitors
    Enalapril (Vasotec)
    Lisinopril (Zestril)
    Ramipril (Altace)
α_2-*Adrenergic agonists*
    Clonidine (Catapres)
    Guanfacine (Tenex)
α_1-*Adrenergic antagonists*
    Doxazosin (Cardura)
    Phentolamine (Regitine)
    Prazosin (Minipress)
    Terazosin (Hytrin)
β-*Blockers*
    Atenolol (Tenormin)
    Betaxolol (Kerlone)
    Metoprolol (Toprol)
    Propranolol (Inderal)
Calcium channel blockers
    Amlodipine (Norvasc)
    Amlodipine plus atorvastatin (Caduet)
    Isradipine (Dynacirc)
    Nifedipine (Adalat, Procardia)
    Verapamil (Calan, Verelan)

Antimalarial agents
Chloroquine (Aralen)
Mefloquine (Lariam)

Antimanic treatments *(see also certain anticonvulsants)*
Lithium carbonate (Lithobid, Eskalith)

Antineoplastic agents
Chlorambucil (Leukeran)
5-Fluorouracil (Adrucil, Efudex)
Ifosfamide (Ifex)
Procarbazine (Matulane)
Rituximab (Rituxan)

Antiparkinsonian agents
Amantadine (Symmetrel) [dopamine and norepinephrine agonist]
Biperiden (Akineton) [antimuscarinic]
Pramipexole (Mirapex)
Ropinirole (Requip)

Anxiolytics (nonbenzodiazepine)
Buspirone (Buspar)

Attention-deficit/hyperactivity disorder treatments (nonstimulant)
Atomoxetine (Strattera)
Guanfacine (Tenex) [α_2-agonist]

Bronchodilators (beta agonists)
Albuterol (Ventolin)

Calcimimetics
Cinacalcet (Sensipar)

Cholinergic agonists
Bethanechol (Urecholine) [muscarinic]
Cevimeline (Evoxac)
Pilocarpine (Salagen)

Diabetes insipidus treatments
Desmopressin intranasal spray (DDAVP)

Diuretics
Amiloride (Midamor)
Hydrochlorothiazide (Microzide, Oretic, Apo-Hydro)
Hydrochlorothiazide plus triamterene (Dyazide)

First-generation antipsychotics
Chlorpromazine (Thorazine)
Haloperidol (Haldol)
Mesoridazine (Serentil)
Molindone (Moban)
Perphenazine (Trilafon)
Pimozide (Orap)
Thioridazine (Mellaril)
Thiothixene (Navane)

Gastrointestinal agents
Antispasmodics
    Dicyclomine (Bentyl)
    Pirenzepine (Gastrozepin) [muscarinic antagonist, reduces
       gastric acid secretion]
Other agents for minor gastrointestinal distress
    Bismuth subsalicylate (Pepto-Bismol, Kaopectate)

Histamine H$_2$ inhibitors
Cimetidine (Tagamet)
Nizatidine (Axid)
Omeprazole (Prilosec)
Ranitidine (Zantac)

HIV treatments
Antiretroviral agents
  Zidovudine or azidothymidine (AZT) (Retrovir)
Nonnucleoside reverse transcriptase inhibitors
  Efavirenz (Sustiva)

Hypoglycemic Agents
Biguanidines
  Metformin
Dipeptidyl peptidase–4 (DPP-4) inhibitors
  Alogliptin (Nesina)
  Linagliptin (Tradjenta)
  Saxagliptin (Onglyza)
  Sitagliptin (Januvia)
Glucagon-like peptide–1 agonists
  Albiglutide (Eperzan, Tanzeum)
  Dulaglutide (Trulicity)
  Exenatide (Byetta)
  Liraglutide (Victoza)
  Lixisenatide (Adlyxin)
Thiazolidinediones
  Pioglitazone (Actos)
  Rosiglitazone (Avandia)

Immunosuppressants
Azathioprine (Imuran)
Basiliximab (Simulect)
Cyclosporine (Neoral, Sandimmune)
Muromonab-CD3 (Orthoclone OKT3)
Mycophenolate mofetil (CellCept)
Rapamycin or sirolimus (Rapamune)
Tacrolimus (Prograf)

Lipid-lowering agents
Inhibitors of intestinal cholesterol absorption
  Ezetimibe (Zetia)
  Ezetimibe plus Simvastatin (Vytorin)

Lipid-lowering agents *(continued)*
Statins (HMG-CoA reductase inhibitors)
Atorvastatin (Lipitor)
Fluvastatin (Lescol)
Lovastatin (Mevacor)
Pravastatin (Pravachol)
Rosuvastatin (Crestor)
Simvastatin (Zocor)

Migraine headache treatments
Eletriptan (Relpax)
Sumatriptan (Imitrex)
Zolmitriptan (Zomig)

Miscellaneous central nervous system agents
Deutetrabenazine (Austedo)
Piracetam (Nootropil)
Tetrabenazine (Xenazine)
Valbenazine (Ingrezza)

Muscle relaxants
Baclofen (Lioresal)
Carisoprodol (Soma)
Cyclobenzaprine (Flexeril)

Narcolepsy treatments and wakefulness-promoting agents
Armodafinil (Nuvigil)
Modafinil (Provigil)
Sodium oxybate (Xyrem)

Nasal decongestants
Phenylephrine (Dimetapp) [α_1-agonist]
Pseudoephedrine (Sudafed) [indirect nonspecific alpha agonist]

Opiate analgesics
Oxycodone (Oxycontin, Roxicodone)
Oxymorphone (Numorphan, Opana ER, Opana IR)

Opiate partial agonists
Buprenorphine (Subutex)
Buprenorphine plus naloxone (Suboxone)

Polymerase inhibitors
Sofosbuvir (Sovaldi)

Protease inhibitors
Boceprevir (Victrelis)
Simeprevir (Olysio)
Telaprevir (Incivek)

Second-generation antipsychotics
Aripiprazole (Abilify)
Asenapine (Saphris)
Brexpiprazole (Rexulti)
Cariprazine (Vraylar)
Clozapine (Clozaril)
Iloperidone (Fanapt)
Lurasidone (Latuda)
Olanzapine (Zyprexa)
Paliperidone (Invega)
Pimavanserin (Nuplazid)
Quetiapine (Seroquel)
Risperidone (Risperdal)
Ziprasidone (Geodon)

Sedative-hypnotics
Benzodiazepines
 Alprazolam (Xanax)
 Chlordiazepoxide (Librium)
 Clorazepate (Tranxene)
 Diazepam (Valium)
 Flurazepam (Dalmane)
 Lorazepam (Ativan)
 Oxazepam (Serax)
 Temazepam (Restoril)
 Triazolam (Halcion)
Nonbenzodiazepines
 Eszopiclone (Lunesta)
 Ramelteon (Rozerem)
 Tasimelteon (Hetlioz)
 Zaleplon (Sonata)
 Zolpidem (Ambien)
Orexin receptor antagonists
 Suvorexant (Belsomra)

Sexual dysfunction treatments
Flibanserin (Addyi)
Sildenafil (Viagra) [phosphodiesterase type 5 inhibitor]
Tadalafil (Cialis) [phosphodiesterase type 5 inhibitor]
Vardenafil (Levitra) [phosphodiesterase type 5 inhibitor]
Yohimbine (Yocon) [an α_2-adrenergic antagonist]

Smoking cessation aids
Varenicline (Chantix)

Stimulants and stimulant-like drugs
Amphetamine (Dexedrine, Adderall [mixed amphetamine salts])
Methylphenidate (Concerta, Focalin, Methylin, Ritalin)
Phentermine (Adipex-P)

Sympathomimetics (β_1-agonists)
Dobutamine (Dobutrex)

Tocolytics
Terbutaline (Brethine, Bricanyl)

Vasopressors/Antihypotensive agents
Fludrocortisone (Florinef) [a mineralocorticoid]
Midodrine [an α_1 agonist]
Pyridostigmine [a reversible cholinesterase inhibitor]

PART I

General Considerations

The Psychiatrist as Physician

Primary Care Psychiatry

Adverse effects from psychotropic medications account for approximately 90,000 emergency department visits annually (Hampton et al. 2014) and arguably pose the greatest obstacle to implementing pharmacotherapies that are safe, effective, and appropriate. Although the mandate *primum non nocere* remains axiomatic throughout medicine, the practical management of serious illnesses demands that physicians recognize and appreciate the risks and benefits of available treatment options relative to alternative treatments — or no treatment. All therapies, including placebo, involve hazards that could worsen a clinical condition either directly (usually because of side effects) or indirectly (due to inappropriate use of an otherwise efficacious therapy or the decision to forgo a treatment for fear that the cure might be worse than the disease). Expertise in clinical psychopharmacology depends heavily on knowledge and experience about how best to balance the risks and benefits of a given treatment relative to its alternatives.

The symbol ■ is used in this chapter to indicate that the FDA has issued a boxed warning for a prescription medication that may cause serious adverse effects.

The tremendous growth in the number of available psychotropic agents has contributed profoundly to the pharmacologically oriented practice of psychiatry. The use of combination drug therapy regimens has become increasingly commonplace, informed at least theoretically by complementary mechanisms of action, potential pharmacodynamic synergies, and concepts such as "breadth of spectrum" to describe psychotropic drugs in analogous fashion to antimicrobials or antineoplastics. Yet, despite the fervor with which psychiatrists often devise complex drug regimens or undertake novel pharmacotherapies for conditions that respond poorly to traditional agents, many practitioners are often remarkably uncomfortable confronting and managing unintended drug effects. Such hesitation may stem in part from the comparatively lower diversity of adverse effects from pharmacologies of generations past, coupled with a historically lower need on the part of psychiatrists than many other medical subspecialists to maintain a working knowledge of basic primary care medicine. Such a medically hands-off model has become increasingly untenable given the diverse end-organ effects of newer psychotropic drugs, coupled with growing awareness of the medical comorbidities associated with depression, bipolar disorder, schizophrenia, and other serious forms of mental illness. Moreover, psychiatrists possess a unique knowledge base among physicians from which to understand the relative benefits of a psychotropic medication for a given patient and to determine when the unique merits of a drug outweigh the risks—and manageability—of a potential adverse effect.

Good psychopharmacotherapy presumes a general appreciation and working knowledge of all end organs potentially affected by a pharmacological intervention. One need not be an endocrinologist to identify and manage lithium-induced hypothyroidism or glycemic dysregulation caused by SGAs, but competency requires a basic awareness of major organ system physiology and the ways in which commonly used medications exert their pharmacokinetic and pharmacodynamic effects. The "remedicalization" of psychiatry has made it more commonplace, if not routine, for contemporary psychiatrists to conduct focused physical examinations that include in-office measurement of weight or body mass index, measurement of abdominal girth, monitoring of blood pressure and heart rate (including orthostatic measurements when appropriate), basic neurological examinations (assessing pupillary responses, extraocular movements, cranial nerves, sensation, motor strength, deep tendon reflexes, gait, and tremor or other movement disorders), detection of thyromegaly or lymphadenopathy, assessment of skin rashes (including those rashes affecting the sclerae and other mucocutaneous tissues, as well as the back, trunk, and extremities), cardiac auscultation, and assessment of fluid volumes (e.g., when evaluating a patient for peripheral edema).

Active collaboration with primary care physicians has never been more fundamental than in the present era, in which patients with significant psychiatric conditions are especially vulnerable to health problems related to both lifestyle (e.g., overweight and obesity, hypertension, sexually transmitted diseases) and iatrogenic factors (e.g., psychotropic-induced weight gain or metabolic dysregulation). No medical subspecialty other than psychiatry bears responsibility for possessing the knowledge base necessary to gauge the relative risks and benefits of treatments that may literally be lifesaving but nevertheless can carry substantial side-effect burdens. Subspecialists from other areas of medicine may be useful resources to help psychiatrists reason through risks, benefits, and available alternatives to a given treatment; but these subspecialists, in turn, may look to psychiatrists for similar guidance.

The presence of certain medical comorbidities may pose relative (if not absolute) contraindications to the use of specific psychotropic agents. Representative examples are summarized in Table 1–1.

Appropriate medical monitoring of psychotropic agents involves an awareness of abnormalities detectable by history or physical examination, as well as pertinent laboratory parameters. Table 1–2 provides a summary of laboratory measures that warrant monitoring or consideration in the course of treatment with specific psychotropic compounds. Recommendations for laboratory monitoring that are presented in Table 1–2 are collectively derived from manufacturers' package insert information for specific agents, as well as from published practice guidelines.

Differentiating Adverse Drug Effects From Primary Illness Symptoms or Nonpsychiatric Medical Problems

One of the greatest challenges in treating disturbances of mood, behavior, thinking, or perception involves the discrimination between symptoms that are intrinsic to a disorder and potential side effects of somatic therapies. Treatment with antipsychotic drugs may induce akathisia, which can sometimes be difficult to distinguish from anxiety or hypomania (necessitating the broader assessment of additional symptoms, such as a sleep disturbance or increased goal-directed activity, to help clarify differential diagnosis). In the case of depression, the presence of reverse

TABLE 1–1.   Medical conditions that may contraindicate specific psychotropic agents

Medical condition	Pharmacotherapy implication
Asthma, chronic obstructive pulmonary disease	β-Blockers are relatively contraindicated.
Chronic kidney disease	Lithium is relatively contraindicated depending on severity and chronicity.
Bradycardia (e.g., sick sinus syndrome)	β-Blockers are relatively contraindicated.
Hepatitis	Carbamazepine or divalproex should be administered with caution.[a]
Hypertension (poorly controlled)	Strongly adrenergic agents, including SNRIs, TCAs, or stimulants, should not be initiated until hypertension is treated.
Hypothyroidism	Lithium is *not* contraindicated.
Neutropenia	Carbamazepine and clozapine are contraindicated.
Seizure disorder	Bupropion and clozapine are relatively contraindicated. Caution should be exercised with use of antipsychotics and maprotiline.

Note.   SNRI=serotonin-norepinephrine reuptake inhibitor; TCA=tricyclic antidepressant.
[a]See the sections "Hepatic Impairment and Transaminitis" and "Hyperammonemia" in Chapter 12, "Gastrointestinal System."

neurovegetative signs (e.g., lethargy, hypersomnia, hyperphagia) — which are typical in bipolar depression — may confound impressions about the emergence of these features as being likely attributable to an antidepressant (e.g., sedation), or rather, to symptoms of the illness itself. Similarly, if symptoms (e.g., agitation, insomnia, suicidal features) worsen after a patient starts a treatment, it may be difficult to differentiate whether they reflect an adverse drug reaction or simply an exacerbation of illness symptoms (and a failure of the intervention, at least at that point, to remedy them).

Clinicians also must be keenly aware of alleged side effects that could actually be manifestations of an underlying nonpsychiatric medical co-morbidity. Clues suggesting the latter may include

- Atypical symptoms or time course.
- Unilateral rather than bilateral neurological signs (e.g., diplopia, weakness) or systemic phenomena (e.g., edema).
- Known medical conditions (e.g., headaches in migraine sufferers or individuals with poorly controlled hypertension).
- Genitourinary complaints in patients with known diabetes.
- Palpitations or chest discomfort in patients with an existing arrhythmia.
- Involvement of multiple organ systems.
- Known infections; allergic, toxic, or other environmental exposures.

Several general principles can help to differentiate side effects from illness symptoms. First, before any treatment is started, it is useful to have cataloged the baseline target symptoms for which a medication is being used.

Second, and perhaps most fundamentally, when a patient reports a presumed side effect, it is obviously essential to clarify whether the phenomenon was absent before treatment. In the case of illness symptoms that may intensify during (or despite) pharmacotherapy, this differentiation can be especially difficult. Consider the example of insomnia or suicidality that predates the initiation of an SSRI for major depression, which then worsens in the week following treatment initiation. The co-occurrence of additional new side effects, particularly those that are not common in depression (Figure 1–1), may help to corroborate the hypothesis that a complaint more likely represents an adverse drug effect than a symptom of depression.

A third consideration involves gathering historical information about previous medication trials and noteworthy past adverse effects. It is often helpful before or during an initial evaluation to have patients construct a summary of past medications they have taken with approximate dates, dosages, benefits (if any), and any recollection of adverse effects. Such a summary holds obvious value not only for capturing complications of previous treatments, but also for distinguishing past treatment nonresponses from intolerances, identifying the adequacy (dose and duration) of past treatments, discovering reasons for discontinuation, gauging an individual patient's capacity to tolerate medically benign side effects, and recognizing potential patterns or sensitivities that may heighten expectations about future potential side-effect susceptibilities or concerns. Finally, and perhaps most obviously, an awareness of particular side-effect

TABLE 1–2. Routine laboratory monitoring for commonly used psychotropic agents

Medication	Parameter	Frequency of measurement and target ranges	Rationale
Carbamazepine	Serum carbamazepine level	No known validity relative to therapeutic effect in mood disorders; nevertheless, some clinicians measure serum levels despite the absence of research. Expert Consensus Guidelines (Keck et al. 2004) identify a favored acute level range (6.5–11.6 µg/mL) and a maintenance dose level range (6.1–11.0 µg/mL). Autoinduction of blood levels.	May be measured periodically in setting of clinical concerns about toxicity or adherence.
	CBC with platelets	Baseline and periodically thereafter (more often in the presence of signs suggestive of bone marrow suppression).	Carbamazepine induces benign and transient myelosuppression in about 10% of patients but very rarely may cause sustained aplastic anemia.
	Electrolytes	Baseline and periodically thereafter.	Carbamazepine can cause age-associated hyponatremia (often modest and benign) in up to 40% of recipients.

TABLE 1–2. Routine laboratory monitoring for commonly used psychotropic agents (*continued*)

Medication	Parameter	Frequency of measurement and target ranges	Rationale
Carbamazepine (*continued*)	Liver enzymes	Baseline and periodically thereafter (more often in the presence of hepatic impairment). (*Note:* Some experts cast doubt on the practical utility and cost-effectiveness of routine laboratory monitoring and instead favor clinical monitoring for signs of hepatotoxicity; see the section "Hepatic Impairment and Transaminitis" in Chapter 12, "Gastrointestinal System").	Carbamazepine can cause hepatotoxicity.
Clozapine	Serum clozapine level	Serum clozapine levels >350 ng/mL likely offer no therapeutic advantage (VanderZwaag et al. 1996); optimal response in schizophrenia appears to occur in range of 200–300 ng/mL.	Serum clozapine levels are not routinely measured, but determining a serum level of the parent compound (clozapine without norclozapine) may sometimes help to inform risk-benefit decisions about further dosage increases when symptoms persist.

TABLE 1–2. Routine laboratory monitoring for commonly used psychotropic agents *(continued)*

Medication	Parameter	Frequency of measurement and target ranges	Rationale
Divalproex	Serum valproate level	In acute mania, steady-state levels achieved after five half-lives (about 3–4 days).	Levels of 50–125 µg/mL are associated with acute antimanic response (Bowden et al. 2006b); no levels have been established for maintenance therapy or acute bipolar depression, although practitioners often extrapolate from levels in acute mania.
	Liver enzymes	Some authorities advise monitoring every 6 months, whereas others regard continued monitoring unnecessary in stable patients (Pellock and Willmore 1991). We advocate semiannual or annual assessment in stable patients.	Divalproex may cause hepatotoxicity.
	Platelet count	Periodic CBC.	Divalproex may cause thrombocytopenia.
	Serum ammonia level	Not routinely measured in the absence of clinical signs of hepatic encephalopathy.	Divalproex can deplete carnitine.

TABLE 1–2. Routine laboratory monitoring for commonly used psychotropic agents *(continued)*

Medication	Parameter	Frequency of measurement and target ranges	Rationale
Divalproex *(continued)*	Serum lipase and amylase	Not routinely measured in the absence of clinical suspicion of acute pancreatitis.	Divalproex recipients who present with an acute abdomen should be evaluated for possible acute pancreatitis, a clinical assessment that includes measurement of serum lipase and amylase.
Lamotrigine	Serum lamotrigine level	No established validity in association with therapeutic effect in mood disorders; toxicity correlates with drug levels (more than one-third of epilepsy patients demonstrate neurotoxicity at levels >15 µg/mL) (Hirsch et al. 2004).	Although lamotrigine blood levels can be lower during pregnancy, oral contraceptive use, and cotherapy with carbamazepine, measurement of lamotrigine blood levels has no known clinical relevance outside of epilepsy.
Lithium	Serum calcium and parathyroid hormone	Annual monitoring is advisable.	10%–25% of patients taking lithium >10 years may show elevated ionized serum calcium levels and hyperparathyroidism (Albert et al. 2013; Meehan et al. 2015; Shapiro and Davis 2015).

TABLE 1–2. Routine laboratory monitoring for commonly used psychotropic agents (*continued*)

Medication	Parameter	Frequency of measurement and target ranges	Rationale
Lithium (*continued*)	Serum lithium level	By convention, measure serum levels obtained approximately 8–12 hours after the previous dose.[a] Steady state is achieved five half-lives (5 days) after dosage changes. Frequent monitoring may be useful after each dosage change in the acute setting. In stable patients, levels are usually measured at least twice a year (Jefferson 2010). (*Note:* Manufacturers' product information for all formulations of lithium advise the monitoring of serum lithium levels "at least every 2 months," although such an onerous schedule has never been adopted by practice guidelines as the standard of care.)	Acute antimanic efficacy is generally associated with serum levels of 0.6–1.2 mEq/L; Expert Consensus Guidelines advise levels of 0.7–1.1 mEq/L (Keck et al. 2004). Maintenance prophylaxis is associated with levels of 0.8–1.0 mEq/L (Gelenberg et al. 1989); Expert Consensus Guidelines advise levels of 0.6–1.0 mEq/L (Keck et al. 2004).

TABLE 1–2. Routine laboratory monitoring for commonly used psychotropic agents *(continued)*

Medication	Parameter	Frequency of measurement and target ranges	Rationale
Lithium *(continued)*	Renal function (typically includes serum creatinine to calculate estimated GFR and urinalysis to measure specific gravity and assess for proteinuria) (Jefferson 2010)	Every 2–3 months during the first 6 months of treatment, and every 6–12 months thereafter (or more often in the setting of rising creatinine).	Lithium may cause nephrotoxicity.
	Thyroid function tests	Once or twice during the first 6 months of treatment; every 6–12 months thereafter.	Lithium-induced hypothyroidism (see the section "Thyroid Abnormalities" in Chapter 11, "Endocrinopathies"): In recipients of thyroid hormone therapy, optimal reassessment of thyroid function should occur ~8 weeks after a T_4 or T_3 dosage adjustment. (*Note:* If a patient is also taking supplemental calcium or iron, a constant temporal relationship should be maintained when measuring thyroid hormone due to binding of these minerals.)

TABLE 1–2. Routine laboratory monitoring for commonly used psychotropic agents (*continued*)

Medication	Parameter	Frequency of measurement and target ranges	Rationale
Lithium (*continued*)	12-lead ECG	Before treatment initiation in adults over age 40.	Lithium, particularly at high dosages, may cause ECG abnormalities (see Table 7–1 in Chapter 7, "Cardiovascular System"). In the absence of heart disease, serial ECG monitoring during lithium therapy is unnecessary.
	CBC	Occasionally recommended by some authorities before lithium initiation; not routinely monitored in serial fashion.	Baseline assessment can help to interpret whether any subsequent leukocytosis is likely iatrogenic.
SGAs	Fasting blood sugar	At baseline, 12 weeks, and annually thereafter.	SGAs may cause glycemic dysregulation.
	Hemoglobin A_{1c}	Levels ≥ 6.5 are definitional of diabetes; levels of 5.7–6.4 identify patients at increased risk for diabetes.	Hemoglobin A_{1c} is an acceptable indicator of diabetes risk.

TABLE 1–2. Routine laboratory monitoring for commonly used psychotropic agents *(continued)*

Medication	Parameter	Frequency of measurement and target ranges	Rationale
SGAs *(continued)*	Fasting lipid profile	At baseline, 12 weeks, and every 5 years thereafter.	SGAs may cause elevation of serum triglycerides and LDL cholesterol.
	12-lead ECG	No formal recommendation. In older patients, or those for whom concerns may exist about conduction delays (e.g., risk factors for QTc prolongation; see Table 7–3), a baseline ECG may be advisable.	Some antipsychotics may cause arrhythmias or conduction delays (see Tables 7–1 and 7–2).
	CBC	All SGAs can rarely cause leukopenia, but routine monitoring of blood counts is unnecessary in the absence of clinical signs.	In patients who present with leukopenia or neutropenia, clinicians should be aware that SGAs as a class may contribute to etiology.

TABLE 1–2. Routine laboratory monitoring for commonly used psychotropic agents (*continued*)

Medication	Parameter	Frequency of measurement and target ranges	Rationale
TCAs	Serum drug levels	Serum nortriptyline levels within an established therapeutic window are associated with antidepressant efficacy (see Table 2–5 in Chapter 2, "Pharmacokinetics, Pharmacodynamics, and Pharmacogenomics").	In the setting of an inadequate clinical response, dosages may be increased until achievement of a therapeutic level. Dosing beyond a therapeutic window likely yields no greater efficacy but more adverse effects.

Note. CBC=complete blood count; ECG=electrocardiogram; GFR=glomerular filtration rate; LDL=low-density lipoprotein; SGA= second-generation antipsychotic; T_3=triiodothyronine; T_4=thyroxine; TCA=tricyclic antidepressant.

[a]The rationale for timing of the measurement of serum lithium levels is based on the assumption of twice-daily dosing, with a "trough" level being measured immediately before the next dose. In practice, however, some experts advocate once-daily dosing of all preparations of lithium carbonate based on 1) the 24-hour half-life of lithium carbonate and 2) the lesser risk for causing glomerulosclerosis when lithium is dosed once daily rather than multiple times per day (see the section "Nephrotoxicity and Nephrogenic Diabetes Insipidus" in Chapter 13, "Genitourinary and Renal Systems"). Serum lithium levels that are obtained 8–12 hours after a once-daily dose are not trough levels, but are considered meaningful for assessing serum concentrations relative to lithium's therapeutic window.

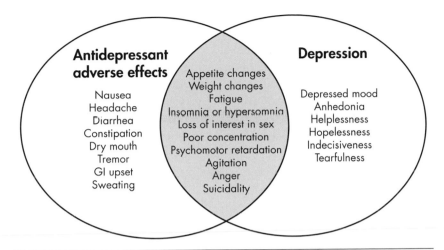

FIGURE 1–1. Overlap between symptoms of depression and common adverse effects of antidepressants.

GI = gastrointestinal.

sensitivities or concerns can and should inform joint deliberations between the prescriber and patient about possible future treatments. (For example, past sexual dysfunction would probably dissuade most practitioners from advocating an SSRI or TCA trial when other viable options for depression or anxiety exist, and past cognitive dulling or sedation would favor the avoidance of benzodiazepines or antihistaminergic or anticholinergic agents if practicable.)

The Nocebo Phenomenon and Proneness to Adverse Effects

Nonspecific side effects that occur during treatment with inert compounds (placebos) have been described as *nocebo effects*. Predictors of the nocebo phenomenon have been shown to include patients' expectations of adverse effects, past experience of adverse somatic effects of treatments that may foster conditioned expectations, and clinical phenomena such as depression, anxiety, or a predisposition to somatization. Alexithymic traits — that is, an impaired capacity to put emotional states into words — may also increase the likelihood for certain individuals to express internal distress through somatic complaints.

Patients who identify themselves as being especially sensitive to side effects are communicating important information about their likely expectation of somatic problems. By definition, physical complaints from a placebo are not pharmacodynamic in origin, yet the prospect that they *might* be linked to treatment can provide validation and legitimacy to an individual's subjective sense of suffering. Clinicians should be especially attuned to the context in which patients may communicate excessive nonspecific or ill-defined complaints (e.g., malaise, "just not feeling right") in connection with treatment, particularly to the extent that they may feel poorly cared for or cared about by others. In such instances, physical complaints may serve to legitimize the occasion for greater contact with the treater and may fundamentally represent the expression of unmet emotional needs.

Clinical trials in major depression report that about two-thirds of subjects will report at least one significant adverse effect from taking a placebo (Dodd et al. 2015). Personality characteristics, particularly neuroticism, have been found to correlate with the number of reported side effects, whereas phobic, obsessive, and hypochondriacal symptoms have been associated with placebo-induced drowsiness. Factors such as suggestibility and expectancy regarding outcomes also may contribute to placebo effects (both good and bad) within psychiatry, as has been demonstrated in studies of analgesia for chronic pain. The phenomenon of "somatosensory amplification," in which an individual experiences normal bodily sensations as unusually intense and noxious, has been linked with an increased perception and reporting of adverse treatment effects.

Certain adverse effects tend to be especially likely during treatment with placebo in clinical trials for particular disorders. For example, across randomized controlled trials in various phases of bipolar disorder or major depression, incidence rates of ≥10% with placebo have been reported for dizziness, headache, nausea, diarrhea, sedation, insomnia, anorexia, nervousness, anxiety, and asthenia (i.e., weakness or lack of strength and energy). Some psychiatric disorders also appear more likely than others to incur nocebo effects. For example, more varied and higher rates of side effects with placebo have been reported in drug trials for patients with anxiety disorders, whereas less extensive or diverse side effects from placebo are typically observed in trials for patients with schizophrenia. Interestingly, a number of reported side effects (i.e., dry mouth, nausea, headache, insomnia, somnolence, and sexual dysfunction) occurred at least twice as often with placebo (in a comparison with sertraline) in patients with dysthymic disorder as was seen in trials of acute major depressive disorder (Thase et al. 1996). These findings further suggest that nocebo effects may be higher among more chronically ill mood disorder patients.

From a psychodynamic perspective, practitioners might consider the idea that a medicine can pose a kind of projective stimulus, one that patients can imbue with malevolent qualities literally capable of destroying them from the inside when ingested. Exposing oneself to a medication can create a psychologically vulnerable and regressive experience that taps early developmental processes, such as the defense mechanism of splitting, in which an individual's internal experience of people and things becomes divided into good or bad psychological objects. Especially in patients with traumatic childhood experiences, bad objects are projected out onto others and then psychologically internalized (i.e., reintrojected) in an effort to gain mastery over them. A medication can lend itself as a convenient psychological nidus for the projection of the bad object (encompassing a range of unconscious or preconscious fears and anxieties about danger and harm caused by the supposed caregiver); thus, medication may conceptually represent both external and internal persecutory forces, creating an array of harmful effects that may not necessarily have any bearing on the pharmacodynamic properties of the actual substance being taken.

Patients sometimes perceive and report what they believe to be adverse drug effects using dramatic language that communicates their feeling harmed (e.g., "It's as if I was being choked" or "I felt like someone was driving a screwdriver into my bones"). True adverse effects may also be described with a histrionic, exaggerated intensity (e.g., "My brain went numb" or "I felt electrical shocks all over my body") that sometimes may even verge on delusional perception or dissociation (e g , "I could feel the blood rushing through my body" or "I could see my skin moving"). The context of a possible adverse effect may be hard to understand without an appreciation for a given patient's psychiatric disorder or cognitive style of processing information. Therefore, practitioners need to clarify the meaning of self-reported adverse effects that may be ill defined, histrionic, or psychotic to determine whether they are meant to communicate true iatrogenic events (e.g., paresthesias, laryngeal dystonias, antihistaminergic cognitive dulling, autonomic activation) or are simple manifestations of underlying psychopathology.

For everyday practitioners, awareness of the potential for nocebo effects (and their differentiation from adverse pharmacodynamic effects) is fundamental to optimal care. The following are some strategies to help minimize nocebo effects and to differentiate them from true drug effects.

- On initial encounters with patients who are already on complex drug regimens or who have baseline somatic complaints, avoid making any pharmacological changes unless an existing drug intolerance or toxicity state is unambiguous, or unless an existing drug is highly suspected of worsening the clinical presentation.

- Identify baseline patient characteristics or diagnostic features (notably, anxiety or proneness to somatic symptoms) that may predispose to nocebo effects.
- Tell patients directly that even placebos can cause side effects, and ask if they think they might be vulnerable to the power of suggestion if they should hear about a particular side effect through the popular media or Internet.
- Resist the temptation to overrespond to frequent complaints or symptoms with excessive dosage changes or medication starts and stops, which may serve mainly to heighten a sense of anxiety or chaos for both the patient and the practitioner.
- Recognize the plausibility between reported adverse effects and the time course for their emergence or relationship to incremental dosing changes; pay particular attention to patients who report "dramatic" effects (either beneficial or adverse) within hours or days of taking a medication if the pharmacodynamic profile of a drug is unlikely to produce effects on so rapid a timescale.
- Avoid multiple changes (drugs, doses, timing) simultaneously, whenever feasible.

Negative Therapeutic Reactions

To borrow a concept from classical psychoanalysis, the notion of a *negative therapeutic reaction* is meant to describe instances in which patients develop a paradoxical worsening of symptoms in response to accurate treatment interventions. Freud originally described and regarded this phenomenon as an unconscious expression of guilt or masochism on the part of the patient, whose symptoms worsened because the prospect of improvement was contrary to an unconscious investment in his or her own suffering. The same mechanism may have similar bearing on psychopharmacology, inasmuch as some symptoms—particularly those with ambiguous etiologies that could reflect either medication or the primary psychiatric problem—may at times worsen in response to treatment. Such a process might be considered when patients report extensive or persistent adverse treatment effects that may not have a clear pharmacodynamic basis—for example, an intensification of depressed mood, guilty ruminations, or anhedonia during antidepressant therapy.

A related concept involves the potential for apparent side effects—or worsening symptoms—in patients who may have a profound sense of resentment and bitterness toward early caregivers, and who may take either conscious or unconscious sadistic pleasure in thwarting the efforts of their psychiatrist. The operative process can involve a powerful drive to defeat the helping efforts of a prescribing clinician as an unconscious means of revenge against internalized representations of early caregivers as having been ineffective or malicious. Patients who articulate a seemingly endless stream of physical complaints related to treatment, with little or no apparent benefit, may engender in the treater a parallel sense of resentment, frustration, and eventual loss of empathy for the plight of the patient. Such encounters between patient and treater can become interpersonally and psychodynamically complex, and they may often go unnoticed and unaddressed when the framework of treatment is focused mainly or exclusively around brief, infrequent encounters for "medication management." Without the treater's appreciation for the psychological context of symptoms, treatment may become a relentless and seemingly fruitless effort either to combat side effects or to identify more benign pharmacotherapies, while yielding minimal if any fundamental improvement. To break such cycles and gain a broader perspective, the treater may sometimes benefit from obtaining consultations. Instances may also arise in which the treater may honestly acknowledge to himself or herself, and to the patient, that existing pharmacologies may not be capable of providing discernible benefits that outweigh, or justify, the toll of side effects. In such situations, alternative treatment strategies, including psychotherapy, may hold greater promise and warrant deeper consideration as a potential route toward improvement.

Attribution and Causality

A fundamental consideration in managing adverse drug effects involves recognizing causal relationships between drug administration and effects (whether beneficial or adverse). Often, short of imposing randomized, blinded, placebo-controlled conditions, clinicians cannot know with certainty whether a change in clinical presentation can reasonably be attributed to a change in pharmacotherapy. Factors that impinge on the attribution of causality include recognizing the natural course of illness, the effects of having discontinued a previous drug, the potential for pharmacokinetic and pharmacodynamic interactions among two or more psychotropic agents, the potential for poor or erratic treatment adherence, medical comorbidities, and the presence of alcohol or illicit substances. The so-called Bradford-Hill criteria for causation identify factors such as the following:

- Temporality between drug exposure and observed effect
- Plausibility of a mechanism to account for an association between a given drug and a suspected effect
- Strength of association between drug and effect (e.g., effect size)
- Consistency or reproducibility of observed effects
- Specificity of a suspected association between a drug and a putative effect
- An observable gradient between extent of exposure and the suspected effect
- Coherence between an observed effect and laboratory parameters (if measurable)
- The presence of experimental evidence to support a drug-effect association

One factor relevant to evaluating a possible drug side effect involves whether a pharmacokinetic or pharmacodynamic rationale can explain an effect, or rather, whether a drug's mechanism of action fails to explain (or even contradicts) a suspected end-organ effect. In the case of highly nonspecific side effects—such as those that may occur as often with placebo as with an active drug (e.g., headache or insomnia), or those that may in reality simply reflect untreated illness features (e.g., agitation or anxiety)—pharmacodynamic mechanisms are unnecessary to account for side-effect plausibility. In other instances, drawing a causal link between a possible side effect and a drug may be mechanistically implausible (e.g., elevation of liver enzymes after lithium administration, nausea from prochlorperazine, a fever increase from acetaminophen). Equally challenging can be idiosyncratic or bizarre adverse effects that do not follow from the known pharmacodynamic properties of a drug, such as tremors caused by propranolol or clonazepam (in the absence of withdrawal), sexual dysfunction with psychostimulants, or lethargy caused by modafinil.

Another pertinent factor when judging likely causality involves the time course for the emergence of a suspected side effect relative to initial drug exposure. For example, rashes attributable to medications typically occur within the first few weeks or months after initiation; it is implausible to construe a rash that arises years after taking a medication as being a likely side effect. Similarly, hypersensitivity reactions to anticonvulsants (see the section "Antiepileptic Hypersensitivity Reactions" in Chapter 20, "Systemic Reactions") seldom if ever arise more than 8 weeks after a treatment has begun. Other potential adverse effects are characteristically encountered only after long-term exposure. Perhaps the best-known example is tardive dyskinesia, which, by conventional definition, does not develop until after at least 3 months of exposure to an antipsychotic in patients < age 60 years (or after at least 1 month in patients ≥ age 60), although acute or withdrawal dyskinesias can occur at any time after exposure.

Naranjo and colleagues (1981) described a rating system for judging the likelihood that adverse drug reactions were attributable to a suspected medication. In their classification scheme (the Naranjo Scale), numerical values are assigned for individual criteria so that the clinician can judge the probability of causal association (definite, probable, possible, or doubtful) between an adverse drug effect and a given medication. These criteria are summarized in Table 1–3. The basic principles incorporated in this rating system are of value for conceptualizing suspected adverse effects outside of research settings.

In practice, clinicians may find the following basic concepts helpful to minimize some of the confusion that can otherwise occur when attempting to draw causal inferences about drug effects.

- Whenever feasible, make only one change to a medication regimen at a time.
- Allow for steady-state pharmacokinetics to occur (typically, after five to six half-lives) before forming conclusions about adverse drug effects (unless they are time independent and emergent, such as allergic reactions, dystonias, or serious rashes; see Chapter 22, "Emergency Situations").
- Impose a method for systematically tracking target symptoms as well as potential side effects of concern (e.g., weigh patients at each visit, devise visual analog scales for patients to track the evolution and severity of a suspected side effect).
- Inquire about missed medication dosages in an inquisitive, nonjudgmental manner; neither take treatment adherence for granted nor routinely assume its absence.

Paradoxical Adverse Effects

Although it is probably a truism that virtually any side effect can happen with any drug at any time, clinicians are always struck by the unambiguous worsening of a symptom in response to a medication intended to ameliorate it. Clinicians usually presume, rightly or wrongly, that such occurrences typically reflect the mere lack of efficacy of a prescribed treatment to effectively counter the symptom being targeted rather than a true and paradoxical iatrogenic worsening of the symptom in question (e.g., when a patient reports feeling more depressed after starting an antidepressant, or when the intensity of hallucinations or delusional thinking worsens during treatment with an antipsychotic).

TABLE 1–3.   Naranjo scoring system for rating the likelihood of adverse drug reactions

Item	Score[a]
1. Are there previous conclusive reports on this reaction?	0 = No, or do not know, or no information +1 = Yes
2. Did the adverse event appear after the suspected drug was given?	0 = Do not know or no information −1 = No +2 = Yes
3. Did the adverse reaction improve when the drug was discontinued or a specific antagonist was given?	0 = No, or do not know, or no information +1 = Yes
4. Did the adverse reaction appear when the drug was readministered?	−2 = No 0 = Do not know, or no information +2 = Yes
5. Might alternative causes have caused the reaction?	−1 = Yes 0 = Do not know, or no information +2 = No
6. Did the reaction reappear when a placebo was given?	−1 = Yes 0 = Do not know, or no information +1 = No
7. Was the drug detected in any body fluid in toxic concentrations?	0 = No, or do not know, or no information +1 = Yes

TABLE 1–3. Naranjo scoring system for rating the likelihood of adverse drug reactions (*continued*)

Item	Score[a]
8. Was the reaction more severe when the dose was increased, or less severe when the dose was decreased?	0 = No, or do not know, or no information +1 = Yes
9. Did the patient have a similar reaction to the same or similar drugs in any previous exposure?	0 = No, or do not know, or no information +1 = Yes
10. Was the adverse event confirmed by any objective evidence?	0 = No, or do not know, or no information +1 = Yes

[a]Scoring is based on a total rating of 0 = doubtful adverse drug reaction; 1–4 = possible adverse drug reaction; 5–8 = probable adverse drug reaction; and 9–13 = definite adverse drug reaction.

Source.   Naranjo et al. 1981.

Among the most vivid examples of unexpected or paradoxical adverse effects is the development of mania or hypomania soon after starting an SGA, or the emergence of suicidal thoughts or behaviors during treatment with an antidepressant. Differentiating suspected iatrogenic reactions from the coincidental introduction of treatment in a still-emerging illness is often difficult. Nonetheless, hypotheses have been offered to explain causal links in certain instances (e.g., linking antipsychotic-induced mania with psychomotor activation caused by noradrenergic and serotonergic effects; or posing the suspicion that agitation, insomnia, akathisia, or unrecognized bipolar disorder may contribute to clinical worsening with antidepressants). Some medications have known mechanisms that may incur paradoxical adverse effects, as in the case of highly GABAergic anticonvulsants such as tiagabine for causing new-onset absence seizures or status epilepticus, even in hitherto non-epileptic patients.

In the setting of frankly implausible adverse effects, there is little value in challenging the validity of a dubious self-report, other than to assure the patient that the phenomenon poses no medical hazard — or when the adverse effect is associated with significant distress, to discontinue the agent, allow for the resolution of the perceived side effect, and consider alternative therapies as appropriate.

Extrapolating "Evidence-Based Research Findings" to "Real-World" Patients

Treatment outcomes for patients seen under ordinary clinical conditions often vary substantially from those reported in controlled trials. Pivotal randomized controlled trials that are designed to attain approvable drug indications from a regulatory agency such as the FDA have typically involved idealized circumstances; hence, drug effects (both beneficial and untoward) may generalize poorly to patients treated under more routine circumstances. Numerous factors likely contribute to the so-called gap between treatment efficacy (i.e., optimal results) and effectiveness (i.e., customary results), including 1) enrollment of "pristine" cases that rigorously meet nosological criteria (e.g., DSM-5; American Psychiatric Association 2013) for a specific disorder (e.g., bipolar I but not bipolar II disorder or unspecified bipolar and related disorder), 2) absence of comorbid psychiatric or substance use disorders or medical conditions, 3) absence versus allowance of adjunctive pharmacotherapies, 4) excellent treatment adherence with close supervision, 5) high motivation and reliable attendance for close monitoring of treatment effects, and 6) the tendency for adverse drug effects to be registered passively and incompletely in randomized controlled trials.

Another relevant consideration when evaluating adverse effects reported from controlled trials involves the illness state under investigation. FDA registration studies typically focus on patients experiencing acute episodes of illness, or those who have initially responded to a short-term treatment for an acute illness, who then enter continuation or maintenance phases of therapy focused on the prevention of relapses and recurrences. In routine practice, however, clinicians may very often initiate a pharmacotherapy for subsyndromal symptoms of a subacute or even chronic illness state, or may undertake the substitution of one drug for another in the absence of acute symptoms, in the hopes of alleviating the side-effect burden associated with an existing medication. Unique side-effect concerns may arise in such novel settings (e.g., withdrawal effects of a first drug, or the reemergence of psychiatric symptoms if a new drug is less effective than the one being discontinued), for which data from controlled trials may offer little or no guidance.

Research trials assess adverse effects either through subjects' spontaneous reporting or, less often, through systematic inventories of possible side effects. Spontaneously reported adverse effects are typically coded using a standardized cataloging system, such as the FDA's Coding Symbols for a Thesaurus of Adverse Reaction Terms (COSTART), which has been superceded by the Medical Dictionary for Regulatory Activities (MedDRA; www.meddramsso.com), developed by the International Conference on Harmonisation (ICH) and maintained by the International Federation of Pharmaceutical Manufacturers and Associations (IFPMA). Generally, MedDRA and COSTART terms capture the occurrence of an event during the course of a clinical trial but do not provide information on the intensity or severity of an event or its transience versus longevity. These reporting systems also carry a higher risk of undercounting rather than overcounting of adverse drug effects. Clinical trials also often report rates of dropout or premature study termination due to adverse events but do not necessarily stratify premature dropout by specific reasons, including particular adverse effects. Moreover, clinical trials seldom if ever permit the use of additional medications to counteract an adverse effect (with few notable exceptions, such as benztropine to treat extrapyramidal side effects from an antipsychotic drug, or benzodiazepines for insomnia or agitation).

A further challenge for interpreting adverse effects as reported in clinical trials involves differentiating a possible negative drug effect from simple lack of efficacy against a target symptom related to the illness being treated, or the persistence of symptoms from a comorbid condition—as exemplified by clinical trials that report fairly uninterpretable phenomena, such as "personality disorder" or "schizophrenia" or "nervousness," as adverse drug effects without commenting on their likely association to the drug.

In clinical trials, adverse events recorded in Phase II and Phase III studies do not necessarily attempt to ascribe causality or even plausibility when subjects report problems (e.g., the emergence of respiratory infections or accidental injuries) that may be entirely unrelated to drug effects. Making such distinctions is often quite complex, may depend on small and statistically underpowered subsample sizes (especially for rare adverse drug effects), and may also pertain selectively to distinct subpopulations of study subjects. Prominent examples of rare adverse drug effects include the potential for antidepressants to induce or exacerbate suicidal features in youth (<age 24) but not older adults, for SGAs to increase the risk for all-cause mortality in elderly dementia patients, and for antidepressants to induce manic or hypomanic symptoms in a minority of depressed patients.

For clinicians, perhaps a greater practical problem involves reconciling low reported rates of adverse effects in randomized trials with much higher rates of an adverse effect under routine conditions. Notable examples include the often relatively low incidence rates of sexual dysfunction reported in clinical trials with serotonergic antidepressants, the low expectation for significant weight gain with serotonergic antidepressants, or underappreciation for the risk of akathisia with some SGAs.

Dose Relationships and Adverse Effects

Clinicians often presume that many if not most adverse drug effects can be diminished by reducing the dosage of a drug. Such assumptions often derive more from anecdotal experience or expectations than from empirical data. One obstacle to generalizable information about relationships between dosage and side effects comes from the rarity of fixed-dose comparative studies and the risk of drawing wrong inferences from flexible-dose studies; another constraint involves factors other than dosage that can influence drug tolerability, such as medical comorbidities (e.g., pretreatment obesity), concomitant drugs, or confusion between drug effects and illness features (e.g., hypersomnolence, hyperphagia, or loss of libido in depression). Other limitations involve unknown assumptions about whether dose relationships, if existent, are predictably linear or nonlinear (as limited by narrow dosing ranges) and whether such relationships are equally true across all dosing ranges (e.g., as may arise for linear vs. curvilinear associations).

Some psychotropic agents that have curvilinear dose-response curves may demonstrate inverse relationships between dosage and adverse effects, as has been proposed with mirtazapine, in which sedation at lower dosages (presumably resulting from the drug's antihistaminergic properties) has been suggested to attenuate at higher dosages (e.g., >30 mg/day) due to more prominent noradrenergic effects (Preskorn 2000).

Data exist regarding dose relationships and adverse effects for a select number of psychotropic agents. For example, in the case of quetiapine, incidence rates of sedation, somnolence, and orthostatic hypotension were similar within a narrow dosing range that compared either 300 or 600 mg/day in trials for acute bipolar depression. The magnitude of weight gain caused by olanzapine has been shown not to correlate at a statistically significant level with drug dose in schizophrenia (Kinon et al. 2001), but possible dose relationships with weight gain and other SGAs are less established. Time on drug may represent a confounding factor with respect to dose (i.e., longer duration of treatment may increase the likelihood and extent of weight gain; moreover, clinicians may be inclined to raise the dosage of a medication over time in the setting of incomplete remissions or breakthrough signs of relapse). By contrast, toxicity related to dosing appears to account for thrombocytopenia with divalproex or for seizures with bupropion or clozapine. Table 1–4 provides a summary of known dose relationships with specific adverse effects identified in manufacturers' product information materials.

A clinical dilemma that arises when considering the relationship between drug dosing and adverse events involves the mediating effects of exposure time. When tolerance to an adverse effect is known to occur over time (as in the case of headaches or nausea during treatment with SSRIs), it can be difficult to know if and when dosage increases would worsen adverse effects without taking into account exposure time. Some psychotropic agents are known to recruit different transmitter systems at different dosages — for example, greater noradrenergic effects are thought to occur with mirtazapine when dosed above 30–45 mg/day or with venlafaxine dosed above 150 mg/day — and as such, dosing may account for adverse-effect profiles (e.g., resolution of fatigue or sedation at higher doses), irrespective of time on drug. Because clinicians are often inclined to raise drug dosages after initial exposure to a lower dosage, the clinician could mistakenly presume that the eventual resolution of an initial side effect was due to prolonged time on drug rather than increased dosing, unless the clinician was aware of dose-related noradrenergic receptor profiles.

Most pharmaceutical trials conducted for the purposes of regulatory agency approval do not track or report the evolution of adverse effects

TABLE 1–4.   Common side effects with dose relationships reported by manufacturers from U.S. Food and Drug Administration registration trials

Adverse effect	Medications with known dose relationships[a]
Ataxia	Gabapentin, lamotrigine, oxcarbazepine
Blurry vision or diplopia	Lamotrigine, oxcarbazepine
Complex sleep behaviors	Zolpidem
Constipation	Duloxetine, escitalopram
Dizziness	Iloperidone, lamotrigine, oxcarbazepine, risperidone, topiramate, ziprasidone
Dry mouth[b]	Escitalopram, nortriptyline, ziprasidone
Dyslipidemias	Desvenlafaxine
Extrapyramidal symptoms, including akathisia	Most FGAs and SGAs
Fatigue	Citalopram, escitalopram, risperidone, topiramate
Headache	Modafinil
Hyperprolactinemia	Lurasidone, risperidone
Hypertension	Venlafaxine
Hypothyroidism	Quetiapine
Insomnia	Citalopram, escitalopram
Nausea or gastrointestinal upset[b]	Divalproex, escitalopram, iloperidone, lamotrigine, oxcarbazepine, paroxetine, quetiapine, topiramate
Orthostatic hypotension	Paliperidone, MAOIs, ziprasidone
Paresthesias	Topiramate
QTc prolongation on ECG	Citalopram, FGAs, SGAs
Rashes	Lamotrigine (based on rapidity of dosing titration)
Sedation or somnolence	Aripiprazole, citalopram, divalproex, escitalopram, gabapentin, lurasidone, oxcarbazepine, paliperidone, paroxetine, risperidone, topiramate, ziprasidone
Seizures	Bupropion, clozapine

TABLE 1–4. Common side effects with dose relationships reported by manufacturers from U.S. Food and Drug Administration registration trials *(continued)*

Adverse effect	Medications with known dose relationships[a]
Sexual dysfunction[c]	Citalopram, nefazodone, paroxetine, sertraline, venlafaxine, risperidone
Sweating	Citalopram, escitalopram, paroxetine
Tachycardia	Iloperidone
Thrombocytopenia	Divalproex
Tremor	Divalproex, paroxetine, ziprasidone
Weight gain	Iloperidone, quetiapine, risperidone
Yawning	Citalopram

Note. ECG=electrocardiogram; FGA=first-generation antipsychotic; MAOI= monoamine oxidase inhibitor; SGA=second-generation antipsychotic.
[a]Within usual therapeutic ranges.
[b]The duloxetine package insert originally also included nausea, dry mouth, and hyperhidrosis as dose-related phenomena in major depression; these three items were removed as dose-related events after safety data were pooled for major depression and generalized anxiety disorder.
[c]No clear dose relationship was found for sexual dysfunction with bupropion, fluoxetine, or mirtazapine (Clayton et al. 2002).

over time, but rather report only the sheer occurrence of an adverse event during the course of a drug trial. Study durations are often too short to provide sufficient exposure time to capture all pertinent adverse effects. Therefore, it is difficult to project when an adverse effect is likely to attenuate with prolonged exposure or how much time should elapse before anticipating that an adverse effect warrants intervention. An example of this conundrum involves the antihistaminergic effects of quetiapine relative to the time course for persistence or resolution of sedation and somnolence. Prolonged blockade of histamine H_1 receptors should produce tachyphylaxis or rapid tolerance (i.e., sedation or somnolence would presumably occur at the outset of treatment and then plateau or diminish over time following receptor saturation; see also the section "Fatigue and Sedation" in Chapter 17, "Neurological System"); indeed, this explanation has been invoked by some practitioners, rightly or wrongly, to reassure patients and prescribers that sedation or somnolence generally does not persist and may not worsen at higher dosages. However, this theoretically plausible concept has not, as of yet, been empirically demonstrated.

A further consideration involves the observation that some adverse effects (e.g., extrapyramidal effects of antipsychotics) may occur at higher receptor saturations (e.g., dopamine D_2 receptor occupancy in the striatum), whereas beneficial effects (e.g., antipsychotic efficacy relative to mesolimbic D_2 receptor occupancy) may occur at lower receptor saturations. In some instances, the relationship between adverse effects and receptor saturation may be relatively linear, whereas the relationship between pharmacodynamic benefits and receptor binding may be sigmoidal rather than linear.

From the standpoint of clinical care, a final point involves managing complaints of adverse effects at extremely low drug dosages. Such events can be vexing not only for patients but especially for prescribers, in that clinicians may feel an urgency to press forward in raising a drug dosage to usual therapeutic levels, making the distress of an early adverse effect seem like an impediment to the common goal of doctor and patient. Such complaints also may sometimes seem ill founded from a pharmacodynamic standpoint (analogous to self-reported improvement within hours of starting an SSRI for depression) and incur the prescriber's suspicion about a patient's suggestibility, histrionic features, tendencies toward somatization, or even possible psychosis. Bearing in mind factors such as the potential existence of a slow metabolizer genotype, pharmacokinetic inhibition from a coadministered agent, possible hepatic or renal insufficiency, excessive self-dosing by a patient, or simply a heightened sensitivity to drug effects, it usually behooves the prescriber to follow the lead of the patient; when a patient's investment in continuing an appropriate treatment is tenuous, clinical wisdom may dictate proceeding slowly with dosage increases, despite a belief on the part of the clinician that true side effects at a low dosage are improbable.

FDA Warnings and Precautions

The FDA tiers its mandated cautionary statements about the severity and importance of adverse events related to medications. *Boxed warnings* (formerly referred to as "black box warnings") carry the highest level of concern and typically pertain to a proved or suspected risk for medically serious or potentially life-threatening side effects. *Warnings* are statements communicating that serious adverse events or potential safety hazards have been observed with a particular drug. *Precautions* indicate that consideration must be taken in special situations or patient groups. *Contraindications* are statements included in manufacturers' product information that a drug should not be used in certain clinical situations because its risks significantly outweigh its projected benefits. Contraindications may be relative or absolute. Table 1–5 provides a summary of boxed warnings associated with commonly prescribed psychotropic medications. Throughout this book, adverse effects that reflect FDA boxed warnings are also designated symbolically (■).

Notably, class warnings impart no information about possible relative differences among agents within a given class (e.g., the potential for glycemic dysregulation may vary considerably among SGAs; suicidal thinking and behavior can differ across drugs that possess antidepressant properties).

All antipsychotics carry a boxed warning (■) regarding a small but significant increased risk for all-cause mortality in elderly patients with dementia-related psychosis. This warning derives from an analysis of 17 placebo-controlled trials conducted over an approximate 10-week period, which found a 1.6- to 1.7-fold increased risk for all-cause mortality (4.5% among subjects taking an SGA compared with 2.6% among those taking placebo), on the basis of safety data analyzed by the FDA.

Risk-Benefit Analyses

The extent to which patients or clinicians prioritize tolerability over efficacy likely varies as a function of illness severity and disease consequences (exemplified perhaps most dramatically in the case of choosing antineoplastics for a malignancy). Remarkably, in psychiatry, doctors and patients seldom discuss how to strike a balance between sufficient efficacy and acceptable adverse effects, despite the high degree of functional disability and excess mortality due not only to suicide, but also to medical comorbidities in people with significant mood or psychotic disorders. Yet, studies of treatment effectiveness point to the relevance of both dimensions. For example, in the National Institute of Mental Health–funded CATIE study in schizophrenia, 15% of subjects discontinued their participation because of drug intolerance, whereas 24% discontinued because of lack of efficacy (Lieberman et al. 2005).

As described below, a number of points merit consideration regarding the balance between risks and benefits of any treatment within the context of a doctor-patient relationship.

Shared Decision-Making With Patients

The notion of shared risk and shared decision-making between doctor and patient is in many respects the hallmark of an effective therapeutic

TABLE 1–5.   U.S. Food and Drug Administration boxed warnings (■) related to adverse drug effects

Warning or precaution	Agents	Practical implications
Agranulocytosis	Clozapine, carbamazepine (alone and especially combined)	REMS (Risk Evaluation and Mitigation Strategies) registry-based CBC and ANC monitoring for clozapine is weekly for the first 6 months, then (if stable) biweekly for the next 6 months, then (if stable) every 4 weeks thereafter. Specific information regarding acceptable CBC and ANC levels and management guidelines are available at https://www.clozapinerems.com/CpmgClozapineUI/home.u.
Serious cardiovascular events and sudden death	All formulations of amphetamine or methylphenidate	The American Heart Association recommends baseline ECGs in children before initiating a stimulant (Vetter et al. 2008).
Serious and potentially fatal dermatological reactions, including toxic epidermal necrolysis and Stevens-Johnson syndrome	Carbamazepine, lamotrigine	Carbamazepine risk is higher in patients with Asian ancestry who carry the *HLA-B*1502* allelic variant of the *HLA-B* gene.
Hepatic failure	Nefazodone	Nefazodone has been observed to cause life-threatening hepatic failure in 1 of 250,000 exposed cases. Preexisting liver disease does not predispose to this occurrence. Nefazodone should not be administered if serum liver enzymes (AST or ALT) exceed three times the upper limit of normal.

TABLE 1–5. U.S. Food and Drug Administration boxed warnings (■) related to adverse drug effects *(continued)*

Warning or precaution	Agents	Practical implications
Hepatotoxicity	Divalproex	Divalproex carries an increased risk for potentially fatal hepatotoxicity, particularly in infants given multiple anticonvulsants, and usually during the first 6 months of treatment. Liver function tests should be monitored on a regular basis.
Increased mortality in elderly patients with dementia-related psychosis	All antipsychotics	Risks must be weighed against potential benefits; caution is necessary in patients with known cardiovascular or cerebrovascular disease.
Myocarditis	Clozapine	Reported incidence is approximately 1%, typically arising within the first few weeks of clozapine initiation. CRP levels >100 mg/L may be an early diagnostic indicator (Ronaldson et al. 2010), as is occasionally eosinophilia.
Pancreatitis	Divalproex	Pancreatitis should be considered in the differential diagnosis of patients who develop signs of an acute abdomen while taking divalproex.
Other serious cardiovascular and respiratory effects	Clozapine	Includes orthostatic hypotension with or without syncope.
QTc prolongation (dose related)	Mesoridazine, methadone, thioridazine	Use of mesoridazine or thioridazine is reserved for schizophrenia that is refractory to other treatments.

TABLE 1–5.   U.S. Food and Drug Administration boxed warnings (■) related to adverse drug effects (*continued*)

Warning or precaution	Agents	Practical implications
Seizures	Clozapine	Seizures are usually dose related or the result of rapid dosing titration; some practitioners advocate cotherapy with an anticonvulsant (e.g., divalproex, carbamazepine, gabapentin) when clozapine is used at high dosages (Toth and Frankenburg 1994; Usiskin et al. 2000).
Increased risk for suicidal thinking and behavior (but no proven increased risk for suicide deaths)	Atomoxetine, all antidepressants, quetiapine, olanzapine-fluoxetine combination, deutetrabenazine	In patients <age 24, especially close attention is needed to the paradoxical worsening or emergence of suicidal thinking during antidepressant therapy in the first few weeks of treatment, in which case drug cessation may be appropriate. Deutetrabenazine risk for depression and suicidality is based on data for patients with Huntington's disease.
Teratogenicity	Divalproex	Divalproex is associated with a 1%–5% incidence of neural tube defects in the developing fetus; use during pregnancy requires that the benefits of use outweigh the potential risks to fetal development.

Note.   ALT=alanine aminotransferase; ANC=absolute neutrophil count; AST=aspartate aminotransferase; CBC=complete blood count; CRP=C-reactive protein; ECG=electrocardiogram; FDA=U.S. Food and Drug Administration.

alliance. Because treatment outcomes are often difficult if not impossible to predict, it can be argued that the most any health care provider can do beyond offering an educated opinion about preferred treatment options is articulate the likely risks and benefits of a given therapy and provide an informed estimate of the probabilities attached to both of these core facets of treatment.

One area that is particularly emblematic of shared risk and decision making is the approach to planned pregnancy in women taking psychotropic medications. As described more fully in Chapter 21, "Pregnancy and the Puerperium," most commonly used psychotropic drugs lack known risk for human teratogenicity, but the potential for unknown risk remains a concern; such uncertainties must be balanced against the more tangible and often known certainties related to symptomatic or syndromal relapse with treatment discontinuation during pregnancy in many individuals with significant psychiatric disorders.

Known Versus Unknown Drug Risks

A reality of medicine involves the accrual of new information about a drug after it is made available for marketing by the FDA. Postmarketing experience provides the essential opportunity to determine experiences with a treatment under more ordinary or routine clinical conditions than is otherwise the case in randomized trials.

Despite the rigors of all phases of safety testing for a drug, pharmacovigilance data at times emerge in ways that could not be anticipated initially in the absence of more extensive exposure to larger segments of the population. Postmarketing surveillance findings sometimes lead to changes in the labeling or categorization of a drug (e.g., warnings regarding the risk for suicidal thoughts or acts with anticonvulsants in epilepsy patients in nonbipolar, nonepileptic patients [Arana et al. 2010]; hepatic failure with nefazodone or pemoline; the reappraisal of paroxetine's safety in pregnancy after postmarketing drug monitoring cases revealed a small but significantly increased risk for atrial or ventricular septal defects during first trimester exposure in pregnancy). Any clinician can report an adverse drug effect to the FDA through its MedWatch program, also known as the FDA Adverse Event Reporting System (FAERS; http://www.fda.gov/Drugs/GuidanceComplianceRegulatory Information/Surveillance/AdverseDrugEffects/default.htm). Under the Freedom of Information Act, clinicians also can request a summary FAERS report for a particular medication by contacting the Division of Freedom of Information at the FDA (or online at http://www.accessdata. fda.gov/scripts/foi/FOIRequest/index.cfm).

Some clinical trials have begun to express the incidence of specific adverse effects as the *number needed to harm* (NNH), defined as the number of patients who need to be exposed to a treatment for an increased risk of an adverse event in one individual. NNH is computed as follows:

$$\frac{1}{\text{event rate among exposed subjects} - \text{event rate among subjects not exposed}}$$

In clinical trials, this proportion typically reflects 1 / (drug rate) – (placebo rate). The denominator in the equation above might, for example, refer to the proportion of patients who develop weight gain exceeding 7% of their pretreatment weight with an SGA less the same proportion among those who took placebo. NNH, analogous to the *number needed to treat* (NNT), expresses the magnitude of effect of an active drug versus a placebo, or of one treatment relative to another. In practical terms, a high NNH indicates that many patients would need to be exposed to a given therapy before one would incur an adverse event of interest. (For further discussion on calculating and using NNT and NNH, see Citrome 2011a.)

When considering the risks versus benefits of a particular treatment, a low NNT (meaning that few patients need to be treated before one responds) with a high NNH suggests an optimal balance. By way of example, in the above instance, an NNH-NNT analysis (i.e., risk-benefit ratio) comparing olanzapine to lithium or divalproex during maintenance treatment for bipolar I disorder yielded NNHs for olanzapine of 5–8, relative to NNTs of 4–10 for preventing symptomatic relapse into mania, depression, or a mixed episode (Tohen et al. 2009). Elsewhere, studies of discontinuation due to adverse events in randomized trials of olanzapine found an NNH of 24 in bipolar depression and 9 in major depression; discontinuation attributable to adverse events in trials of quetiapine XR found NNHs of 9 in bipolar depression and in major depression, 8 in refractory major depression, and 5 in generalized anxiety disorder (Gao et al. 2011). The NNH:NNT ratio has also been described as the *likelihood of being helped or harmed* (LHH).

Risk-benefit analyses that consider drug tolerability versus efficacy often may also be usefully informed by appreciating the magnitude or clinical meaningfulness of a drug's beneficial effect. In addition to NNT, the clinician might consider the concept of *effect size* — a statistic derived from the observed difference in mean scores divided by their pooled standard deviation. Also known as Cohen's *d*, effect sizes are generally ranked as being small (≤0.20), medium (~0.50), or large (~≥0.80) (Cohen

1992). Clinicians might wisely be more inclined to encourage patients to tolerate or manage adverse effects when a drug's expected benefits correspond to a larger rather than a smaller effect size. Drugs that exert only a small effect, or merely a "just noticeable difference" from placebo, may not possess a sufficiently clinically meaningful impact to justify their adverse effects.

Watchful Waiting

It is fundamental for practitioners to know when adverse drug effects are usually transient and typically resolve with time through the process of accommodation to a medication (e.g., nausea after starting an SSRI) and when a given side effect is likely to endure (e.g., as is common with medication-induced weight gain). Elements of decision making in this domain involve an awareness not only of drug exposure time as contributing to tolerability but also an awareness of association (or lack of association) between a side effect and progressive dosage increases. In the latter instance, the clinician might consider the example of sedation with mirtazapine as being purportedly more common at low rather than high dosages due to the drug's greater noradrenergic effects at higher dosages; and in the former instance, the frequent transience of nonspecific CNS effects, such as headache or dizziness, experienced by a patient soon after beginning an antidepressant. By contrast, weight gain caused by psychotropic agents has rarely been shown to diminish with dosage reductions, and the hope that weight gain will spontaneously halt or reverse itself either with time alone or with a lowered dosage is usually unrealistic. Possession of a fairly strong working knowledge of the time course, dose relationships, risk factors, and clinical relevance of common side effects allows the practitioner to make more informed recommendations and forecast outcomes more effectively when anticipating and managing the potential emergence of adverse effects.

Deciding When to Pursue Antidotes and When to Switch Medicines

In some respects, practitioners rely more on art than science when deciding whether to actively manage an adverse effect (either by dosage adjustments or the addition of other medications intended to counteract adverse effects) or to discontinue a treatment because of its adverse effects. Some unpredictable or idiosyncratic yet adverse effects obviously defy management; these include agranulocytosis, NMS, and serious rashes. Other adverse effects may clearly pose more of an annoyance than a danger to physical well-being. In such instances, there may be a compelling rationale to introduce additional medicines to remedy an adverse effect while preserving a benefit (as in the case of β-blockers or benzodiazepines to diminish akathisia). Still other adverse effects may signal probable drug toxicities that may be dose related (e.g., tremor caused by lithium, thrombocytopenia caused by divalproex). A further conundrum can arise when a particular side effect has been suggested to correlate with a favorable treatment response (as in the reported predictive value of weight gain with use of antipsychotics or the antimanic efficacy of some SGAs); such correlations may be spurious artifacts of drug exposure time or dosage.

"Antidote" drugs that may counteract a psychotropic drug's adverse effects could themselves have adverse effects that further bear on risk-benefit analyses. For example, anticholinergic drugs such as benztropine, trihexyphenidyl, or oxybutynin may in themselves cause cognitive impairment, sedation, and visual or gastrointestinal problems. Clinicians choosing from among several viable antidote drugs should consider these medications' relative risks and benefits. (For example, amantadine may offer a more cognitively benign remedy than anticholinergic drugs to counteract antipsychotic-induced extrapyramidal adverse effects.) Prescribers should be familiar with possible adverse effects of a given nonpsychotropic drug before prescribing it as an intended remedy to counteract adverse psychotropic drug effects.

Practitioners might consider adverse drug effects as falling along a continuum of severity that can range from "minimal or mild" to "annoying but medically inconsequential" to "serious" or even "life threatening." Table 1–6 lists the levels of difficulty and severity in managing psychotropic side effects. Practitioners can counsel patients on the likelihood that a given side effect is transient or dose related and advise conservative management strategies (e.g., taking acetaminophen for headaches when starting an SSRI), assuming that the clinician understands the typical time course for the emergence and resolution of a particular medication side effect. Sometimes, nuisance side effects can be averted or at least minimized by changing a medication dosage, formulation (e.g., extended release), cotherapy, or timing of administration (e.g., giving sedating drugs at night).

Treatment Adherence and Adverse Effects

Randomized studies that report premature dropouts due to adverse effects can be difficult to extrapolate to real-world treatment settings for a variety of reasons. Research trial subjects typically have only one diag-

TABLE 1–6. Levels of difficulty and severity in managing psychotropic side effects

Relatively simple to manage	Often difficult to manage	Medically serious
Anticholinergic effects (e.g., dry mouth, constipation)	Alopecia	Neuroleptic malignant syndrome
	Cognitive complaints	Serotonin syndrome
	Insomnia	Severe cutaneous reactions
Extrapyramidal side effects	Nephrogenic diabetes insipidus	
Gastrointestinal upset	Sedation	Severe metabolic dysregulation (e.g., hyperosmotic nonketotic coma)
Headache	Sexual dysfunction	
Tremor	Sialorrhea	
	Tardive dyskinesia	Substantial weight gain
	Mild to moderate weight gain	

nosis that conforms more closely to DSM-IV-TR or DSM-5 criteria than may be the case in routine practice (where patients with poorly defined conditions may encounter different beneficial or adverse drug effects). Also, nonresearch patients often take more than one medication at a time, and their motivations and expectations may differ during a time-limited clinical trial than is the case for patients in more open-ended routine treatment. Some researchers point out that in a double-blind trial, research subjects often will tolerate adverse effects in the context of clinical response and be less likely to prematurely leave a clinical trial because of adverse effects than subjects who encounter adverse effects but minimal or no improvement. One problem when interpreting such observations involves determining whether the presence of adverse effects in and of themselves may inadvertently allow patients to discern whether they are taking an active drug or placebo, which in turn may influence their decision to remain in a double-blind study if they believe they are improving while receiving an active therapy.

A frequent, intuitively logical assumption is that medication adherence wanes in the setting of cumulative or substantial adverse drug effects. However, surprisingly little research has addressed the extent to which patients across psychiatric disorders are inclined to tolerate adverse effects and remain in treatment if efficacy is robust, or rather, how much a potential side-effect burden drives adherence and retention with treatment irrespective of drug efficacy. Some pharmacotherapy studies suggest that less premature study termination occurs due to adverse effects when efficacy is high relative to placebo, but the balance between tolerability and efficacy is difficult to express in either a quantitative or generalizable format.

Clinicians cannot assume that side-effect burden necessarily drives medication nonadherence. For example, in the 2000 British National Psychiatric Morbidity Survey, concerns about psychotropic drug side effects were identified by only 14% of 634 respondents as a reason for incomplete adherence with medications (Cooper et al. 2007). Those who linked side effects with poor adherence were younger, had histories of psychosis, and had lower intellectual functioning. Elsewhere, Agosti et al. (2002) found that depressed patients who stopped antidepressant therapy during randomized placebo-controlled trials with various antidepressants were more likely to have high baseline somatization.

In an interesting study of mood stabilizer adherence among individuals with bipolar disorder, Scott and Pope (2002) found that patients' apprehension or perceptions about possible adverse drug effects, rather than the actual occurrence of adverse effects, contributed to nonadherence. A corollary to these observations is that patient adherence to pharmacotherapy may improve if prescribers are better able to anticipate and desensitize fears about potential drug side effects before they occur. Clinicians sometimes think that when they disclose possible side effects to a patient, they are mainly performing an act of due diligence by discharging a medicolegal obligation, with the presumption that providing more than the minimum necessary amount of information would heighten fears and inspire nonadherence. In fact, little evidence supports this notion. Many patients also poorly retain such information after only a single presentation.

An alternative perspective is that patients may respond more to the sense of factual openness and confidence with which a practitioner forecasts likely outcomes, both good and bad. Physicians who impart their perspective not only on the likelihood of occurrence of an adverse event but also on the ability to anticipate and actively manage a side effect if it arises, are likely to strengthen rather than weaken the therapeutic alliance—which may in turn serve to minimize patients' fears about unknown consequences of treatment. Patients, in turn, may also be grateful for honest appraisals coupled with a sense of empowerment from their treaters who indicate that no matter what could happen, the patients' care will fall under a watchful eye and a proactive guardianship.

Patients and prescribers have been shown to differ in their perceptions about drug side effects. Over 60% of survey respondents with self-identified bipolar disorder in the British Manic Depression Fellowship reported feeling dissatisfied with the level of information their physicians provided to them regarding the nature and extent of medication side effects, especially potential sexual adverse effects (Bowskill et al. 2007).

A final consideration relating to medication adherence involves the potential negative impact of underdosing, potentially as an effort by prescribers to minimize side-effect burden. A study of 312 individuals with bipolar disorder found that the number of daily medications or pills did not correlate with medication adherence but that low adherence was significantly associated with taking smaller dosages of mood-stabilizing drugs (Bauer et al. 2010), although that study did not account for the potential moderating effects of illness severity on treatment adherence.

General Approach to Assessing Adverse Drug Effects

Perhaps a first consideration regarding the assessment of drug side effects involves differences in their recognition by patients versus psychiatrists, and the extent to which patients spontaneously report or even recognize possible side effects. Given pharmacodynamic and pharmacokinetic synergies that occur from combination drug regimens, it is pointless for a psychiatrist to ask a patient if he or she is aware of any possible side effects from one drug out of many. It is crucial for practitioners to *assess*, rather than merely *note*, suspected adverse drug effects, because patients' physical complaints may, in actuality, be communications of subjective distress that is unrelated to medications. Implausible adverse effects or nocebo responses are psychiatric phenomena that require exploration—for example, sedation or cognitive problems from non-antihistaminergic, nonanticholinergic drugs. Astute clinicians also recognize the presence of pharmacodynamic inconsistencies, as when patients report co-occurring problems that involve opposing mechanisms, such as dry mouth with diarrhea, or sialorrhea with constipation. Rather than dispute the validity of a patient's experience (e.g., "That's impossible! This medicine doesn't have anticholinergic effects!"), the clinician would be wise to validate the patient's distress and adopt a more psychotherapeutic stance (e.g., "We will figure this out together; let's go back and examine more closely what's been happening since the time you began this medicine").

Clinicians sometimes proactively assess adverse drug effects but must be even more alert to patients' spontaneous symptom complaints that require probing to differentiate iatrogenic from illness-based etiologies (e.g., insomnia, anxiety, agitation). Practitioners vary in how they track adverse effects using a systematic versus an ad hoc approach. A minimum standard of care has yet to be established in psychiatry for the surveillance monitoring of adverse drug effects in clinical practice. Perhaps two of the greatest considerations in monitoring drug safety involve the sheer identification of side effects (i.e., sensitivity to recognizing when a side effect may be present) and the ability to attribute proper causality to a possible side effect (i.e., deducing the specificity or likelihood that the cause of a potential side effect is indeed a particular medication). The former responsibility involves a strong knowledge of common side effects of all medications being prescribed (and the resourcefulness to investigate whether or not an uncommon side effect has been linked with a particular medication), and their active (rather than passive) recognition. The latter becomes especially challenging when a patient takes a variety of medications and attempts are made to discern which one (or which combination) is most likely producing a given effect.

Practitioners assess potential side effects with great variability. Some choose not to bring up side effects altogether unless patients do so themselves for fear of inspiring nonadherence. Others adopt a rather businesslike stance in disclosing to patients (and documenting) mainly the potentially serious side effects listed in a manufacturer's package insert, largely as a matter of medicolegal due diligence. The use of systematic rating scales (see "Rating Scales for Measuring Adverse Drug Effects" in Appendix 3) offers one means for delineating and quantifying the extent of certain adverse drug effects, providing a method for prospectively tracking potential worsening from baseline. From the standpoint of providing good medical care, the proverbial middle ground likely involves assessing an individual patient's attitudes and beliefs about medications, both beneficial and harmful, and tailoring an informed discussion accordingly. Patients with diffuse anxiety and trepidation about possible hazardous results would be ill served and cognitively flooded by a recitation of any and all possible side effects; such individuals likely respond better to the fostering of an emotionally safe and secure environment in which the prescriber projects a stance of vigilance on behalf of the patient, guarding against the intrusion of side effects that lurk beyond the safe confines of the consultation room. By contrast, obsessional or paranoid patients — who may be inclined to research any and all possible side effects, regardless of their plausibility or likelihood — may need their safety concerns validated and fare best when engaged as their own sentries poised to safeguard their own welfare. Individuals with histrionic or dramatic presentation styles may exaggerate their experience of suspected adverse effects, and clinical wisdom often demands exploring such patients' subjective complaints and concerns beyond their face value.

For the majority of patients, perhaps the most honest and reasonable approach for anticipating side effects is to proactively inform patients of the most common and medically important side effects to watch for and to provide some sense of context and proportion about their likelihood, seriousness, and time course (e.g., "Nausea is the most common side effect of SSRIs; it typically passes shortly after starting a drug. It is less likely to occur if the medicine is taken with food than on an empty stomach. If it occurs and is bothersome, an over-the-counter medication such as famotidine may be helpful until the nausea eventually goes away."). Sometimes, such information can also empower patients to know the parameters under which side effects may happen, especially if clinicians can impart a sense of predictability and control over an otherwise random-risk event. For example, when prescribing lamotrigine, the clinician might inform patients that the greatest risk window for developing a serious rash during treatment is from weeks 2 through 8, that serious rashes have a characteristic appearance, and that the risk can be minimized by taking precautions such as avoiding new environmental exposures.

A related point for engaging patients as collaborators in risk-benefit decision making involves the ability to forecast the probability that a side effect will occur and to describe a management strategy before it is needed. For example, in the case of weight gain caused by olanzapine, patients with bipolar mania who gain 1.8–2.3 kg in the first 2–3 weeks of treatment have a significantly greater risk for eventual substantial weight gain (≥9.9 kg) after 30 weeks of continued therapy, as contrasted with a much smaller risk (~10%) of substantial weight gain later developing in patients without such increases in the first few weeks (Lipkovich et al. 2006). Speaking from that database, a clinician might suggest to a patient who is concerned about possible weight gain that within the first few weeks of treatment, a reasonable estimate can be made on both the potential for improvement and the likelihood for later weight gain. In that sense, clinical decision making becomes a nonstatic process, informed by successive (and changing) risk-benefit analyses over time.

Pharmacokinetics, Pharmacodynamics, and Pharmacogenomics

Pharmacokinetics and Pharmacodynamics

Pharmacodynamics refers to the effects of a drug on the body, whereas *pharmacokinetics* refers to the effect of the body on a drug (absorption, distribution, metabolism, and elimination).

Drug absorption becomes relevant to pharmacodynamic effects mainly when external factors exist that hasten or delay absorption, which in turn may affect the bioavailability of a compound. Malabsorption syndromes (e.g., dumping syndrome after gastric bypass surgery) may slow drug absorption or pose implications for the utility of certain drug formulations (e.g., after gastric bypass, extended-release formulations that are absorbed more distally in the gastrointestinal tract are generally less well absorbed than are immediate-release formulations).

The absorption of some psychotropic drugs also may vary greatly when ingested with or without food. Drugs that are administered parenterally (by injection), transdermally, or sublingually avoid first-pass hepatic metabolism and may reach maximal blood concentrations (Cmax) faster than orally ingested formulations, although time until achieving Cmax does not necessarily translate to faster or more substantial therapeutic efficacy or an altered side-effect burden.

Important concepts related to drug absorption, distribution, metabolism, and elimination are summarized in Table 2–1. Manufacturers' suggested dosing for many pharmaceutical agents is based on the plasma elimination half-life rather than terminal elimination half-life.

Clinicians sometimes assume (and drug manufacturers sometimes intimate) that Tmax (time to Cmax) reflects a maximal pharmacodynamic drug effect (whether beneficial or adverse), but such a simple association cannot necessarily be presumed. Drugs exert different effects at different sites of action (e.g., in the case of TCAs, α_1-adrenergic receptor blockade mediates orthostatic hypotension while central cholinergic receptors mediate adverse cognitive effects), yet such regional differences in concentration may not accurately be reflected by the maximal plasma level. Some adverse effects also occur only after chronic administration of a drug (e.g., tardive dyskinesia or metabolic syndrome arising from antipsychotics; secondary hypothyroidism due to lithium; osteoporosis from anticonvulsants or SSRIs) and are not clearly related to plasma blood levels or maximal concentrations.

Known effects of drug administration on absorption with or without food are summarized in Table 2–2.

Orodispersible (i.e., orally disintegrating) forms of a medication dissolve supralingually and are then swallowed (rather than absorbed to any appreciable degree through the oral-buccal mucosa). Orally disintegrating preparations require the same gastrointestinal (nonbuccal) absorption as oral tablet formulations, and do not demonstrate appreciable pharmacodynamic differences from nonorodispersible forms of these drugs.

Drug metabolism becomes especially pertinent when it may account for drug side effects. For example, *Phase I* metabolism refers to the effects of hepatic microsomal CYP enzymes on drug substrates and includes chemical reactions such as oxidation (e.g., of carbamazepine to its epoxide metabolite, as illustrated in Figure 2–1) or reduction (e.g., the reduction of the keto group at the 10-carbon position of the middle ring structure of oxcarbazepine to generate its metabolite monohydroxy-oxcarbazepine, as illustrated in Figure 2–2). Similarly, Phase I demethylation of tertiary amine TCAs (e.g., amitriptyline or imipramine, via CYP2C19) derives their secondary amine metabolites (nortriptyline and desmethylimipramine [desipramine], respectively); the latter are often thought to cause fewer anticholinergic (e.g., cognitive) and sedative effects—although potentially greater cardiotoxicity—than their tertiary amine parent compounds.

TABLE 2–1.   Key concepts related to pharmacokinetic effects

Term	Definition
Area under the curve (AUC)	Plasma concentration of a drug plotted against time after administration; relevant for estimating drug bioavailability and clearance
Bioavailability	Extent to which a drug is absorbed and becomes available to its target tissue; formally defined as the AUC for a given dose
Cmax	Maximum plasma concentration of a drug (*Note:* This does not necessarily reflect drug concentration at the drug's site of action— e.g., maximal plasma concentrations of lithium may not necessarily reflect brain lithium levels in patients with bipolar disorder; Sachs et al. 1995)
Plasma elimination half-life ($t_{1/2}$)	Time required until the plasma concentration of a drug is reduced by half; often taken as a proxy for the half-life at end-organs of interest (e.g., brain), following an exponential decay process (see also Table 2–2)
Steady-state concentration (C_{ss})	An equilibrium state in which a stable concentration of a drug is achieved, typically after the passage of five half-lives
Therapeutic index	Amount of a drug that causes death (i.e., a lethal dose for 50% of the population, or LD_{50}) relative to the amount that causes a therapeutic effect (i.e., the minimum effective dose for 50% of the population, or ED_{50}); defined as the ratio of LD_{50}/ED_{50}
Therapeutic window	Range between an effective dose (ED_{50}) and the median toxic dose (TD_{50}, the dose at which toxicity occurs for 50% of the population)
Tmax	Time to Cmax

TABLE 2–2. Mean half-life and differential absorption of psychotropics under fasting conditions versus with food

Agent	Mean $t_{1/2}$	Does food alter drug absorption and bioavailability?		
		No	Yes	Comment
Atomoxetine	5 hours	✓		
Buspirone	2–3 hours		✓	Administration either with or without food should be consistent.
Anticonvulsants and lithium				
Carbamazepine	25–65 hours	✓		
Divalproex	9–16 hours		✓	Food slows rate but not extent of absorption.
Eslicarbazepine	20–24 hours	✓		
Gabapentin	5–7 hours		✓	High-protein meals may increase absorption via intestinal transport (Gidal et al. 1996).
Lamotrigine	25–33 hours	✓		
Lithium	24 hours		✓	Lower absorption occurs on an empty stomach.
Oxcarbazepine	30 hours	✓		
Topiramate	21 hours	✓		

TABLE 2–2. Mean half-life and differential absorption of psychotropics under fasting conditions versus with food (*continued*)

Agent	Mean $t_{1/2}$	Does food alter drug absorption and bioavailability?		
		No	Yes	Comment
Antidepressants				
Bupropion	14 hours (IR) 21 hours (SR or XL)	✓		
Mirtazapine	20–40 hours	✓		
Nefazodone	2–4 hours		✓	Food decreases absorption and bioavailability by ~20%.
SNRIs	Desvenlafaxine=11 hours	✓		
	Duloxetine=12 hours	✓		
	Levomilnacipran=12 hours	✓		
	Venlafaxine=5 hours	✓		
SSRIs	Citalopram=35 hours		✓	Modest increased bioavailability and higher Cmax with food for sertraline; otherwise, no known associations with other SSRIs.
	Escitalopram=27–32 hours		✓	
	Fluoxetine=4–6 days (norfluoxetine=9 days)		✓	
	Fluvoxamine=15 hours		✓	
	Paroxetine=21 hours		✓	
	Sertraline=26 hours		✓	

TABLE 2–2. Mean half-life and differential absorption of psychotropics under fasting conditions versus with food *(continued)*

Agent	Mean $t_{\frac{1}{2}}$	Does food alter drug absorption and bioavailability?		
		No	Yes	Comment
Antidepressants *(continued)*				
TCAs	Amitriptyline=10–50 hours	✓		
	Clomipramine=19–37 hours	✓		
	Desipramine=7–60 hours	✓		
	Imipramine=6–18 hours	✓		
	Nortriptyline=16–90 hours	✓		
Vilazodone	25 hours		✓	Should be taken with food; absorption and bioavailability are reduced by ~50% when taken on an empty stomach.
Vortioxetine	66 hours	✓		
SGAs				
Aripiprazole	75 hours	✓		
Asenapine	24 hours		✓	Optimal bioavailability (~35%) via sublingual absorption; declines to ~28% with food or liquid ingested within 10 minutes of administration; ~2% bioavailability if swallowed.
Brexpiprazole	91 hours	✓		
Cariprazine	48–120 hours	✓		

TABLE 2–2. Mean half-life and differential absorption of psychotropics under fasting conditions versus with food *(continued)*

Agent	Mean $t_{1/2}$	Does food alter drug absorption and bioavailability?		
		No	Yes	Comment
SGAs *(continued)*				
Iloperidone	18–26 hours		✓	Slightly delayed Tmax if taken with food; manufacturer advises twice-daily dosing to minimize risk for orthostatic hypotension.
Lurasidone	18 hours		✓	Cmax reduced 3-fold and bioavailability markedly reduced if administered without food; should be administered within 30 minutes of at least a 350-calorie small meal.
Olanzapine	30 hours	✓		
Paliperidone	23 hours		✓	54%–60% less under fasting conditions.
Pimavanserin	57 hours		✓	Negligible effect in Cmax (~9% decrease in Cmax with high-fat meal).
Quetiapine	7 hours		✓	Food modestly increases absorption and Cmax.
Risperidone	24 hours	✓		
Ziprasidone	7 hours		✓	~2-fold increased absorption when administered with food.

TABLE 2–2.   Mean half-life and differential absorption of psychotropics under fasting conditions versus with food (*continued*)

Agent	Mean $t_{1/2}$	Does food alter drug absorption and bioavailability?		
		No	Yes	Comment
Sedative-hypnotics				
Alprazolam	11 hours	✓		
Clonazepam	18–50 hours	✓		
Diazepam	20–100 hours	✓		
Lorazepam	12–15 hours	✓		
Eszopiclone	6 hours		✓	Administration with a high-fat meal does not affect AUC but does reduce Cmax by 21% and delays Tmax by 1 hour.
Suvorexant	12 hours		✓	A high-fat meal does not affect Cmax or AUC but delays Tmax by ~ 1.5 hours.
Tasimelteon	1.3 hours		✓	A high-fat meal lowers Cmax by 44% and delays Tmax by ~1.75 hours.
Zaleplon	1 hour		✓	A high-fat meal does not affect Cmax or AUC but delays Tmax by ~2 hours.
Zolpidem	2–3 hours		✓	AUC and Cmax decrease by 15% and 25%, respectively, when administered with food.

TABLE 2–2. Mean half-life and differential absorption of psychotropics under fasting conditions versus with food (*continued*)

Agent	Mean $t_{1/2}$	Does food alter drug absorption and bioavailability?		Comment
		No	Yes	
Miscellaneous CNS agents				
Deutetrabenazine	9–10 hours		✓	When deutetrabenazine is taken with food, AUC is unchanged but Cmax is ~50% greater.
Valbenazine	15–22 hours		✓	Administration with a high-fat meal decreases AUC by 47%.

Note. Information based on manufacturers' product information.
AUC=area under the curve; CNS=central nervous system; Cmax=maximal drug plasma concentration; IR=immediate release; SGA=second-generation antipsychotic; SNRI=serotonin-norepinephrine reuptake inhibitor; SR=sustained release; SSRI=selective serotonin reuptake inhibitor; $t_{1/2}$=plasma elimination half-life; TCA=tricyclic antidepressant; Tmax=time until Cmax; XL=extended release.

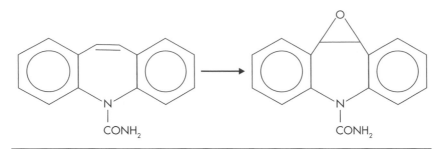

FIGURE 2–1.   Epoxidation of carbamazepine to its 10,11-epoxide metabolite via CYP3A4.

Phase II drug metabolism involves conjugation of a drug substrate with a moiety such as glucuronidation, methylation, acetylation, or sulfation. An important example of Phase II metabolic effects with respect to adverse drug effects would be the delayed metabolism of lamotrigine resulting from divalproex-induced delayed glucuronidation of lamotrigine—and the consequent increased risk for serious drug rashes unless lamotrigine dosing is halved in the presence of divalproex.

The rate at which a particular individual acetylates a substrate during Phase II metabolism is mediated by genetic factors, giving rise to so-called slow acetylators or fast acetylators. The former group may be especially prone to develop adverse effects at relatively low medication doses due to slow metabolism, whereas the latter group may have minimal or no adverse effects (or efficacy) at usual dosages and may require what would otherwise be considered supratherapeutic dosages, either to achieve a clinical response or incur side effects.

Pharmacokinetic interactions represent an extensive subject unto themselves (for a full review, see Preskorn and Flockhart 2009; Wynn et al. 2009). However, for the current purposes, it is important to recognize the potential for drug interactions that may cause one agent to inhibit the CYP enzymes responsible for metabolizing another agent, thereby increasing serum levels and, in turn, side-effect burden. For example, fluvoxamine—a potent inhibitor of CYP1A2 metabolism—may increase blood levels of coadministered psychotropics that are also metabolized (at least in part) by the same enzyme, such as clozapine, olanzapine, and asenapine. Although some practitioners capitalize on this phenomenon for the sake of therapeutic efficacy (e.g., boosting clozapine levels by deliberately coadministering fluvoxamine with low-dose clozapine), the clinician must be cognizant of the potential for more pronounced adverse effects (e.g., sedation) or even frank toxicity, inasmuch as CYP1A2 inhibition by fluvoxamine can cause a 4- to 5-fold increase in serum clozapine levels.

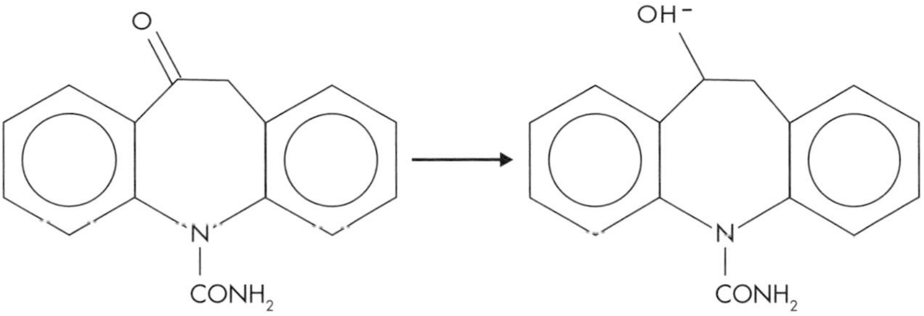

FIGURE 2–2.   Reduction of oxcarbazepine carbonyl group (10-position) to monohydroxy-derivative oxcarbazepine.

Long-acting (e.g., extended-, controlled-, or sustained-release) preparations of a medication often involve slow-release absorption mechanisms (e.g., osmotic pumps or gel matrix coatings) that do not necessarily alter plasma half-life or pharmacodynamic properties of a psychotropic compound. They may produce differences from immediate-release formulations in Tmax or Cmax, but the clinician cannot assume that such altered pharmacokinetics will necessarily lead to pharmacodynamic differences in efficacy or side-effect profiles.

Manufacturers seldom if ever conduct direct, head-to-head comparisons of immediate-release versus long-acting preparations of a given compound for the purposes of prospectively identifying differences in safety or efficacy in a randomized controlled fashion; therefore, potential differences in adverse-effect profiles across formulations must be interpreted with caution. Lack of direct head-to-head comparisons also prevents consideration of drug-placebo differences that may vary across different studies. Nevertheless, if the clinician were to compare side by side the incidence rates of common adverse drug effects from manufacturers' product information on immediate-release versus long-acting drug preparations, he or she would find only a limited number of noteworthy differences. These are summarized in Table 2–3.

Pharmacodynamic adverse effects of a medication sometimes can be anticipated based on drug receptor profiles, as summarized in Table 2–4.

Toxic Polypharmacy

Although thoughtful combination pharmacotherapy regimens seek to capitalize on pharmacodynamic synergies and complementary mechanisms of action, chaos may result from the more haphazard accrual of multiple (or redundant) agents — or medications with opposing pharma-

TABLE 2–3. Noteworthy incidence rates of common adverse effects in short- and long-acting drug preparations

Medication	Indication	Side effect(s)	Recipients (%) reporting side effects[a]	
			Short-acting agent	Long-acting agent
Bupropion	Major depression, smoking cessation	Agitation	32% (IR)	2% (XL) 3%–9% (SR)
		Decreased appetite	18% (IR)	4% (XL) 3%–5% (SR)
Divalproex	Acute mania	Dyspepsia	9% (DR)	23% (ER)
Quetiapine monotherapy	Bipolar mania	Somnolence or sedation	18% (IR)	50% (XR)
	Bipolar depression	Somnolence or sedation	57% (IR)	52% (XR)
	Schizophrenia or bipolar mania	Agitation	20% (IR)	<1% (XR)

Note. DR=delayed release; ER=extended release; IR=immediate release; SR=sustained release; XL=extended release; XR=sustained release.
[a]Based on respective product FDA registration trials, as reported in manufacturers' product information.

codynamic profiles (e.g., stimulants plus sedative-hypnotics, dopamine agonists plus antagonists). Consider, for example, the precarious combination of multiple SGAs that bind tightly to the dopamine D_2 receptor—such as risperidone plus ziprasidone or lurasidone—resulting in an increased potential for adverse extrapyramidal effects or dystonias. Consider also the effects of combining partial agonists with full antagonists (e.g., the μ-opioid receptor partial agonist buprenorphine plus the full antagonist methadone; the tight-binding D_2 partial agonist brexipiprazole with any full D_2 antagonist neuroleptic or with a D_2 agonist such as amphetamine or methylphenidate), which at least theoretically may lead to displacement of receptor binding. For example, buprenorphine added to methadone might be expected to displace the binding of methadone and trigger opiate withdrawal; coadministration of brexipiprazole with another SGA would virtually dominate the D_2 receptor and might therefore at least theoretically prevent or minimize binding of coadministered dopaminergic agents, resulting either in lack of efficacy or simply additive adverse effects (e.g., changes in appetite, sedation, or level of alertness) without a rationale-based benefit. Noncontrolled studies of two or more SGAs used in combination have demonstrated greater anticholinergic and other side-effect burdens, but no greater efficacy, than single-agent SGAs in the case of bipolar disorder or other serious mental illness (Megna et al. 2007). Weight gain does not necessarily appear to be more substantial with the use of one versus two or more SGAs. Risks must be carefully weighed against observable benefits when such combination pharmacotherapy approaches are undertaken.

Gender and Racial Differences in Adverse Effects

Sex differences in pharmacokinetic parameters include slower absorption due to lower gastrointestinal blood flow in women than men, a relatively smaller V_d and higher percentage of body fat in women, sex differences in drug metabolism, and lower glomerular filtration rates in women. Determinants of V_d by sex may sometimes also further stratify by weight, as observed in the case of suvorexant, where plasma AUC and Cmax are 46% and 25% greater, respectively, in obese females as compared with nonobese females. With respect to rates of drug metabolism, at least some reports suggest that women have higher activity of CYP2D6 and CYP3A4, with relatively lesser activity of CYP2C19 and CYP1A2; no sex differences have been identified in Phase II metabolism.

TABLE 2–4.   Common adverse effects associated with specific drug receptor targets

Receptor	Examples	Common adverse events
Adrenergic		
α₁ Agonism	Phenylephrine, modafinil	Headache, restlessness, mydriasis, reflex bradycardia, tremor
α₁ Antagonism	Prazosin	Hypotension and orthostatic hypotension (by vasodilating vascular smooth muscle), lightheadedness, reflex tachycardia, nasal congestion
α₂ Agonism	Clonidine, guanfacine	Hypotension (by vasodilating vascular smooth muscle), sedation (by inhibiting norepinephrine release from noradrenergic autoreceptors in locus coeruleus), initial hypertension with reflex bradycardia, first-degree AV block
α₂ Antagonism	Yohimbine, idazoxan, phentolamine	Anxiety or panic, tachycardia, hypertension, insomnia, headaches, dizziness, skin flushing
β₁ Agonism	Dobutamine	Tachycardia, hypertension, angina, arrhythmia
β₁ Antagonism	Atenolol, metoprolol	Hypotension, bradycardia, fatigue, dizziness, headache, cold extremities, diarrhea, sedation
β₂ Agonism	Albuterol, terbutaline	Nausea, headache, tremor, rhinorrhea, nervousness, palpitations
β₂ Antagonism	Propranolol	Nausea, diarrhea, insomnia
Histaminergic		
H₁ blockade	Diphenhydramine, TCAs, most antipsychotics	Sedation, weight gain, cognitive dulling

TABLE 2–4. Common adverse effects associated with specific drug receptor targets (*continued*)

Receptor	Examples	Common adverse events
Cholinergic		
M_1 blockade	Benztropine, trihexyphenidyl	Blurry vision, dry mouth, constipation, urinary retention, reduced REM sleep
Dopaminergic		
D_2 blockade—nigrostriatal	All antipsychotics	Parkinsonian symptoms, akathisia
D_2 blockade—mesocortical	All antipsychotics	Exacerbation of negative symptoms; cognitive dulling
D_2 blockade—tuberoinfundibular	All antipsychotics with pure D_2 antagonism[a]	Hyperprolactinemia, galactorrhea, amenorrhea, sexual dysfunction
Serotonergic		
$5\text{-}HT_{2A}$ agonism	SSRIs, SNRIs; not mirtazapine (which antagonizes $5\text{-}HT_{2A}$)	Agitation, sexual dysfunction
$5\text{-}HT_{2C}$ agonism	*m*-Chlorophenylpiperazine (m-CPP)	Appetite increase
$5\text{-}HT_3$ agonism	SSRIs, SNRIs; not mirtazapine (which antagonizes $5\text{-}HT_3$)	Nausea, increased gastrointestinal motility

Note. AV=atrioventricular; REM=rapid eye movement; SNRI=serotonin-norepinephrine reuptake inhibitor; SSRI=selective serotonin reuptake inhibitor; TCA=tricyclic antidepressant.

[a]D_2 partial agonists, such as aripiprazole, are unlikely to increase prolactin levels.

Some adverse drug effects are known to be more pronounced among women than men, most notably hyperprolactinemia from antipsychotic medications and a greater incidence of sexual dysfunction (particularly anorgasmia) from serotonergic antidepressants. Another common adverse effect that may stratify by sex includes antipsychotic-associated weight gain, with a higher risk among women reported for at least some SGAs (notably, olanzapine, risperidone, and clozapine).

Racial differences in drug effects can occur as a result of variations in CYP isoforms. For example, in a pooled analysis of trials involving SGAs, African Americans appeared more likely than other racial groups to develop hyperglycemia and possible diabetes, whereas East Asians were more likely than other groups to develop extrapyramidal side effects (Ormerod et al. 2008). Among children and adolescents, African Americans appear more likely than other racial groups to develop obesity, sexual side effects, or dyslipidemias during treatment with SGAs, antimanic agents, or antidepressants (Stauffer et al. 2010).

Alcohol

Manufacturers' product information for virtually all psychotropic drugs includes cautionary language warning that patients should be advised to avoid alcohol, or that the concomitant use of alcohol with a given psychiatric medication is not recommended. Such admonitions largely reflect the absence of controlled data on the safety and efficacy of most psychotropic drugs with alcohol, as well as the potential for additive sedative or adverse cognitive effects from alcohol in combination with a psychotropic medication.

Brand Versus Generic Formulations

The FDA requires that generic formulations of approved compounds must have between 80% and 125% of the bioavailability of the proprietary (branded) compound. Bioavailability is determined by calculating a 90% confidence interval for Cmax and area under the curve (see Table 2–1); that confidence interval must thus fall entirely within the range of 80% and 125%. Determinations of bioequivalence are based solely on a drug's pharmacokinetic profile (e.g., the comparable achievement of plasma drug levels between two different preparations of the same drug) rather than its clinical properties (e.g., the measurement of intended therapeutic efficacy or drug safety). In the case of some medications, brand-name compounds have better efficacy or tolerability over generic formulations (e.g., Tegretol over carbamazepine [Borgheini 2003], Synthroid over levothyroxine [Stoffer and Szpunar 1980]). Additionally, variations in generic medications across manufacturers lead to further interindividual pharmacodynamic variation among generic products.

In some patients with epilepsy, seizure frequency has been shown to increase after substitution of generic for branded anticonvulsant formulations (Borgheini 2003). Less systematic information exists on the substitution of generic for branded psychotropic agents. Notable examples include reports of patients with anxiety disorder stably maintained with long-term brand-name Celexa who relapse after generic citalopram substitution, then recover after having the brand-name drug reintroduced (Van Ameringen et al. 2007), and case reports of depression relapse when patients switch from brand-name Paxil to generic paroxetine (Borgheini 2003). Usually, generic psychotropic drugs are reasonable cost-efficient treatments for many patients, although some may carry the price of more "nuisance" side effects, such as poorer gastrointestinal tolerability. Because bioequivalence studies of brand versus generic drugs do not compare their relative pharmacodynamic efficacies or adverse-effect profiles, clinicians should be mindful of the possibility that a generic drug may sometimes prove to be less desirable than its brand-name counterpart for a given patient.

Enantiomeric Versus Racemic Agents, and Parent Versus Metabolite Compounds

A number of psychotropic agents are racemic (mirror-image) mixtures of the *S* (dextrorotatory [+]) and *L* (levorotatory [−]) enantiomeric forms of a drug. Resolution of those chiral molecules creates enantiopure drugs that may have biological activity and may (or may not) differ from their racemic mixture formulations in efficacy, potency, or adverse effects. "Inactive" enantiomers can diminish the activity of pure "active" isomers (e.g., as in the case of *d*-threo-methylphenidate (dexmethylphenidate), the active isomer of methylphenidate) so that potency may differ by varying degrees. A comparison of reported adverse drug effects between racemic and enantiopure forms, as reported in FDA registration trials, yields few meaningful differences. For example, armodafinil was associated with a lower incidence of headache (17%) than was modafinil (34%), although doses are not directly comparable between the racemic and enantiopure compounds. Insomnia was somewhat more prevalent with venlafaxine (15%–24% across dosages) than with desvenlafaxine (9%–15% across dosages). Also noteworthy is the lesser incidence of specific subtypes of sexual dysfunction with desvenlafaxine than venlafaxine, particularly at the more commonly used dosages of 50–100 mg/day (e.g., delayed ejaculation in 1%–5% and erectile dysfunction in 3%–6% of subjects taking desvenlafaxine, as contrasted with abnormal ejaculation occurring in 16% of subjects with major depression taking venlafaxine XR).

Drug Blood Levels

Clinicians often express interest in the measurement of serum levels of a drug or its metabolite, although the research base to support the clinical utility of drug-level monitoring is variable, largely inconclusive, and not always adequate to guide clinical treatment. Important caveats that may limit the clinical relevance of monitoring serum drug levels include the extent of intraindividual and interindividual variability and possibly invalid assumptions about pharmacokinetic dose relationships. (For example, the C_{max} for nefazodone after a single 100-mg dose can vary from 29% to 131% [Barbhaiya et al. 1996], precluding generalizations about relationships between dosing and blood level.)

In general, the measurement of serum drug levels may be useful for one of several reasons:

- To detect the presence or absence of a prescribed agent (i.e., as an indicator of treatment adherence).
- As a possible marker for drug toxicity, especially in the case of medications that have a narrow therapeutic index.
- As a potential correlate of therapeutic efficacy (as has been established for a handful of psychotropic compounds with an established therapeutic window, described in Table 2–5).
- To gauge the pharmacokinetic impact of clinical situations (e.g., lamotrigine in pregnancy) or additional drug cotherapies (e.g., carbamazepine) that might induce or inhibit a drug's metabolism.
- For some agents, as a means to gauge whether "room" exists to increase a drug dose in the setting of an incomplete response when adverse effects are not in themselves apparent or limiting. The dosing of divalproex ER in acute mania represents a ready example, inasmuch as serum valproate levels exceeding 105 µg/mL incur more extensive gastrointestinal adverse events with no greater efficacy as compared with levels below this threshold (Bowden et al. 2006b).

Serum levels of a drug also may not extrapolate from one clinical setting to another. For example, although serum levels of valproate have been correlated with acute antimanic response, no data exist to inform optimal levels for the use of divalproex in acute bipolar depression, maintenance phases of therapy for bipolar disorder, or off-label use for impulsive aggression in disorders other than bipolar illness. Similarly, in the case of other anticonvulsants, established therapeutic ranges for epilepsy (as exist for carbamazepine or lamotrigine) usually have no known relevance to the psychotropic properties of these agents, apart from affirming possible toxicity states.

Psychotropic agents for which measurement of serum levels hold established value (for efficacy and/or safety) are summarized in Table 2–5.

Pharmacogenomic Predictors of Adverse Effects

As advances have occurred in the recognition of functionally significant single nucleotide polymorphisms (SNPs) within the human genome, interest has grown in examining potential associations between genetic markers and adverse drug effects. Within psychiatry, it has been suggested that *pharmacogenomics* (i.e., the study of genome-wide targets that may contribute to explain variation on drug response) and *pharmacogenetics* (a subset of pharmacogenomics, focusing on individual candidate genes or combinations of individual alleles at different sites for a given SNP [haplotypes] that are thought to confer risk for particular drug effects) may hold particular value for predicting adverse drug effects in predisposed groups of individuals.

Perhaps the best-known example of pharmacogenetic testing with respect to predicting adverse drug effects (sometimes termed "safety pharmacogenetics") lies in the identification of individuals who are so-called poor metabolizers (PMs) of drugs that are substrates for CYP enzymes (resulting in elevated drug levels and potentially more side effects) and those patients considered to be ultrarapid metabolizers (URMs, for whom higher medication dosages may be necessary to achieve therapeutic responses). Up to about 20% of the general population, depending on race and ethnicity, may be genetically predisposed to poorly metabolize drugs that undergo Phase I oxidation by the CYP system. Table 2–6 describes known genetic variants that correspond to phenotypic status for drug metabolism involving CYP2D6, which contributes in whole or part to the metabolism of a majority of psychotropic agents (based on rates reported by Bernard et al. [2006] and Bertilsson [1995]), alongside exam-

TABLE 2–5. Clinical relevance of serum drug levels

Agent	Known relevance
Anticonvulsants and lithium	
Carbamazepine	No established correlation between the serum levels used in epilepsy and psychotropic effects (though typical reference ranges are 4–12 mg/L).
Divalproex	Acute antimanic efficacy associated with serum levels of 50–125 ng/mL; optimal levels not established for maintenance therapy.
Gabapentin	None.
Lamotrigine	None.
Lithium	Acute antimanic efficacy associated with serum levels of 0.6–1.2 mEq/L; maintenance efficacy generally associated with serum levels of 0.8–1.0 mEq/L.
Topiramate	None.
Antidepressants	
Bupropion	Possibly better antidepressant response associated with blood levels of 10–29 ng/mL than with higher levels in adults based on preliminary open label data (Goodnick 1992), although there is no well-established association between blood levels and therapeutic efficacy.
Duloxetine	Serum duloxetine levels above 58 ng/mL have been proposed, based on ROC curve analysis, to predict substantial improvement (Waldschmitt et al. 2009).
Levomilnacipran	None.
MAOIs	No established relationship between blood levels and psychotropic effects (although the degree of MAO inhibition can be estimated from platelet MAO-B levels).
Mirtazapine	None.
Nefazodone	None.

TABLE 2–5.   Clinical relevance of serum drug levels *(continued)*

Agent	Known relevance
Antidepressants *(continued)*	
SSRIs	Fluoxetine and norfluoxetine levels, or their ratios, are not associated with acute antidepressant response (Amsterdam et al. 1997) or with relapse prevention during maintenance treatment for depression (Brunswick et al. 2002); lack of C_{ss} from long $t_{1/2}$ also impedes assessment of relationships between dose and levels.
TCAs	*Amitriptyline:* No definitive association between serum levels and response in major depression, although some experts consider the range of 150–300 ng/mL to be therapeutic. *Desipramine:* No clear association between serum levels and response in major depression. *Imipramine:* Established therapeutic window (sum of imipramine + desipramine) between 175 and 350 ng/mL. *Nortriptyline:* Established therapeutic window between 50 and 150 ng/mL; levels >500 ng/mL are considered toxic, and dosages > 150 mg/day are not recommended.
Venlafaxine and desvenlafaxine	Magnitude of desmethylvenlafaxine serum levels, and lower ratios of enantiomeric [+]/[–] venlafaxine ratios, may predict speed of antidepressant response (Gex-Fabry et al. 2004); a therapeutic range of 125–400 ng/mL for the sum of venlafaxine and desmethylvenlafaxine levels has been proposed (Charlier et al. 2002), although not widely adopted.
Vilazodone	None.
Vortioxetine	None.

TABLE 2–5.   Clinical relevance of serum drug levels *(continued)*

Agent	Known relevance
SGAs	
Aripiprazole	None.
Asenapine	None.
Brexpiprazole	Not studied.
Cariprazine	Not studied.
Clozapine	Greater efficacy with serum clozapine levels in the range of 200–300 ng/mL (VanderZwaag et al. 1996); higher likelihood of drug toxicity >1,000 ng/mL (Freeman and Oyewumi 1997); monitoring of serum clozapine levels may be useful only in specific situations, including poor response with routine dosages, signs of toxicity (e.g., seizures), cotherapy with CYP1A2 inhibitors (e.g., fluvoxamine, fluoroquinolones) or inducers (e.g., tobacco, omeprazole), presence of liver disease, changes in caffeine or nicotine consumption, or nonadherence.
Iloperidone	None.
Lurasidone	None.
Olanzapine	12-hour serum olanzapine levels >23.2 ng/mL have been reported in association with therapeutic response in acutely ill patients with schizophrenia (Perry et al. 2001), but measurement is uncommon in clinical practice.
Pimavanserin	Not studied.
Quetiapine	None.
Risperidone	None.
Ziprasidone	Large interindividual variation; no established relationship between blood levels and psychotropic effects.

Note. C_{ss}=steady-state concentration; MAOI=monoamine oxidase inhibitor; ROC=receiver operating characteristic; SGA=second-generation antipsychotic; SSRI=selective serotonin reuptake inhibitor; $t_{1/2}$=plasma elimination half-life; TCA=tricyclic antidepressant.

ples of major psychotropic drugs that are CYP substrates, inhibitors, or inducers (Preskorn and Flockhart 2009).

Provisional studies in major depression have suggested possible links between side-effect burden and CYP2D6 PM status, and nonresponse with the URM phenotype (Rau et al. 2004). Case reports of drug toxicity reactions with drugs such as risperidone (Strauss et al. 2010) have identified the presence of the CYP2D6 PM phenotype as causing markedly elevated blood levels at usual doses, leading to excessive adverse effects. However, some CYP2D6 PMs show fewer adverse effects than would be expected from their genotype. Notably, because the incidences of both the PM and URM genotypes are rare in the general population (see Table 2–6), it is unlikely that this feature accounts for adverse effects (or lack of therapeutic efficacy) in the majority of patients encountered by a clinician.

PMs may not derive pharmacodynamic benefits from pro-drugs that must be converted to active metabolites (e.g., codeine's conversion to morphine, or tamoxifen's conversion to its active metabolite, endoxifen, both via CYP2D6). However, most psychiatric pro-drugs become activated not by Phase I or Phase II hepatic metabolism but by peripheral hydrolytic enzymes (as in the removal of a lysine moiety to liberate free dextroamphetamine from lisdexamfetamine, or the cleavage of valine from valbenazine to liberate dihydrotetrabenazine). PMs in general may avoid adverse effects if the clinician chooses medications cleared by pathways other than CYP2D6. Major enzyme pathways of cytochrome P450 or UGT substrates are summarized in Table 2–7.

In the case of metabolic dysregulation associated with the use of many SGAs, the literature contains very preliminary reports of a number of candidate genes possibly associated with iatrogenic weight gain, as summarized in Table 2–8.

In addition to the foregoing, other provisional findings on possible pharmacogenetic predictors of adverse effects of psychotropic drugs include the following:

- A Ser9Gly variant of the dopamine D_3 receptor gene *DRD3* was associated with an increased risk for developing tardive dyskinesia in patients taking antipsychotics (Lerer et al. 2002).
- Discontinuation of paroxetine due to adverse effects in a randomized clinical trial was significantly predicted by allelic variants in the serotonin type 2A (5-HT$_{2A}$) locus (Murphy et al. 2003).
- Schizophrenia patients with the D_2 receptor gene allele *DRD2*A1* show a greater risk for developing antipsychotic-induced hyperprolactinemia when compared with patients without this allele (Young et al. 2004).

TABLE 2–6. Cytochrome P450 (CYP) metabolizer subtypes with known inhibitors and inducers

CYP family	Poor metabolizers	Ultrarapid metabolizers	Psychotropic inhibitors	Psychotropic inducers
CYP2D6	Whites: 6%–10% Blacks: 2%–7% (South African blacks: 29%) Asians: 0%–2% Hispanics: 2%–6%	Whites: 4% Blacks: 5% (Ethiopians: 29%) Asians: 1% Hispanics: 1%–2%	Bupropion Citalopram Doxepin Duloxetine Fluoxetine Fluvoxamine (weak) Imipramine Paroxetine Risperidone	None
CYP1A2	Not well characterized	Not well characterized	Fluvoxamine	Modafinil
CYP3A4/5	Whites: 5%	Not well characterized	Fluvoxamine Nefazodone	Carbamazepine Modafinil Oxcarbazepine
CYP2C19	Whites: 3%–5% Asians: 15%–20%	Not well characterized	Fluoxetine Fluvoxamine Moclobemide Modafinil Oxcarbazepine Topiramate	Carbamazepine

TABLE 2–7. Metabolic hepatic enzyme pathways of psychotropic drugs

Agent	Cytochrome P450 enzymes				UGT	Known implications for poor metabolizers (PMs)
	2D6	3A4/5	2C19	1A2		
Amitriptyline[a]	(✓)	✓	✓	✓		
Amphetamine-dextroamphetamine	✓					
Aripiprazole	✓	✓				Halve dose in CYP2D6 PMs; quarter dose in CYP2D6 PMs taking CYP3A4 inhibitors.
(Ar)modafinil		✓				
Asenapine				✓	✓ (1A4)	
Atomoxetine	✓					5-fold higher peak concentrations.
Brexpiprazole	✓	✓				Halve dose in CYP2D6 PMs; quarter dose in CYP2D6 PMs or patients taking 3A4 inhibitors.
Bupropion[b]		✓				
Buspirone		✓				
Carbamazepine		✓			(✓) (2B7)	
Cariprazine		✓				Halve dose in patients taking CYP3A4 inhibitors.
Citalopram		✓	✓			Dosing should not exceed 20 mg/day in CYP2C19 PMs.

TABLE 2–7. Metabolic hepatic enzyme pathways of psychotropic drugs (continued)

Agent	Cytochrome P450 enzymes					Known implications for poor metabolizers (PMs)
	2D6	3A4/5	2C19	1A2	UGT	
Clozapine	(✓)		(✓)	✓		
Clomipramine[c]						
Desvenlafaxine					✓ (1A1)	
Deutetrabenazine	✓	(✓)		(✓)		Maximum daily dose = 36 mg/day in CYP2D6 PMs.
Dextromethorphan	✓					
Divalproex[d]					✓	
Duloxetine	✓			✓		
Escitalopram	✓		✓			
Eszopiclone[e]		✓				
Fluoxetine	✓					
Fluvoxamine	✓			✓		
Gabapentin[f]						
Iloperidone	✓	✓				Halve dose in CYP2D6 PMs.
Lamotrigine					✓ (1A4)	
Levomilnacipran[g]	✓	✓	✓			

Pharmacokinetics, Pharmacodynamics, and Pharmacogenomics 73

TABLE 2–7.   Metabolic hepatic enzyme pathways of psychotropic drugs (continued)

Agent	Cytochrome P450 enzymes				UGT	Known implications for poor metabolizers (PMs)
	2D6	3A4/5	2C19	1A2		
Lurasidone		✓				
Mirtazapine	✓	✓		✓		
Nefazodone		✓				
Nortriptyline	✓	✓	✓	✓		
Olanzapine		(✓)		✓	✓ (1A4)	
Paliperidone[f]	(✓)	(✓)				
Paroxetine	✓					
Pimavanserin[h]	(✓)	✓				Recommended dosage is 17 mg/day when coadministered with strong 3A4 inhibitors.
Pregabalin[f]						
Quetiapine		✓				
Risperidone	✓	(✓)				
Sertraline[i]	(✓)	(✓)	(✓)			
Suvorexant		✓				
Tasimelteon		✓		✓		
Topiramate[f]						

TABLE 2–7. Metabolic hepatic enzyme pathways of psychotropic drugs (continued)

Agent	Cytochrome P450 enzymes				UGT	Known implications for poor metabolizers (PMs)
	2D6	3A4/5	2C19	1A2		
Trazodone		✓				
Valbenazine	✓	✓				
Venlafaxine	✓	✓				
Vilazodone		✓				
Vortioxetine[j]	✓	(✓)	(✓)			
Ziprasidone		✓				
Zolpidem		✓			(✓)	Halve dose in CYP2D6 PMs.

Note. Minor metabolic pathways are identified in (parentheses).

[a]Amitriptyline is also metabolized (demethylated to nortriptyline) via CYP2C9 and likely also CYP2B6 and CYP2C8.
[b]Bupropion is primarily metabolized (hydroxylated to hydroxybupropion) by CYP2B6.
[c]Clomipramine is metabolized by CYP2C19, CYP1A2, CYP3A4, and *N*-demethylation to form desmethylclomipramine. Imipramine is metabolized by CYP2D6, CYP3A4, CYP1A2, and CYP2C9 to desipramine and 2-hydroxydesipramine.
[d]Minor metabolic pathways of divalproex (15%–20%) include CYP2C9, CYP2A6, CYP2B6, and CYP3A5.
[e]Eszopiclone is also metabolized by CYP450 2E1.
[f]Gabapentin is not extensively metabolized and is largely excreted renally unchanged.
[g]Levomilnacipran is desethylated to form desethyl levomilnacipran additionally via CYP2C8 and (minor pathway) CYP2C8.
[h]CYP2J2 is an additional minor metabolic pathway of pimavanserin.
[i]Sertraline is *N*-demethylated primarily via CYP2B6.
[j]Vortioxetine is also metabolized by CYP2C8, CYP2C9, CYP2A6, and CYP2B6.

TABLE 2–8. **Pharmacogenetic correlates of antipsychotic-associated weight gain**

Polymorphism	Findings
Adrenergic receptor beta 3 (ADRB3) 64Trp/Arg	Arg/Arg homozygosity linked with olanzapine-related weight gain (Ujike et al. 2008)
5HT2C -759 C/T	"CC" homozygosity associated with weight gain from risperidone or chlorpromazine (Reynolds et al. 2002) or from clozapine (Reynolds et al. 2003), though not from olanzapine (Ujike et al. 2008).
5HT2C Cys23/Ser23	23 Cys allele associated with olanzapine-induced weight gain (Ujike et al. 2008).
Dopamine DR*D2 rs2440390	"A" allele associated with greater risk for weight gain with olanzapine in adult white nonschizophrenia patients (Houston et al. 2012).
5HTR2A 102T/C	"CC" homozygotes have greater risk for olanzapine-associated weight gain (Ujike et al. 2008).
Leptin -2548 A/G (rs7799039)	Presence of "G" allele confers greater risk for weight gain with clozapine (Zhang et al. 2007) and other atypical antipsychotics among Europeans (Shen et al. 2014).
MTHFR 677C/T	"CC" genotype associated with greater increase in body mass index (Srisawat et al. 2014).
G-protein Beta3 Subunit (GNB3) gene	C825T variant associated with weight gain from olanzapine (Ujike et al. 2008).

- A 120-bp tandem repeat sequence in the promoter region of the *DRD2* gene was associated with an approximate threefold increased likelihood of developing sialorrhea during clozapine therapy (Rajagopal et al. 2014).
- Severe hypercholesterolemia or hypertriglyceridemia arising during treatment with SGAs appears significantly more likely in patients with identified variants in the acetyl-coenzyme A carboxylase alpha gene (Diaz et al. 2009).

- The emergence of sexual dysfunction during citalopram treatment for depression was associated with variants in glutamatergic genes (*GRIA3* and *GRIK2* with decreased libido, *GRIA1* with difficulty achieving orgasm, and *GRIA2* and *GRIN3A* with erectile dysfunction) (Perlis et al. 2003).
- Increased likelihood of insomnia and agitation during fluoxetine treatment occurred among major depression patients with the homozygous "short/short" genotype of the serotonin transporter gene polymorphism (locus SLC6A4) (Perlis et al. 2003).
- The development of suicidal ideation during antidepressant pharmacotherapy was associated with markers that reside within specific genes that encode the sulfated glycoprotein papilin *(PAPLN)* and the interleukin 28 receptor *(IL28RA)* (Laje et al. 2009).
- An increased risk for antidepressant-induced mania occurs among patients with bipolar disorder who receive an SSRI and carry the short allelic variant of the serotonin transporter gene polymorphism SLC6A4 (Mundo et al. 2001).

It must be emphasized, however, that the extent to which pharmacodynamic drug effects are in fact heritable or otherwise under genetic control remains uncertain, relative to other, nongenetic, factors. Findings from most studies of safety pharmacogenetics, such as those mentioned above, are preliminary and await replication with larger and more racially diverse samples. It should also be noted that correlations between a PM or URM genotype and phenotype may not always be reliable. For example, about one in four individuals with the CYP2D6 non-PM genotype may "phenoconvert" to a PM phenotype, suggesting that genotyping results can be misleading for purposes of clinical decision making and, if obtained, should be considered with caution (Preskorn et al. 2013).

3

Vulnerable Populations

Patients' Diverse Proneness to Drug Side Effects

Limited data are available from studies that track the course of adverse effects from psychotropic drugs and that seek to identify risk factors for their development. Although efforts to identify robust predictors of adverse effects (or for that matter, efficacy) represent a clinically and scientifically important research goal, there is frankly little incentive for pharmaceutical manufacturers to identify such factors because they would unavoidably limit the potential market share of a proprietary compound. From the clinician's and patient's perspective, however, the ability to anticipate risk factors for specific adverse effects only enhances confidence in treatment and might help deter fear of adverse effects as a reason to avoid otherwise highly effective medications. Predictors of adverse effects may include both clinical and biological characteristics. For example, one large study of depressed outpatients treated with fluoxetine or paroxetine found that those who were more severely depressed were especially likely to report significant adverse effects, although the reporting of adverse effects diminished over time in similar fashion for both high- and low-severity depressed groups (Demyttenaere et al. 2005). This study

---

The symbol ■ is used in this chapter to indicate that the FDA has issued a boxed warning for a prescription medication that may cause serious adverse effects.

also found that eventual habituation to side effects was faster in men than in women, in study completers than in early terminators, and in men with recurrent rather than first-episode depression.

As described in Chapter 2, "Pharmacokinetics, Pharmacodynamics, and Pharmacogenomics," individuals who are PMs of CYP isoenzymes may expectably be more prone to the known adverse effects of drugs that are substrates for a given CYP enzyme if it is the drug's primary or sole metabolic pathway. Apart from individuals with genetic predispositions for poor drug metabolism, other patient subgroups may have heightened sensitivities to the adverse drug effects of psychotropic agents. In this chapter, we focus on broad concepts and issues regarding adverse psychotropic drug reactions that are unique or especially pertinent to populations with heightened vulnerabilities or sensitivities to untoward drug effects.

Children

The potential for SGAs to cause weight gain and metabolic dysregulation appears especially high in children and adolescents, even after a first-time course of treatment (Correll et al. 2009). In the case of short-term trials of olanzapine for pediatric mania or schizophrenia, for example, weight gain was reported in 30% of such subjects, as contrasted with 6% of adults. The magnitude of weight gain reported in short-term controlled studies of SGAs among pediatric patients varies by agent: mean weight changes from baseline range as follows: 3.6–16.2 kg with olanzapine, 0.9–9.45 kg with clozapine, 1.8–7.2 kg with risperidone, 2.3–5.9 kg with quetiapine, and 0–4.5 kg with aripiprazole (Fraguas et al. 2011). Children and adolescents may differ from adults in their susceptibility to a number of other specific adverse effects, including the following:

- Markedly increased risk for severe skin rashes in children and adolescents during treatment with lamotrigine, and moderately increased risk with (ar)modafinil.
- Weight gain from psychotropics other than SGAs (e.g., venlafaxine XR and mirtazapine; see Chapter 15, "Metabolic Dysregulation and Weight Gain") appears greater in children <age 12 than in adolescents ≥age 12 or in adults.
- Greater sensitivity to somnolence and sedation in children and adolescents (e.g., in 22%–30% of subjects taking risperidone for pediatric mania and in 49% of risperidone monotherapy–treated children in FDA registration trials for autism, in contrast to an incidence of <7% in

adults with schizophrenia or of 5% in adults with bipolar mania taking risperidone).

- A significantly increased risk for the induction or exacerbation of suicidal thinking or behavior during treatment with antidepressants among individuals <age 24 (■); this risk has not been demonstrated in patients >age 24, and in fact antidepressants demonstrate a protective effect against suicidal behavior in adults >age 65.

Medically Ill Patients

Issues of particular concern to people with chronic medical conditions involve an increased potential for pharmacokinetic interactions with other medications, greater difficulty in parsing side effects and their attribution to specific agents, and increased sensitivity to side effects of psychotropic medications.

Liver Disease

For individuals with hepatic impairment, drugs that are metabolized by Phase I or Phase II metabolism often may be administered with caution, depending on the extent of hepatic dysfunction. The Child-Pugh classification for liver disease (Pugh et al. 1973; Table 3–1) was devised as a prognostic estimate for survival in patients with chronic liver impairment, with progressive classification ratings (A, B, and C) reflecting increasingly low 1-year and 5-year survival rates. Scores of 5–6 are designated as Class A liver failure, scores of 7–9 indicate Class B failure, and scores of 10–15 are termed Class C. Dosing adjustments in patients with liver disease are often recommended based on Child-Pugh classification.

HIV/AIDS

Because HIV/AIDS preferentially affects subcortical CNS structures, including the basal ganglia, patients are especially susceptible to adverse drug effects related to motor coordination and cognition (such as akathisia and other extrapyramidal side effects) as well as NMS. This susceptibility includes dopamine-blocking drugs, which typically should be administered at dosages lower than they might be otherwise. Relatedly, by virtue of their immunosuppressed status, patients with HIV/AIDS who are given drugs that can lower white blood cell counts (e.g., carbamazepine, SGAs) should be monitored with particular vigilance. A further concern regarding heightened susceptibility to psychotropic drug effects stems from pharmacokinetic interactions with antiretroviral and

TABLE 3–1. **Child-Pugh score for assessing the severity of liver disease**

Measure	1 point	2 points	3 points
Total bilirubin (μmol/L [or mg/dL])	<34 (or <2)	34–25 (or 2–3)	>50 (or >30)
Serum albumin (g/L)	>35	28–35	<28
INR[a]	<1.7	1.71–2.20	>2.20
Ascites	None	Mild	Severe
Hepatic encephalopathy	None	Grade I–II[b]	Grade III–IV[c]

[a]INR, or international normalized ratio, accounts for prothrombin time relative to an international sensitivity index.
[b]Or suppressed with medication.
[c]Or refractory.
Source.   Pugh et al. 1973.

antimicrobial agents, which can induce or inhibit CYP enzymes. Protease inhibitors such as ritonavir exert numerous and extensive pharmacokinetic interactions, serving as an inducer, inhibitor, and substrate of various CYP effects. Similarly, CYP inducers such as carbamazepine may diminish the efficacy of antiretroviral drugs.

Psychiatrists who treat individuals with HIV or AIDS should be especially attentive to obtaining a careful history of psychiatric problems that predate the suspected onset of HIV and its treatments, reviewing all medications within a global regimen that may contribute to psychiatric symptoms, and differentiating probable iatrogenic from primary psychiatric disturbances. The psychiatrist and the patient's primary medical doctor should collaborate in making decisions about "treating through" the suspected psychiatric side effects of antiretroviral agents (see section "Antiretroviral Agents" in Chapter 4, "Adverse Psychiatric Effects of Nonpsychotropic Medications"), considering the severity of a suspected side effect (e.g., insomnia vs. suicidality), the patient's capacity to tolerate an adverse psychiatric effect, the presence or absence of realistic alternative HIV therapies, and the degree to which a psychiatric side effect can be successfully and safely managed with psychotropic drugs.

When prescribing psychiatric medications to patients with HIV or AIDS, clinicians must also be cognizant of potential pharmacokinetic interactions with antiretroviral agents (for review, see Repetto and Petitto 2008), as well as the frequent necessity to use low medication dosages (e.g., in the case of antipsychotics, given the high penetrance of HIV in the basal ganglia, which can render patients especially susceptible to adverse motor and other dopaminergically based side effects). Patients with HIV nephropathy or coinfection with hepatitis also may require dosing adjustments based on impaired renal function (see Table 13–2 in Chapter 13, "Genitourinary and Renal Systems") or hepatic dysfunction (see Table 12–1 in Chapter 12, "Gastrointestinal System").

Older Adults

A general rule of thumb among psychiatrists who treat older adults is that low dosages (even dosages that sometimes might otherwise seem inadequate) are the usual standard. Renal clearance declines with age; for every decade beyond age 40, glomerular filtration rate declines by about 10 mL/min. Accordingly, some (but not all) psychotropic agents require downward dosing adjustments in elderly patients, usually when there is evidence of reduced hepatic metabolism or renal clearance. Hepatic dysfunction is typically a more salient contributor than renal impairment to drug tolerability. Very few controlled studies have been conducted with most psychotropic agents specifically in geriatric patients with mood, anxiety, or psychotic disorders, and inferences about safety and tolerability often are drawn from post hoc analyses of enrolled subjects usually ≥ age 65 (and seldom >age 75). (Notable exceptions include FDA registration trials of vortioxetine in major depression up to age 88 and lurasidone in schizophrenia up to age 85.) However, some controlled trials specifically in geriatric settings have yielded several important observations. For example, a multisite placebo-controlled trial of divalproex ER for agitation in elderly patients with dementia (mean age=83) that used a relatively high dose (20 mg/kg, titrated by increments of 125 mg/day) yielded excessive somnolence, dehydration, and reduced nutritional intake (manufacturer's product information, Abbott Laboratories). Manic older adults may poorly tolerate divalproex doses exceeding ~15 mg/kg (Tariot et al. 2001).

Studies addressing the management of psychosis or disruptive behaviors in elderly patients with dementia have found significant adverse effects, as exemplified most dramatically in the 1.6-fold increased risk for all-cause mortality with antipsychotic drugs. The review of findings by the FDA that led to a boxed warning (■) of increased risk for death dovetailed with a meta-analysis of 15 randomized placebo-controlled trials involving aripiprazole (3 trials), olanzapine (5 trials), quetiapine (3 trials), and risperidone (5 trials) for the treatment of dementia-related psychosis, encompassing a collective group of 3,353 subjects receiving active drug and 1,757 randomly assigned to placebo (Schneider et al. 2005). That meta-analysis identified an odds ratio of 1.54 (95% CI, 1.06–2.23) for increased risk of death, with no observed differences among individual drugs. In calculating NNH and NNT, the authors determined that one death would likely occur for every 9–15 elderly dementia patients helped by an SGA, but predictors of that increased risk among antipsychotic recipients were not identified.

Presumably, cumulative risk factors for cardiovascular or cerebrovascular disease may play a contributing role, as would other preexisting conditions, such as esophageal dysmotility (with consequent risk for aspiration pneumonia). All of these concerns must be weighed against the risks posed by untreated psychosis or agitated behavior, as well as findings from other studies, which suggest that even FGAs (particularly at high dosages) may carry a risk for excess mortality in older adults that is at least as high as that seen with SGAs (Schneeweiss et al. 2007). (Hence, in June 2008, the FDA extended its boxed warning (■) for increased mortality in elderly dementia patients to FGAs as well as SGAs.)

General considerations for the dosing and monitoring of adverse effects with psychotropic drugs used in older adults are summarized in Table 3–2.

Generally, the types of adverse effects that become of particular concern for older adults include the following:

- Cognitive effects of anticholinergic drugs
- Greater risk for syndrome of inappropriate antidiuretic hormone secretion (SIADH) during treatment with SSRIs or some anticonvulsants (notably, oxcarbazepine)
- Greater risk for orthostatic hypotension from drugs with α_1-adrenergic blocking properties
- The potential for disinhibition with the use of benzodiazepines
- Excessive somnolence from antihistaminergic agents or other possible sedative agents

Other well-recognized concerns relevant to adverse drug effect sensitivities in elderly patients include decreased protein binding (hence the potential for more circulating unbound drug fractions) and the greater likelihood of multiple drug interactions.

TABLE 3–2. Dosing considerations for psychotropic drug use in geriatric populations

Medication	Manufacturer's dosing recommendation in geriatric patients
Atomoxetine	None.
Buspirone	No special dosing is recommended, although known renal insufficiency can increase plasma half-life (see Table 13–2 in Chapter 13, "Genitourinary and Renal Systems").
Antipsychotics	Boxed warning (■) for use in elderly patients with dementia-related psychosis is unrelated to drug dose.
Anticonvulsants	
Carbamazepine	No studies exist in geriatric patients to guide dosing recommendations.
Divalproex	The manufacturer advises a reduced starting dosage and more gradual dosage increases. Monitor for a greater potential for somnolence than in younger patients.
Gabapentin	Dosage selection should be cautious, usually starting at the low end of the dosing range. Higher incidence of peripheral edema and ataxia found in older adults.
Lamotrigine	Formal studies do not exist in adults over age 65. The manufacturer recommends dosage initiation at the low end of the dosing range due to the potential for decreased hepatic, renal, or cardiac function in older adults.
Oxcarbazepine	Observed increases in plasma levels among older adults (>age 60) are attributable to decreased CrCl. There are otherwise no formal recommendations for dosage reductions in elderly patients.
Topiramate	No age-related differences in adverse effects are known. Dosage reductions are advised when CrCl is <70 mL/min.

TABLE 3–2. **Dosing considerations for psychotropic drug use in geriatric populations *(continued)***

Medication	Manufacturer's dosing recommendation in geriatric patients
Antidepressants	
Bupropion	None unless renal function is diminished.
Desvenlafaxine	None unless renal function is diminished (see Table 13–2). Higher risk of orthostatic hypotension in patients≥age 65.
Duloxetine	Dosing adjustment based on age is unnecessary.
Escitalopram	Maximum for elderly patients is 10 mg/day.
Fluoxetine	The manufacturer advises using lower dosages in elderly patients. No age-related differences in adverse effects are known apart from those attributable to decreased renal clearance. FDA registration studies in major depression included 687 drug-treated patients ≥age 65 and 93 drug-treated patients who were ≥age 75.
Fluvoxamine	Mean plasma concentrations in older adults are 40%–50% higher than in younger adults. The manufacturer recommends slower initial dosing increases in geriatric patients. No age-related differences in adverse effects are known apart from those attributable to decreased renal clearance. FDA registration studies included 230 patients ≥age 65 who took immediate-release fluvoxamine and 5 patients ≥age 65 who took the controlled-release formulation.
Levomilnacipran	None.
Mirtazapine	Diminished drug clearance in elderly patients was due to renal insufficiency and was more prominent in men than in women.

TABLE 3–2. Dosing considerations for psychotropic drug use in geriatric populations *(continued)*

Medication	Manufacturer's dosing recommendation in geriatric patients
Antidepressants *(continued)*	
Nefazodone	The manufacturer advises initial dosing at half the usual dosage, although eventual therapeutic dosages may be the same as in younger patients.
Paroxetine	No age-related differences in adverse effects are known apart from greater side-effect burden in cases of known renal insufficiency. FDA registration studies in major depression included approximately 700 drug-treated patients ≥age 65.
Sertraline	No age-related differences in adverse effects are known. FDA registration studies in major depression included 663 drug-treated patients ≥age 65 and 180 drug-treated patients ≥age 75.
Transdermal selegiline	Somewhat higher risk for skin rash reported in patients ≥age 50 (4.4% vs. 0% with placebo); no other age-related adverse effects are known. Recommended dosing in patients ≥age 65 is 6 mg/day. FDA registration studies in major depression included 198 drug-treated patients ≥age 65.
Venlafaxine	None.
Vortioxetine	None.

Note. CrCl=creatinine clearance; FDA=U.S. Food and Drug Administration.

Patients Prone to Somatization

Special consideration is warranted when anticipating and evaluating possible adverse drug effects in individuals prone to somatization. It has been estimated that about 20% of the population self-identifies a high PSM, even at small doses, and such individuals tend to utilize health care services more extensively than those with low PSM (Faasse et al. 2015). Relatedly, the phenomenon of *somatosensory amplification* describes the experience of normal bodily sensations as being excessively intense, noxious, or distressing; it tends to be linked with illness anxiety disorder (formerly referred to as *hypochondriasis*) as well as trait alexthymia, and in turn may predispose some individuals to misidentify normal somatic sensations as adverse effects caused by a medication (Doering et al. 2015).

Clinical wisdom would dictate several basic principles when prescribing psychotropic medications to people with somatic preoccupations. To minimize the potential for further (or paradoxical) side effects, the following principles are recommended:

1. Use the smallest effective dosages possible.
2. Make changes to a medication regimen very gradually.
3. Minimize the cumulative number of medications to the extent that is feasible.
4. Make an extra effort to avoid medications that involve more extensive or severe possible side effects.
5. Change no more than one medication at a time to minimize pharmacodynamic and pharmacokinetic confusions.
6. Reduce dosages or eliminate medications rather than add additional drugs as intended antidotes.

From a diagnostic standpoint, practitioners also may wish to consider whether somatic preoccupations suggest the presence of a psychotic process or body dysmorphic disorder that may warrant treatment with low-dose antipsychotics having the fewest potential adverse effects.

Nonpharmacological approaches may be especially important in the comprehensive treatment of individuals with somatic preoccupations or conversion disorders, conditions that may be suspected when extensive complaints emerge about multiple perceived side effects. Some awareness of psychodynamic concepts also may help to foster greater tolerability and engagement in the therapeutic alliance. A practical corollary to this approach involves deciding how to share information (and how much to share) with patients in anticipation of the potential for developing adverse drug effects.

Sparse literature exists on the pharmacotherapy of somatization and related disorders (e.g., hypochondriasis). Interestingly, a 12-week placebo-controlled study of fluoxetine for hypochondriasis yielded no differences between drug and placebo in rates of premature discontinuation due to adverse effects, although no significant improvements were observed with active drug versus placebo on outcome measures related specifically to illness concerns or somatization (Fallon et al. 2008). In our experience, preoccupations for some patients about real or imagined side effects (or the sheer prospect of them) can become a distracting pseudofocal point of treatment, one that may altogether derail pharmacologically based efforts to alleviate symptoms. For patients who undergo multiple aborted trials with successive pharmacotherapies that are inevitably deemed intolerable, redirecting efforts to address the capacity to tolerate physical distress often becomes necessary. In the setting of persistent nonpsychotic somatic preoccupations, particularly when they coincide with maladaptive personality traits (conscious or otherwise), iterative pharmacotherapy efforts may at some point become counterproductive and frankly inadvisable. Such circumstances may warrant a reappraisal of realistic therapeutic goals and a shift away from efforts aimed at disease modification and instead toward the improvement of coping skills. The latter sometimes may be pursued more productively through primarily cognitive-behavioral or other purely psychotherapeutic approaches.

4

Adverse Psychiatric Effects of Nonpsychotropic Medications

Contrary to what might otherwise be expected, the majority of people who develop adverse psychiatric effects from nonpsychotropic medications do not have preexisting psychiatric conditions. For example, in a review of manias secondary to medications (e.g., isoniazid or the antineoplastic procarbazine), Krauthammer and Klerman (1978) noted that pretreatment histories of affective illness were not apparent in the majority of cases.

Analgesics

Carisoprodol

Carisoprodol, a combination analgesic and muscle relaxant, is a prodrug of the Schedule IV anxiolytic agent meprobamate and is classified

---

The symbol ■ is used in this chapter to indicate that the FDA has issued a boxed warning for a prescription medication that may cause serious adverse effects.

as a Schedule IV drug in certain states (viz., Alabama, Arizona, Arkansas, Florida, Georgia, Hawaii, Indiana, Kentucky, Louisiana, Massachusetts, Minnesota, Mississippi, New Mexico, Nevada, Oklahoma, Oregon, and Texas). It can cause physical dependence with prolonged use and, because it is a CNS depressant, may cause additive sedating effects when combined with alcohol or other sedating psychotropic drugs.

Opiates

Opiates may show great variability and unpredictability in their psychotropic effects. Anxiety and nervousness are identified as possible adverse effects, occurring in 1%–5% of patients in premarketing studies of most opiates taken for extended periods of time, although it is difficult to know the extent to which preexisting or comorbid psychiatric symptoms account for such occurrences. Acute psychosis and delirium have been reported with synthetic opiates.

Although some clinicians express concern about the potential for long-term opiates to induce anhedonia, there is actually a small, mostly anecdotal literature to suggest that some long-acting semisynthetic opiates such as oxycodone (10–30 mg/day) or oxymorphone (8 mg/day), as well as the partial agonist buprenorphine, can safely and effectively treat depressive syndromes that are unresponsive to more traditional pharmacotherapies (or electroconvulsive therapy) in people with unipolar or bipolar depression.

Tramadol

The centrally acting Schedule IV synthetic opioid analgesic tramadol warrants separate mention from other opiate analgesics by virtue of its inherent noradrenergic-serotonergic reuptake mechanism, which has been known to hinder or prolong efforts to discontinue its use because of withdrawal-like features similar to those reported with pure SNRIs (see the section "Discontinuation Syndromes" in Chapter 20, "Systemic Reactions"). Tramadol has been shown to cause nervousness or anxiety, hallucinations, agitation, and depression (incidence rates of 1%–5% in manufacturer's FDA registration trials).

Anticholinergics

Detrimental psychiatric effects of centrally active anticholinergic drugs can include diffuse cognitive deficits, in addition to somnolence or sedation. Anticholinergic drugs may be especially deleterious in patients with intrinsic cognitive deficits or dementias (in whom cholinomimetic drugs are used in efforts to counteract primary cognitive deficits).

Anticonvulsants

Case reports have described patients with epilepsy or other primary neurological disorders (e.g., essential tremor, neuropathic pain) and no prior psychiatric history who have developed new-onset psychosis with several anticonvulsant agents, including levetiracetam (particularly in children), topiramate, vigabatrin, and lamotrigine, as well as depression in connection with the use of topiramate (Goldberg 2008) or zonisamide (occurring in 6% of epilepsy patients during adjunctive zonisamide FDA registration trials; manufacturer's package insert, Elan Pharma International). It is speculative whether psychotomimetic or other adverse psychiatric effects of anticonvulsants seen in epilepsy patients generalize to other clinical populations, including patients with primary psychiatric disorders. Some authors have suggested that temporal lobe pathology may predispose patients to psychosis from anticonvulsants.

In 2008, the FDA issued a warning (nonboxed) indicating that all anticonvulsant drugs carry an increased risk for suicidal thinking or behavior, although this observation appears to vary based on the clinical population being treated (see the section "Suicidal Thinking or Behavior" in Chapter 5, "Adverse Psychiatric Effects of Psychiatric Medications"). Other possible iatrogenic psychiatric phenomena that have been reported in connection with anticonvulsants include catatonia, agitation, or hostility with levetiracetam.

Antimicrobials

Antibiotics

Psychiatric adverse effects caused by antibiotics are considered to be extremely rare (ranging from 1 per 100 to 1 per 10,000 prescriptions), but case reports have identified dramatic and sudden presentations of depression, psychosis, or suicidal ideation, often in individuals with no psychiatric history. Current or recent use of the antimicrobial agents listed in Table 4–1 should be considered as one possible factor in the etiology of new-onset psychiatric symptoms.

TABLE 4–1.   Adverse psychiatric effects of antimicrobials

Agent	Adverse effects
Antimalarials (e.g., mefloquine, chloroquine)	Reports of secondary psychosis, depersonalization, and anxiety or mania in individuals with no psychiatric history.
Fluoroquinolones (e.g., ciprofloxacin, levofloxacin, rufloxacin, ofloxacin)	Psychosis associated with ciprofloxacin; sudden-onset depressive symptoms and suicidal ideation associated with levofloxacin plus trimethoprim-sulfamethoxazole or lomefloxacin.
Gentamicin	Rare reports of secondary psychosis.
Isoniazid	Reports of secondary mania (Krauthammer and Klerman 1978) or psychosis.
Macrolide antibiotics	Case reports of catatonia with azithromycin; psychosis and dissociation reported with clarithromycin.
Rifampin or sulfonamide antibiotics (e.g., trimethoprim-sulfamethoxazole)	Reports of exacerbation of existing panic disorder; hallucinations rarely associated with trimethoprim-sulfamethoxazole.

Antifungal Agents

Ketoconazole has been described in case reports to cause visual and command auditory hallucinations of self-harm in patients with no prior psychiatric history.

Antineoplastics

In addition to the adverse psychiatric effects that may occur with interferon-α (see the section "Interferon-α" later in this chapter) or systemic corticosteroids (see the section "Steroids" later in this chapter), such as prednisone or dexamethasone used in cancer chemotherapy, untoward psychotropic effects have known associations with several other antineoplastic agents, as summarized in Table 4–2. Antineoplastics known to impair attention, memory, or other cognitive domains without causing psychopathological symptoms are not considered here. Malignancies

TABLE 4–2. Adverse psychiatric effects associated with antineoplastic agents

Agent	Adverse effects	Comments
ʟ-Asparaginase	Dose-related confusion, depression, hallucinations, personality changes	—
Chlorambucil	Agitation, confusion, or hallucinations	—
5-Fluorouracil	Mania, psychosis	—
Ifosfamide	Hypomania, hallucinations	Neurotoxicity involving encephalopathy and confusional states is seen more commonly than affective or psychotic symptoms.
Interleukin-2	Depression, suicidality	—
Letrozole, anostrazole	Mood changes, including mania or anxiety	Aromatase inhibitors used in breast cancer may disrupt mood via anti-estrogen effects, but may do so to a lesser degree than direct estrogen receptor antagonists such as tamoxifen.
Procarbazine	Mania or psychosis	—
Tamoxifen	Depression, psychosis; may have antimanic properties	Antimanic effect is thought to be mediated via protein kinase C inhibition, rather than anti-estrogen effect.

that penetrate the CNS can account for or contribute to acute mental status changes. In the absence of known mechanisms of action to explain iatrogenic psychiatric effects, the clinician must always consider the possibility that spontaneous cases of psychopathology may arise coincidentally with the use of a given agent, and suspected iatrogenic etiologies should not necessarily be assumed with certainty.

The term *chemo brain* has gained popular use to describe the phenomenology of persistent postchemotherapy cognitive impairment and so-called "foggy thinking" that has been observed to occur in 10%–40% of individuals (mainly women) who undergo high-dose antineoplastic chemotherapy, particularly for breast cancer. Although observations of persistent cognitive deficits have been reported following chemotherapy since the 1980s, the validity of chemo brain as a distinct and definable syndrome has been the subject of debate. Measurable cognitive deficits exist in a substantial minority of antineoplastic chemotherapy recipients, although some authors have raised questions as to the relative contribution of depression, anxiety, subjective distress, fatigue, and other emotional and physical experiences that may contribute to the phenomenon. The magnitude of cognitive impairment following chemotherapy has been described as mild in severity. No pharmacological strategies have been reported to counteract cognitive effects attributable to antineoplastic drugs.

Antiparkinsonian Agents

Probably the most well-known adverse psychiatric effects of dopamine agonists used to treat Parkinson's disease are psychotomimetic effects. The dopamine agonists pramipexole and ropinirole are both sometimes used in off-label fashion to treat depression in unipolar or bipolar disorder, to ameliorate cognitive complaints, or to counteract hyperprolactinemia and sexual dysfunction caused by dopamine antagonists. When used in patients with Parkinson's disease or restless legs syndrome, each has been reported to rarely cause pathological gambling, other impulsive and compulsive behaviors, or psychosis. More than 1,500 reports have been identified from the FDA Adverse Event Reporting System regarding new-onset impulse-control disorders (e.g., hypersexuality, compulsive shopping, pathological gambling) during treatment with dopamine agonists such as pramipexole, ropinirole, rotigotine, or the dopamine partial agonist aripiprazole (Moore et al. 2014). Such occurrences, potentially related to D_3 receptor partial agonism, have been reported up to 35 weeks after treatment initiation and appear to resolve after drug cessation. Although incidence rates or predictive factors do not exist for this unusual phenomenon, clinicians should be alert to the possibility for its occurrence.

Antiviral and Antiretroviral Agents

Oseltamivir, marketed as Tamiflu, and used to prevent or treat influenza A and influenza B, carries a manufacturer's warning of rare (NNH=94) psychiatric adverse effects that include confusion, hallucinations, and delirium, particularly in children. Risk factors (including preexisting psychiatric illnesses) have not been identified, although symptoms generally resolve soon after drug cessation.

The majority of adverse psychiatric effects related to pharmacotherapies used in HIV and AIDS have been reported to involve the antiretroviral agent efavirenz. The most common adverse CNS effects of efavirenz reported by patients include sleep disturbances (e.g., vivid dreams, nightmares, insomnia) and dizziness or other vestibular complaints (i.e., imbalance, positional vertigo), which usually resolve after the first few weeks of treatment. Rare complications of efavirenz, as compared with treatment with protease inhibitors, may include increases in somatic concerns, anxiety, depression, and obsessive-compulsive behavior, although many of these effects appear to attenuate with time. Other reports have identified rare cases of mania or psychosis in the short term following treatment initiation. It remains controversial as to whether or not the apparent adverse psychiatric consequences of efavirenz are dose related, and uncertainty persists about differentiating possible dosing effects from the relative contributions of CD4$^+$ (T-cell) count or hepatitis coinfection on psychiatric symptoms. Importantly, neuropsychiatric adverse effects of efavirenz are rare and often mild, and they generally are outweighed by the benefits of efavirenz with respect to HIV treatment.

Early reports exist of mania and psychosis during treatment with nucleoside reverse transcriptase inhibitors such as zidovudine, often among patients with a family history of mood disorders, although the majority of that literature involved mostly monotherapy at higher dosages than are now customarily recommended. Many of the existing reports failed to include adequate information about immune status, comorbidity, substance abuse, and other related factors that may contribute to psychiatric symptoms.

Cardiovascular Drugs

α_2-Adrenergic Agonists

In addition to the potential for causing sedation or fatigue, the centrally acting antihypertensive α_2-adrenergic agonist clonidine has been reported to cause depression in 1%–10% of people treated for hypertension. Other psychiatric adverse effects that have infrequently been reported with clonidine use include irritability, fear, nervousness, "psychic distress," and rare cases of hypomania or paranoia.

α_1-Adrenergic Antagonists

α_1-Adrenergic antagonists such as prazosin, terazosin, or doxazosin tend to be viewed as second- or third-line interventions for hypertension, because of their potential for orthostatic hypotension and risk for sudden falls in blood pressure (so-called first-dose phenomenon), and are more often used to treat benign prostatic hyperplasia. They have rarely been described in case reports to cause hallucinations or other psychotic features.

Antiarrhythmics

A limited number of antiarrhythmic agents have been reported to cause adverse psychiatric effects. Among them are amiodarone, which has been identified in case reports as causing depression secondary to amiodarone-induced hypothyroidism; the hypothyroidism may be ameliorated by supplemental levothyroxine. Digitalis toxicity can be associated with mania, depression, hallucinations, or other acute cognitive changes suggestive of delirium. Paranoia and psychosis have also been associated with toxicities of flecainide, procainamide, or quinidine.

β-Adrenergic Agonists

Psychiatric adverse effects are not mentioned in manufacturers' product information materials for inhaled β-adrenergic agonists, such as albuterol. However, rare postmarketing reports have described either the new onset or worsening of preexisting hallucinations, paranoid thinking, mania, or other psychotic features after excessive use in both children and adults. Predictors of such phenomena have not been identified, although cessation of the probable offending agent generally resolves the disturbance without sequelae.

β-Adrenergic Antagonists

Since early anecdotal case observations, controversy has existed about the potential for centrally acting β-blockers to cause depression based on their antiadrenergic effects. In the late 1960s and early 1970s, depression was spontaneously reported as an adverse effect of propranolol treatment in <6% of hypertensive patients (reviewed by Paykel et al. [1982]). A comprehensive review of 15 randomized trials involving over 35,000 subjects with hypertension who received a β-blocker for at least 6 months found no appreciably increased risk for treatment-related depressive symptoms (6 per 1,000 patients) (Ko et al. 2002). Small, clinically nonsignificant increased rates of fatigue or sexual dysfunction also were identified among β-blocker recipients in this latter study. Nevertheless, mental depression is listed (but without a reported incidence rate) among adverse events identified by the manufacturer in association with propranolol. In addition, propranolol specifically has been linked with depressive symptoms (but not necessarily syndromes) during the first few months of use among elderly patients.

Dermatological Agents

The acne product isotretinoin (Accutane) is reported to confer an increased risk for depression and suicidal thoughts or behaviors and is among the leading medications reported by the FDA as being associated with depression and suicide, although this relationship remains highly controversial. Empirical studies of affective psychosis newly arising after exposure to isotretinoin suggest a greater propensity among individuals with a personal history of obsessive-compulsive disorder or neurological disease, or a family history of major psychiatric illness.

Gastrointestinal Agents

A handful of case reports in the literature suggest that histamine H_2 blockers (e.g., cimetidine or ranitidine) may cause depression, although case-control studies have failed to affirm those reports and instead point to other demographic or clinical factors as more likely proximal contributors to the development of depression in individuals who take H_2 blockers.

Hormone Supplements

A number of synthetic hormones, available either over-the-counter or by prescription, have occasionally been linked with possible psychotropic effects, both beneficial and adverse. Some in particular have gained increasing popularity through advertising as purported "energy boosters," aphrodisiacs, or otherwise enhancers of vitality and virility. Possible adverse psychiatric effects of female gonadal steroid hormones (estrogen, progesterone) are described in a subsequent section ("Oral Contraceptives and Intravaginal Rings"). Adverse psychotropic effects reported with other hormonal agents and supplements are described in Table 4–3.

Immunosuppressants

Immunosuppressants are often administered for inflammatory or other medical conditions that in themselves often involve neuropsychiatric disturbances (e.g., systemic lupus erythematosus). Moreover, coadministration of immunosuppressants with corticosteroids (e.g., prednisone) may further contribute to adverse psychiatric effects. Known adverse psychiatric effects of immunosuppressants are largely identified in case reports, further limiting the ability to draw causal inferences about drug effects versus other possible contributors to psychiatric morbidity. Patients taking immunosuppressants often receive other medications (e.g., corticosteroids, antineoplastics), which can be additional sources for adverse psychiatric effects.

When patients develop new psychiatric symptoms while taking an immunosuppressant (Table 4–4), clinicians should comprehensively assess possible contributing factors—including the coincidental independent presence of a psychiatric disorder or of a psychiatric disturbance secondary to a general medical condition or a substance other than an immunosuppressant—before drawing conclusions about an iatrogenic etiology. When medically feasible, substitution of an alternative immunosuppressant may help to affirm etiology and to resolve symptoms (e.g., anxiety symptoms linked with azathioprine dissipated after substitution of methotrexate [van der Hoeven et al. 2005]). Symptomatic management with antipsychotics—similar to the approach taken with corticosteroid-induced psychosis (see section "Steroids" later in this chapter)—may be necessary for agitation, psychosis, or marked anxiety.

Interferon-α

The antiviral drug interferon-α is widely used in the treatment of chronic hepatitis B or C, certain lymphomas and leukemias, and melanoma. It is known to cause major depression in one-third or more of cases through poorly understood mechanisms that have been hypothesized to include activation of cytokines that in turn may decrease CNS serotonin production and downregulation of dopaminergic tone. About one in three recipients of interferon-α develop new-onset depression. More rarely, new-onset mania or hypomania has been reported in connection

TABLE 4–3.   Psychotropic effects of hormones

Hormone	Common uses	Possible adverse psychotropic effects
Clomiphene	Selective estrogen receptor modulator used for fertility	Case reports of mood swings, mania, psychosis in patients with known bipolar disorder.
Dihydroepi-androsterone (DHEA)	May improve mood and anxiety symptoms; possible utility for negative symptoms of schizophrenia	Case reports of mania induction.
Human chorionic gonadotropin (HCG)	Occasionally used off-label to treat obesity	Case reports of mania.
Melatonin	Treatment of insomnia, REM sleep behavior disorders, jet lag, SGA-associated weight gain; may help protect against delirium in medically ill elderly patients	Dosing of over-the-counter preparations are not well-regulated or -standardized; improperly timed dosing in bipolar disorder patients could exacerbate circadian dysrhythmias.
Testosterone	Treatment of hypogonadism or deficiencies of endogenous testosterone	Supraphysiological doses (e.g., 600 mg/week) can exert variable and unpredictable effects on mood and aggression features in healthy men (Pope et al. 2000). Rare case reports of mania or hypomania with transdermal patch (2–4 mg/day). Postmarketing reports of anxiety, depression, hostility, emotional lability, or nervousness with testosterone gel (20.25–81 mg/day of testosterone).
Thyroid hormone	Adjunct to antidepressants for major depression; replacement therapy in hypothyroidism	Rare case reports of mania during thyroid replacement among hypothyroid patients (typically initiated at >150 µg/day of levothyroxine).

TABLE 4–4.   Adverse psychiatric effects of immunosuppressants

Agent	Adverse effects
Azathioprine	Case reports of obsessive-compulsive behavior and panic attacks
Cyclosporine	Case reports of psychosis
Monoclonal antibodies (e.g., muromonab-CD3, basiliximab, rituximab)	Case reports of psychosis or encephalopathy; anxiety (≤5% incidence) with rituximab in FDA registration trials for non-Hodgkin's lymphoma
Mycophenolate mofetil	None reported
Sirolimus (or rapamycin)	None reported
Tacrolimus	Neurotoxicity at high doses may be associated with psychosis or delirium

Note.   FDA=U.S. Food and Drug Administration; REM=rapid eye movement; SGA=second-generation antipsychotic.

with the use of interferon-α. Advances in knowledge about genotype variants for hepatitis C have led to increasing use of agents other than interferon-α, including ribavirin, nucleoside and nucleotide HS5B polymerase inhibitors (e.g., sofosbuvir), and NS3/4A protease inhibitors (e.g., simeprevir, boceprevir, and telaprevir).

Several small studies have suggested that prophylactic treatment with SSRIs such as citalopram begun before interferon-α therapy may reduce the incidence of subsequent depression, although such findings are difficult to interpret because of small sample sizes, the lack of placebo control groups, and the failure to consider pretreatment risk factors for depression. A review of the collective literature suggests that prophylactic treatment with antidepressants (including paroxetine) is no better than placebo for the prevention of interferon-α–induced depression (Galvão-de Almeida et al. 2010). On the other hand, in prospective trials of antidepressants, including citalopram (Kraus et al. 2008), the drugs appear better than placebo in reducing depressive symptoms among hepatitis C patients who developed depressive symptoms during interferon-α therapy.

The use of psychostimulants such as methylphenidate monotherapy also has been described as a possible rapid, safe, and effective strategy for reducing vegetative symptoms in patients who develop protracted depression in the context of interferon-α therapy.

Oral Contraceptives and Intravaginal Rings

General Recommendations

Oral contraceptives can have variable and unpredictable effects on mood. Adverse mood effects may be more likely with contraceptives containing levonorgestrel than desogestrel. The emergence or exacerbation of mood or anxiety symptoms shortly after beginning an oral contraceptive may warrant its discontinuation.

Oral contraceptives combine an estrogen formulation (typically ethinyl estradiol or mestranol) with a progestin (typically a synthetic progesterone-like compound). Progestins have been associated with dysphoria and anger. Concerns often arise about the extent to which oral contraceptives may exert either a beneficial or an adverse effect on mood, either in the presence or absence of preexisting premenstrual mood disturbances. Indeed, package insert information for all oral contraceptive pills includes the following precaution:

> Patients becoming significantly depressed while taking oral contraceptives should stop the medication and use an alternate method of contraception in an attempt to determine whether the symptom is drug related. Women with a history of depression should be carefully observed and the drug discontinued if depression recurs to a serious degree.

Key points regarding oral contraceptive preparations are as follows:

- Concentrations of ethinyl estradiol range from 20 to 50 µg.
- Synthetic progestins include levonorgestrel, desogestrel, and drospirenone (a spironolactone analogue with antimineralocorticoid and antiandrogenic properties).
- Monophasic oral contraceptives involve the administration of 21 days of estrogen followed by 7 days of placebo, whereas triphasic formulations contain three varying hormone doses across the first 21 days of active treatment.
- Second-generation oral contraceptives combine ethinyl estradiol and a synthetic progestin, with varying concentrations of both hormones.
- Third-generation oral contraceptives use desogestrel as the progestin (e.g., Yasmin, Yaz).

Importantly, monophasic desogestrel oral contraceptives have been associated with less mood dysregulation than monophasic or triphasic levonorgestrel compounds, making Yaz and Yasmin popular among many gynecologists for women with sensitivities to premenstrual or perimenstrual mood disturbances. The pairing of ethinyl estradiol with drospirenone rather than levonorgestrel has been associated with greater improvement in affective symptoms of menstrual distress in healthy women (Kelly et al. 2010). Adverse mood effects associated with oral contraceptives appear higher in women under age 20, women with a history of perinatal depression or dysmenorrhea, women with current postpartum status, and women with a family history of obsessive-compulsive-related mood symptoms (Oinonen and Mazmanian 2002). Although some authors believe that mood worsening from oral contraceptives may vary depending on ratios of ethinyl estradiol to progestin, this theory remains debated.

Notably, a limited number of psychotropic agents are known to induce the metabolism of estrogen-containing oral contraceptives via induction of CYP isoenzymes and may therefore diminish the efficacy for preventing conception. These agents include topiramate, carbamazepine, oxcarbazepine, and modafinil—thus prompting the need to consider the use of contraceptive preparations that contain higher estrogen concentrations for patients also taking these medications. (No reduction in efficacy of oral contraceptives occurs during coadministration with divalproex, gabapentin, lamotrigine, levetiracetam, tiagabine, or zonisamide.) When a hepatic enzyme–inducing agent is taken in conjunction with an oral contraceptive, it may be advisable to use an oral contraceptive with a higher dose of ethinyl estradiol than might otherwise be the case.

In addition, estrogen-containing oral contraceptives may reduce the bioavailability or efficacy of other psychotropic medications. Pharmacokinetic studies show that conjugated estrogens such as those found in oral contraceptives may reduce the bioavailability of lamotrigine, which may prompt the need for modestly increasing the dose of lamotrigine if clinically warranted (i.e., in the setting of breakthrough signs of illness). Oral contraceptives may also diminish the efficacy of (and potential for sedation from) certain benzodiazepines (i.e., lorazepam, oxazepam, and temazepam) but potentiate the effects of others (i.e., alprazolam, chlordiazepoxide, diazepam, flurazepam, and triazolam).

Polymeric intravaginal contraceptive rings that contain and release estrogen and progestin (e.g., NuvaRing, containing etonogestrel [the metabolite of desogestrel] and ethinyl estradiol), considered to be third-generation contraceptives, have been available in the United States since 2002. Depression has been reported as an adverse effect of NuvaRing, although no incidence rate is reported in the manufacturer's product information materials. There is no contraindication to its use in women with a history of depression or other mood disorders.

Smoking Cessation Aids

Oral varenicline is a nicotinic receptor partial agonist smoking cessation aid whose labeling package carries a boxed warning (■) identifying a risk for "changes in behavior, hostility, agitation, depressed mood, and suicidal thoughts" that can develop during treatment in individuals either with or without a history of psychiatric illness. Incidence rates of depression associated with varenicline are not well identified and remain controversial, but the magnitude of risk appears small. Notably, a 12-week manufacturer-sponsored randomized comparison of varenicline or placebo in 110 smokers without past psychiatric histories found no differences in the emergence of depressive, anxiety, or aggressive features (Garza et al. 2011). Similarly, a British cohort study of 80,660 primary care patients revealed no significant increased risk for suicidal thoughts or depression among varenicline recipients; this report identified a possible but statistically nonsignificant 2-fold increased risk for self-harm that could not be ruled out based on the upper limit of observed confidence intervals (Gunnell et al. 2009). More recent randomized controlled trials of varenicline for smoking cessation in bipolar disorder or schizophrenia have revealed no significantly greater risk than with placebo for either worsening of depressive symptoms or emergence of new suicidal thinking (Chengappa et al. 2014; Evins et al. 2014). Hence, a history of depression should not contraindicate the use of varenicline, although all patients who receive varenicline should be monitored for the possible emergence of depressive or suicidal features.

Steroids

Corticosteroids are well known to cause a variety of adverse psychiatric effects, including agitation, psychosis, anxiety, mania, depression, and delirium. Affective symptoms are generally considered to be more common than psychosis as a consequence of steroids, with mania being more common than depression. Adverse psychiatric effects are estimated to occur in approximately 2%–20% of corticosteroid recipients, with increasing likelihood as dosages escalate. (For example, the Boston Collaborative Drug Surveillance Program [1972] identified new-onset affective or psychotic symptoms in 1.3% of recipients taking ≤40 mg/day of prednisone, 4.6% of those taking 41–80 mg/day, and 18.4% of those taking

>80 mg/day.) Symptoms appear unrelated to age, may be somewhat more common in women than men, and usually arise within the first several days after steroid initiation. Importantly, neither preexisting psychiatric conditions nor a history of previous steroid-induced psychiatric symptoms are known to increase the risk for developing steroid-induced psychiatric symptoms. Without intervention, symptoms may persist for several weeks after steroids are tapered off.

Alternatives to steroids may sometimes be feasible in specific clinical settings (e.g., the immunosuppressant mycophenolate mofetil may be used instead of prednisone for patients with systemic lupus erythematosus). In patients who require high-dose or prolonged steroid treatment, symptomatic management of iatrogenic psychiatric symptoms may be necessary. Wada and colleagues (2001) reported efficacy and good tolerability using traditional mood stabilizers (lithium, divalproex, or carbamazepine) to treat steroid-induced mania in patients without bipolar disorder, as permissible based on renal or hepatic function. Adequately dosed antipsychotics are also considered fairly standard for managing steroid-induced mania or psychosis, although the evidence base for their use derives mainly from case reports. Dosing of antipsychotics needs to be based on symptom severity and response to initial dosages, as well as duration of a projected steroid course, balanced against medical comorbidity and tolerability.

5

Adverse Psychiatric Effects of Psychiatric Medications

Activation and Mania/Hypomania or Mixed States

Contemporary meta-analyses of antidepressant-associated mania or hypomania suggest an incidence of only about 10%–15% in patients with bipolar disorder, and coadministration of an antimanic agent does not necessarily and reliably prevent the potential for affective polarity switch (Tondo et al. 2010). However, available studies are limited by their retrospective study designs, variability in treatment regimens, recognition of patient-specific factors that increase risk for antidepressant-induced mania (summarized in Table 5–1), and nonstandardization of definitions and assessments of polarity switch. Clinicians sometimes broadly use the term *activation* as a catchphrase to describe features suggestive of various phenomena, ranging from mania or hypomania to akathisia to anxiety to psychomotor agitation. Regardless of terminol-

---

The symbol ■ is used in this chapter to indicate that the FDA has issued a boxed warning for a prescription medication that may cause serious adverse effects.

ogy, signs of increased psychomotor activity during treatment with any psychotropic drug warrant systematic and thoughtful evaluation by the prescriber. Relevant signs of treatment-emergent mania or hypomania may be subtle and can include new-onset sleep disturbance, anger, and irritability, as well as other DSM-5 (American Psychiatric Association 2013) symptoms of a manic or hypomanic episode. The following are important points to consider:

- How recently a medication was begun or dosages were changed
- Whether or not an apparent dose relationship corresponds to the emergence of symptoms
- The presence or absence of bipolar disorder
- A known history of prior antidepressant-associated mania or hypomania
- The possible contributing role of concomitant medications
- The loss of need for sleep without consequent fatigue (as opposed to simple insomnia or phase advancement of the sleep-wake cycle)
- The absence of alcohol intoxication or withdrawal states, or illicit substance abuse that could mimic psychomotor activation otherwise attributable to a prescribed medication

The emergence of mania or hypomania following exposure to an antidepressant or stimulant touches on the distinction between a frank side effect of a drug and the precipitation of a diathesis (in this instance, to mania or hypomania) that is catalyzed by exposure to a particular medication. DSM-5 (American Psychiatric Association 2013) construes mania arising soon after the initiation or dosing increase of an antidepressant medication as indicative of bipolar disorder only if mania symptoms persist "at a fully syndromal level beyond the physiological effect of that treatment"; antidepressant-associated manias or hypomanias that dissipate before then are considered to be medication-induced adverse effects. Manias or hypomanias that arise beyond 12 weeks after treatment initiation are generally difficult to reasonably attribute to an antidepressant rather than to the natural course of illness.

It is presently unknown whether antidepressant-induced mania or hypomania may be a dose-related (vs. an all-or-none exposure) phenomenon and whether antimanic drugs effectively "counterbalance" or reliably prevent antidepressant-induced mania or hypomania. Psychomotor activation that is possibly caused by a psychotropic agent should be evaluated to differentiate agitation, akathisia, anxiety, and mania or hypomania. Mania or hypomania resulting from psychostimulants remains a theoretical risk that has received remarkably little study in pa-

TABLE 5–1. Risk factors associated with the emergence of mania or hypomania during treatment with antidepressants

Factor	Finding
History of antidepressant-induced mania or hypomania	A 2- to 5-fold increased risk for subsequent antidepressant-induced mania or hypomania, regardless of antidepressant
Recent mania preceding current depressive episode	Higher risk for antidepressant-associated mania if current depressive episode was preceded by manic phase
Bipolar I vs. bipolar II subtype	Greater risk for switch in bipolar I
Comorbid alcohol or substance use disorder	A 5- to 7-fold increased risk for antidepressant-associated mania
Noradrenergic vs. serotonergic antidepressants	Possible higher risk for mania induction with TCAs or SNRIs than with bupropion or SSRIs
Concurrent mania symptoms during a depressive episode	Increased risk for mania in patients with mild or subthreshold mania symptoms during a depressive episode
Hyperthymic temperamental traits	Increased likelihood of antidepressant-induced mania

Note. SNRI=serotonin-norepinephrine reuptake inhibitor; SSRI=selective serotonin reuptake inhibitor; TCA=tricyclic antidepressant.
Source. Adapted from Goldberg JF: "Antidepressants in Bipolar Disorder: Seven Myths and Realities." *Current Psychiatry* 9:41–49, 2010.

tients with known bipolar disorder, limiting the ability to make broad assumptions about either the safety or efficacy of psychostimulants in patients with bipolar disorder. Suspected inductions of true mania or hypomania warrant cessation of the suspected causal agent, and if resolution does not occur, initiation of an antipsychotic or similar antimanic agent may be advisable.

Open trials and cases have reported that new-onset mania results from some SGAs, such as risperidone and ziprasidone, and even lithium. Although various theoretical mechanisms have been proposed to explain the foregoing observations (e.g., mania resulting from the SNRI properties of ziprasidone), it remains difficult to draw generalizable pharmacodynamic inferences about such cases relative to the natural course of illness in bipolar disorder.

Anxiety and Panic

Manufacturers' product information materials for many psychotropic compounds identify anxiety or nervousness as self-reported adverse effects, although it is often difficult to determine whether such phenomena reflect true iatrogenic effects or symptoms of the primary psychiatric disorder being treated. Certain psychotropic drugs, such as bupropion, have acquired popular perceptions that they may be anxiogenic despite a lack of evidence from controlled trials to suggest either lesser efficacy in anxious depression or a higher incidence of treatment-emergent anxiety as compared to SSRIs. For other sympathomimetic psychotropic drugs such as stimulants, incidence rates of anxiety or agitation are typically reported in the range of ~5%–10% of adult subjects.

The possible iatrogenic emergence of panic attacks merits specific consideration with some psychotropics. Most antidepressants carry package insert information indicating that panic attacks have been reported in both children and adults being treated for major depression, although little empirical information exists on the timing, phenomenology, and course of new-onset panic among depressed patients after starting an antidepressant. High baseline comorbidity rates of panic disorder with both major depression and bipolar disorder (about 10% [Kessler et al. 1998] and 20% [Chen and Dilsaver 1995], respectively, based on findings from large-scale epidemiologic studies) also complicate efforts to differentiate iatrogenic from primary panic attacks. Several isolated case reports appear in the literature linking panic attacks with the use of topiramate (50–150 mg/day) in patients with bipolar disorder, drawing on the hypothesis that its carbonic anhydrase activity could potentially induce panic via carbon dioxide retention.

Clinical Trial Subjects With Psychiatric Illness

A dilemma arises when subjects who are psychiatrically ill enroll in clinical trials and then report psychiatric symptoms as adverse effects; it is often difficult if not impossible to discern whether such complaints reflect true iatrogenic phenomena, whether they reflect untreated or undertreated manifestations of the illness state being treated, or whether they are spurious observations that may have no direct bearing either on the target symptoms of the condition being treated or on the effects of treatment itself. Pertinent examples would include purported side effects such as personality disorder or psychosis that may be reported during treatment for schizophrenia.

Discontinuation Phenomena

Abrupt cessation of short-acting serotonergic antidepressants may lead to discontinuation syndromes involving mainly gastrointestinal or neurological (e.g., vestibular) phenomena (see "Discontinuation Syndromes" in Chapter 20, "Systemic Reactions"), although an induction or exacerbation of psychiatric symptoms is rare. Mania has been described following the rapid discontinuation of antidepressants in patients previously identified with unipolar depression (Goldstein et al. 1999); this discontinuation is thought to reflect disruption of a homeostatic state. For patients with major depression or panic disorder, rapid antidepressant cessation (≤7 days) also appears to significantly hasten time to relapse as compared with more gradual discontinuation schedules (>14 days) (Baldessarini et al. 2010). Case reports also exist of new-onset mania, psychosis, or delirium resulting from the abrupt withdrawal of either short- or long-acting benzodiazepines. In patients with bipolar disorder, discontinuation of lithium over less than a 2-week period can markedly hasten the time to affective relapse (Faedda et al. 1993).

Disinhibition and Impaired Impulse Control

Benzodiazepines have been associated with the development of disinhibited behavior or paradoxical aggression in vulnerable populations, particularly in patients who are elderly or patients with preexisting frontal lobe disease. Individuals with a history of impulse control disorders (including substance use disorders and borderline or antisocial personality disorders) are also sometimes considered to be at greater risk for disinhibition with benzodiazepine use.

A chart review of disinhibited behaviors in 323 inpatients found no differences among those receiving alprazolam, clonazepam, or no benzodiazepine (Rothschild et al. 2000), although underlying diagnoses were heterogeneous and patients varied in their use of additional medications. The authors surmised that contrary to some popular impressions, behavioral disinhibition may be no more likely with short-acting than with long-acting benzodiazepines.

Emotional Dulling

SSRIs have been reported, although rarely, to induce a state of emotional indifference or apathy that is sometimes confused with depression. A literature review of this phenomenon in 2004 identified 12 case reports and determined apathy to be a rare, reversible, dose-related side effect (Barnhart et al. 2004). Switching from an SSRI to an SNRI after otherwise successful treatment of major depression has not been shown to ameliorate subsequent apathy symptoms. The ability of SGAs to increase prefrontal dopamine transmission via serotonin type 2A (5-HT_{2A}) blockage has been identified as one possible mechanistic strategy that might counteract avolition or apathy. In an 8-week pilot study of 21 formerly depressed patients who manifested signs of apathy after ≥3 months of treatment with an SSRI (citalopram, fluoxetine, sertraline, or paroxetine), Marangell et al. (2002) found significant improvement in apathy symptoms after the addition of olanzapine (2.5–20 mg/day; mean dosage = 5.4 mg/day), although subjects had a mean weight gain of 3 kg. Other SGAs have not, as yet, been studied for this purpose but may merit consideration.

Psychosis

A limited number of psychotropic medications may have psychotomimetic effects—not to be confused with reports of "psychosis" that become identified in the course of clinical trials of antipsychotic drugs, which usually simply reflect a lack of antipsychotic efficacy against the primary illness being treated. Psychosis is a known risk of psychostimulants, usually in dose-related fashion, as well as from dopamine agonists such as ropinirole, pramipexole, bromocriptine, and amantadine.

Rare case reports of new hallucinations that have been described in association with the use of some SSRIs (notably, fluvoxamine) or SNRIs (venlafaxine) are thought to reflect serotonergic overstimulation, eliminated by dosage reductions or by drug cessation. Cases also exist of new-onset psychosis associated with bupropion, typically within days to weeks of treatment initiation, and observed even at relatively low dosages (100–150 mg/day). Hypothesized mechanisms accounting for rare psychotomimetic effects include the structural similarity of bupropion to amphetamine, and bupropion's putative inhibition of dopamine reuptake.

The use of nonbenzodiazepine hypnotics such as zolpidem has been reported in association with new-onset hallucinations, depersonalization, or dissociation rarely in adults (<1%), but more often in pediatric patients. For example, hallucinations occurred in 7.4% of children or adolescents receiving zolpidem for insomnia associated with attention-deficit/hyperactivity disorder, as reported by the manufacturer.

Suicidal Thinking or Behavior

On January 31, 2008, the FDA issued an alert that all anticonvulsants carried the potential to induce or exacerbate suicidal thoughts or behaviors, based on its review of 199 placebo-controlled trials involving 11 anticonvulsant agents and 43,900 subjects, over a median duration of 12 weeks, that were linked with an overall 1.8-fold increased risk. No boxed warning was imposed despite the concerns raised by the FDA's Scientific Advisory Committee. The FDA ranked agents by risk for suicidal behavior as levetiracetam > topiramate > zonisamide > oxcarbazepine > pregabalin > gabapentin > lamotrigine > divalproex > carbamazepine (Pompili and Baldessarini 2010). Notably, contrary findings that dispute a relationship between anticonvulsant use and suicidal behavior have been reported in patients with bipolar disorder (Gibbons et al. 2009). Similarly, a cohort study of 5.1 million prescription recipients in the United Kingdom found no increased risk for suicide-related events in patients with either epilepsy or bipolar disorder who received anticonvulsant medication; however, anticonvulsant use was associated with a 1.7-fold increased risk for suicidality in patients with major depression and a 2.6-fold increased risk among patients with disorders other than major depression, epilepsy, or bipolar disorder (Arana et al. 2010). The relationship between suicidal thoughts or behaviors and anticonvulsants appears to be complex, with some authors pointing out unexpectedly high risks for suicide among epilepsy patients, likely attributable to psychiatric comorbidity (Pompili and Baldessarini 2010).

Antidepressant medications have come under particular scrutiny since the FDA issued a boxed warning (■) in October 2004 that all antidepressants can increase suicidal thinking or behavior in individuals <age 24; this risk does not apply to individuals >age 24, and antidepressants appear to confer protection against suicidal behavior in adults ≥age 65. These observations derived from an FDA advisory panel that reviewed 25 drug trials (16 in patients with depression) involving approximately 4,000 children or adolescents, in which 109 events were deemed "possibly suicide-related," although no suicide completions occurred. Suicide-related "events" ranged from attempted hangings or overdoses to behaviors such as self-mutilation or self-slapping. Those data were corroborated by an observed 1.5-fold increased risk for suicide attempts and 15.6-fold increased risk for suicide deaths among youth ages 6–18 years in a nationwide Medicaid database case-control study of individuals ages 6–64 who did not have bipolar disorder, schizophrenia, dementia/delirium, or mental retardation and who were not pregnant (Olfson et al. 2006).

Purported links between suicidal behavior and antidepressant use have been challenged by naturalistic population studies, such as the finding that a 1% increase in antidepressant use appears associated with a *decrease* of 0.23 suicides per 100,000 adolescents ages 10–19 per year (Olfson et al. 2003), or National Vital Statistics data from the Centers for Disease Control indicating that use of SSRIs and other newer-generation antidepressants is linked with lower rates of suicide deaths in the general population (Gibbons et al. 2005). Suicide completion rates declined 13% from 1985 to 1999, accompanied by a 4-fold increase in rates of SSRI and other newer-generation antidepressant prescriptions (Grunebaum et al. 2004).

6

What Nonmedical Therapists Should Know About Adverse Drug Effects

Although prescribers often have difficulty discerning the etiology of physical complaints, differentiating their probable associations with treatment versus underlying illness, and recognizing the necessity (or nonnecessity) of interventions, such challenges can be even more daunting for nonmedical psychotherapists. The potential advantages and disadvantages of so-called split or collaborative treatments between two clinicians involve broad issues that fall beyond the scope of this book (but are well addressed by Riba and Balon [2005]; cf. Kelly [1992] on the concept of "parallel" treatments as independent endeavors). However, because nonmedical therapists have a positive role to play as a member of a treatment team, we offer the following cautionary considerations that bear on the assessment of adverse drug effects:

- Nonmedical therapists may not recognize which physical complaints are or are not plausibly iatrogenic and could erroneously reinforce patients' misattributions about etiology.

- Patients who erratically take sedative-hypnotics or opiates or binge on alcohol might describe withdrawal phenomena that could be misconstrued as psychological or psychiatric rather than physical; similarly, patients who abuse controlled substances may complain of symptoms that could be misinterpreted as medication side effects (or primary psychiatric symptoms) that actually reflect intoxication, withdrawal, or neurotoxic states.
- Nonmedical therapists may sometimes unwittingly overstep scope-of-practice boundaries through well-intended but potentially medically inaccurate suggestions about ways to manage adverse effects (e.g., advising a patient to alter the dosage of a medicine, proposing a pharmacological remedy for an adverse effect, or wrongly encouraging patients to "wait out" a serious side effect that they assume will ultimately resolve with time—rather than advising a patient to redirect medication concerns to the prescriber).
- Nonmedical therapists may be unaware of the medical significance of a probable adverse drug effect when addressing physical symptoms that might also have a psychodynamic or behavioral etiology. For example, the therapist may examine loss of libido or sexual dysfunction solely in the context of past conflictual or traumatic intimate relationships, or may perceive complaints of anxiety and restlessness as manifestations of psychic distress surrounding the material under scrutiny in psychotherapy (rather than, perhaps, as manifestations of akathisia or pharmacologically induced psychomotor activation).
- Dynamically oriented psychotherapists also may be unaware of emotional or cognitive phenomena that could be iatrogenic. For example, complaints of apathy during SSRI therapy may be misconstrued either as depression or as a defensive posture against confronting emotionally upsetting material.
- Nonmedical therapists may fall back on personal experience, biases, or secondhand information about drug effects, from which they may make professional or overgeneralized recommendations to patients who, in turn, may misconstrue the accuracy and authoritative nature of medical information they receive from a clinician without medical training. Negative biases on the part of nonprescribing therapists also can inappropriately intrude into the course of a collaborative treatment in ways that are a disservice to the needs of the patient (e.g., telling a patient experiencing adverse effects that he is probably better off if he can get by without a drug, or otherwise implying that pharmacotherapy is an elective accessory to psychotherapy that should ideally be halted as soon as feasible).

- The potential arises for splitting to occur between prescriber and non-prescriber, as well as acting out of relationship dynamics between medical and nonmedical treaters (e.g., Patient: "My therapist says my thinking is less sharp from this medicine and says you should lower the dosage or change it"). Alternatively, nonmedical psychotherapists can strengthen the integrity of a team approach by pointing out the appropriate delineation of roles and responsibilities when patients ask medication questions (e.g., Therapist: "Have you mentioned that concern to Dr. Smith? What information has she given you?").

Nonmedical psychotherapists can provide both patients and pre-scribers with invaluable observations on many levels regarding adverse drug effects. Often, such perspective comes from having more frequent contact with a patient and a more intimate knowledge about the patient's personal habits and coping styles, as well as seemingly routine medical events. For example, consider a patient who remarks to her nonmedical therapist that she has begun an oral contraceptive prescribed by her gyn-ecologist but may not have discussed with the physician whether there may be drug interactions with existing psychotropic medications or whether any subsequent mood changes might be iatrogenic. Patients who have a closer working alliance with a nonmedical therapist also typically provide him or her with more personal information and detail, and con-sequently may be more comfortable (or selective) in sharing sensitive information. Common examples include patients' concerns about sexual functioning, alcohol or substance misuse, or adverse drug effects that be-come fodder for interpersonal or family-based conflicts (e.g., Patient: "My mother says I'm getting too fat; I should stop this medicine").

Nonmedical psychotherapists may have a particular vantage point from which to recognize and intercede when patients are inclined to stop taking medications. Patients, for their part, sometimes may not feel inclined to tell a prescriber about their wish to discontinue a treatment — perhaps because of the fear of admonition or an otherwise judgmental response. By contrast, nonprescribing psychotherapists who are alert to such issues may be able to provide patients with a more impartial envi-ronment in which to discuss thoughts and feelings about medication likes and dislikes. A therapist's ability to help a patient identify his or her own concerns about medication (or other health issues) and articu-late them effectively to the physician is modeling behavior for taking proper care of oneself, while overcoming defeatist expectations (e.g., Pa-tient: "Dr. Jones will just tell me I have to live with the side effects. Why bother complaining to him?") and fostering a sense of responsibility and empowerment over the patient's pursuit of treatment (e.g., Therapist: "You are assuming Dr. Jones won't be sympathetic to the problems you're having, and won't be able to help you find a solution for them").

Finally, although it remains the responsibility of the prescriber to monitor and address adverse drug effects, nonmedical psychotherapists should consider that these actions unfortunately may not always occur routinely and properly. Rather than taking it upon themselves to inventory the presence of potential adverse drug effects or other medication concerns, nonprescribing therapists should periodically ask patients about the status of their pharmacotherapy and medical follow-up. Sample gentle prompts and points for discussion might include the following:

- "How often are you and Dr. Smith in contact with one another? How often has Dr. Smith recommended that you meet with her?"
- "Has Dr. Smith reviewed with you the purpose of the medicines she is prescribing? Has she discussed dosing and possible side effects with you?"
- "Did Dr. Smith tell you whether any lab tests are necessary for the safe use of the medicines you are taking and how often those need to be done?"
- "Have you asked Dr. Smith if that problem could be related to the medicine you're taking?"
- "What did Dr. Smith advise about the effects of alcohol on the medicines you're taking?"
- When poor adherence is suspected, or known: "Many people sometimes have trouble taking their medicines exactly the way their doctors recommend. Do you?" or "Are you comfortable talking with Dr. Smith about your reluctance to take medicine? How do you think she would respond if you brought this up with her?"
- "Have you asked Dr. Smith whether there may be ways to manage possible side effects, or whether there are alternative medicines worth considering?"
- "You should let Dr. Smith know that your internist has prescribed a new medicine to make sure there are no conflicts with the medication she is prescribing for you."
- "Don't forget to tell Dr. Smith that you're having surgery to find out if there might be any special issues for postoperative pain management—or if there might be any other concerns with the medicines you're taking."

It makes sense for two (or more) mental health professionals who share common cases to make clear to their mutual patients the importance of permission for free communication among providers. Such information exchange helps to minimize misunderstandings, miscommunications, and potential hazards about medically or psychiatrically relevant information that might otherwise go unknown by each clinician.

PART II

Organ Systems

7

Cardiovascular System

Arrhythmias and Palpitations

General Recommendations

Arrhythmias may occur as a consequence of treatment with all antipsychotics, TCAs, some SSRIs, lithium, stimulants, and anticholinergic drugs, or in the setting of toxicity states. Clinicians should be familiar with cumulative risk factors for prolonged ventricular repolarization (the QTc interval; see Table 7–3) or ventricular depolarization (in the case of TCAs), and the relevance for baseline electrocardiographic monitoring (e.g., in adults with known or suspected cardiac disease, before starting a TCA, lithium, or in some instances an SGA). Palpitations (the subjective awareness of heartbeats) are usually benign in the absence of underlying structural heart disease, but carry a wide differential diagnosis that involves factors unrelated to psychotropic drugs.

The symbol ■ is used in this chapter to indicate that the FDA has issued a boxed warning for a prescription medication that may cause serious adverse effects.

Overall Considerations

The arrhythmogenic potential of some psychotropic drugs is long established and often poses a significant deterrent to prescribing otherwise effective medications. Examples of these drugs include TCAs by virtue of their anticholinergic effects, α-adrenergic blockade, and quinidine-like effects from the blockade of fast sodium channels in myocardial cells.

Table 7–1 summarizes known relationships between electrocardiographic changes and common psychotropic medications. Some experts advise obtaining a baseline ECG in adults over age 40 (in addition to those with a history of cardiac disease) before beginning a TCA, lithium, and some SGAs (such as those with a greater potential for QTc prolongation, as described in Table 7–2).

Most SGAs carry risks for both tachycardia (presumably due to anticholinergic effects) and orthostatic hypotension (probably due to α_1-adrenergic blockade). Proper management involves measurement of heart rate and blood pressure, including orthostatic measurements, and gradual dosage increases when necessary. If a β-blocker is being used to treat akathisia or tremor, monitoring heart rate and blood pressure is especially important to assure no exacerbation of hypotension from α_1-adrenergic blockade.

Palpitations refer to the awareness or subjective experience of irregular heartbeats. They may or may not reflect actual ectopic beats. Atrial premature complexes (APCs) or premature ventricular complexes (PVCs) that are isolated, intermittent, and arise spontaneously are usually benign and common occurrences in healthy people, unless the contractions are accompanied by other cardiovascular signs (such as chest pain, dizziness, or syncope) or arise in the setting of structural heart disease.

Psychiatrists who evaluate palpitations should review all of a patient's medications (both psychiatric and nonpsychiatric) to identify drugs that may cause tachycardia (e.g., anticholinergics), prolong the QT interval (see Tables 7–2 and 7–3), or pharmacokinetically inhibit the metabolism of anticholinergic or QT-prolonging drugs (see Tables 2–6 and 2–7 in Chapter 2, "Pharmacokinetics, Pharmacodynamics, and Pharmacogenomics"). Pulse rate and regularity should be measured and the heart auscultated to discern premature beats, particularly if occurring as couplets or triplets. Obtaining an electrocardiogram (ECG) is appropriate to assure normal intervals and identify APCs or PVCs. Runs of bigeminy or trigeminy warrant more extensive studies (e.g., Holter monitoring) and referral to a cardiologist. Echocardiography may be indicated for patients with a murmur who complain of palpitations. Iatrogenically, stimulants may cause sinus or supraventricular tachyarrhythmias but not

TABLE 7–1. Electrocardiographic changes associated with psychotropic medications

Medication	Electrocardiographic changes and concerns
Anticonvulsants and lithium	
Carbamazepine	QRS prolongation; heart block and ventricular arrhythmias possible in overdose.
Divalproex	Tachycardia or bradycardia.
Gabapentin	None known.
Lamotrigine	Rare associations reported with lamotrigine overdose and Brugada pattern[a] on ECG, presumably via the effect of lamotrigine on sodium channels, as well as QRS widening; routine ECG monitoring not indicated.
Lithium	Reversible T-wave changes, sinus bradycardia, sick sinus syndrome, heart block, case reports of Brugada pattern[a] on ECG; controversial case reports of QTc prolongation.
Oxcarbazepine	None known.
Topiramate	None known.
Antidepressants	
Bupropion	Tachycardia, premature beats, nonspecific ST-T changes, QRS prolongation in overdose.
Mirtazapine	Possible association with relatively minor increase in heart rate (<5 beats per minute); no other known electrocardiographic abnormalities.
SNRIs	May increase heart rate due to increased noradrenergic tone.
SSRIs	May decrease heart rate; rare increase in QTc intervals with escitalopram, fluoxetine, fluvoxamine, and sertraline; more likely increase in QTc with citalopram (dose related) or in the setting of overdoses or drug interactions.
Vilazodone	No known effects on any ECG parameters when dosed up to 80 mg/day (Edwards et al. 2013).
Vortioxetine	No QTc > 10 msec when dosed up to 40 mg/day.

TABLE 7–1.   Electrocardiographic changes associated with psychotropic medications *(continued)*

Medication	Electrocardiographic changes and concerns
Antidepressants *(continued)*	
TCAs	Tachycardia possible due to vagolytic effects; quinidine-like effects possible (i.e., blockade of fast sodium channels causes prolonged depolarization with decreased myocardial contractility, leading to PR prolongation, QRS widening, right axis deviation, and bradycardia or heart block in overdose); TCAs can inhibit cardiac hERG K^+ channel currents, prolonging action potentials and increasing the risk for QT prolongation.
Antipsychotics	
FGAs	Sinus tachycardia, QTc prolongation (particularly with pimozide, thioridazine, and intravenous haloperidol), ventricular arrhythmias.
Pimavanserin	QTc prolongation.
SGAs	Tachycardia (lurasidone, risperidone), first-degree AV block (lurasidone), QTc prolongation (ziprasidone, iloperidone, and potentially others in dose-related fashion).
Anxiolytics or sedative-hypnotics	
Benzodiazepines	Rare reports of QTc prolongation with lorazepam in patients with underlying arrhythmia.
Buspirone	None known.
Eszopiclone	None known.
Ramelteon	None known.
Suvorexant	No clinically significant QTc prolongation at 12 times the maximal recommended dose.
Tasimelteon	None known.
Zaleplon	None known.
Zolpidem	None known.

TABLE 7–1.	Electrocardiographic changes associated with psychotropic medications *(continued)*
Medication	Electrocardiographic changes and concerns
Psychostimulants	Tachycardia.
Miscellaneous CNS agents	
Deutetrabenazine	Mean 4.5 msec (24-mg single dose) (90% CI=2.4–6.5 msec) increase in QTc interval (healthy volunteers).
Valbenazine	Mean 6.7 msec (40-mg dose) (healthy volunteers); for CYP2D6 PMs, maximally dosed (80 mg/day) ΔQTc=11.7 msec.

Note. AV=atrioventricular; CI=confidence interval; CNS=central nervous system; ECG = electrocardiogram; FGA=first-generation antipsychotic; hERG = human ether-à-go-go-related gene (which codes for the alpha subunit of the K^+ ion channel in cardiac myocytes); SGA=second-generation antipsychotic; SNRI=serotonin-norepinephrine reuptake inhibitor; SSRI=selective serotonin reuptake inhibitor; TCA=tricyclic antidepressant.
[a]The Brugada pattern on ECG involves right bundle branch block with coved-type ST segment elevation (see Figure 7–1).

APCs or PVCs. Rare reports of new-onset PVCs have been described with the use of modafinil (Oskooilar 2005). Clinicians obviously should recognize and consider nonpsychotropic drug causes of a rapid or irregular heart rhythm, including the effects of thyroid hormone, inhaled beta agonists, antihypertensive agents, caffeine, and nicotine, as well as the potential contribution of hyperthyroidism, electrolyte abnormalities, and anxiety, among other possible etiologies.

Psychiatrists (and other health professionals) often rely on computer-read interpretations of ECG parameters, including QTc intervals. However, one must bear in mind the presence of factors that can interfere with accurate reading of QTc intervals (whether computerized or manual), including wide QRS complexes, pacemakers, and rapid heart rates.

Sudden Cardiac Death

General Recommendations

Clinicians should be aware that all antipsychotics and psychostimulants carry a small but statistically significantly increased risk for sudden cardiac death.

TABLE 7–2.   QTc prolongation with FGAs and SGAs (in order of increasing concern by duration)

Agent	Findings in FDA registration trials	Likelihood > placebo (OR, 95% CI)[a]
Clozapine	No known QTc prolongation.	—
Lurasidone	Manufacturer's product information: at dosages of 120 or 600 mg/day, "no patients experienced QTc increases >60 msec from baseline, nor did any patient experience a QTc >500 msec"; 5.1-msec and 4.5-msec increases from baseline at 40 mg/day and 120 mg/day doses (Meltzer et al. 2011).	−0.10 (−0.21 to 0.01)
Aripiprazole	−4.2-msec decrease from baseline (Marder et al. 2003).	0.01 (−0.13 to 0.15)
Paliperidone	12.3-msec increase from baseline (8-mg dose); no subjects had a change exceeding 60 msec or QTc >500 msec (manufacturer's product information).	0.05 (−0.18 to 0.26)
Haloperidol[b]	4.7-msec increase from baseline (Glassman and Bigger 2001).	0.11 (0.03 to 0.19)
Quetiapine	14.5-msec increase from baseline (Glassman and Bigger 2001).	0.17 (0.06 to 0.29)
Olanzapine	6.8-msec increase from baseline (Glassman and Bigger 2001).	0.22 (0.11 to 0.31)
Risperidone	11.6-msec increase from baseline (Glassman and Bigger 2001).	0.25 (0.15 to 0.36)
Asenapine	2- to 5-msec increase from baseline as compared with placebo; no observations of QTc ≥500 msec (manufacturer's product information).	0.30 (−0.04 to 0.65)
Iloperidone	~9-msec QTc prolongation at 12 mg twice daily; ~19 msec if coadministered with CYP2D6 or CYP 3A4 inhibitors (manufacturer's product information).	0.34 (0.22 to 0.46)
Ziprasidone	20.3-msec increase from baseline (Glassman and Bigger 2001).	0.41 (0.31 to 0.51)

TABLE 7–2. QTc prolongation with FGAs and SGAs (in order of increasing concern by duration) *(continued)*

Agent	Findings in FDA registration trials	Likelihood > placebo (OR, 95% CI)[a]
Thioridazine	35.8-msec increase from baseline (Glassman and Bigger 2001).	Not reported
Pimavanserin	~5- to 8-msec increase from baseline (34 mg/day); sporadic observations of QTc (Fridericia-corrected) > 500 msec and increases > 60 msec from baseline, but no reports of TdP (manufacturer's product information)	Not reported

Note. CI=confidence interval; FDA=U.S. Food and Drug Administration; FGA=first-generation antipsychotic; msec=milliseconds; OR=odds ratio; SGA = second-generation antipsychotic; TdP=torsades de pointes.
[a]ORs and 95% CIs based on meta-analysis findings reported by Leucht et al. 2013.
[b]High doses of haloperidol or intravenous haloperidol may carry a greater risk for QTc prolongation than oral or intramuscular haloperidol.

TABLE 7–3.   Factors associated with QTc prolongation

Advanced age

Alcohol

Antifungal agents (e.g., ketoconazole, fluconazole)

Certain antihistamines (astemizole and terfenadine only[a])

Certain antibiotics (including azithromycin, ciprofloxacin, clarithromycin, erythromycin, gemifloxacin, levofloxacin, moxifloxacin, norfloxacin, ofloxacin, rufloxacin) and antimalarials (e.g., chloroquine, mefloquine, halofantrine)

Certain antiemetics (e.g., ondansetron, prochlorperazine)

Certain antifungal agents (e.g., ketoconazole)

Certain antineoplastics (e.g., anthracyclines, 5-fluorouracil, alkylating agents)

Certain SSRIs at high doses (e.g., citalopram and escitalopram), possibly fluoxetine

Class I antiarrhythmics (e.g., quinidine, disopyramide, procainamide) and Class II antiarrhythmics (e.g., amiodarone, sotalol, dofetilide)

Congenital QT prolongation syndrome (arising in ~1/5,000 live births)

Congestive heart failure

Cyclobenzaprine

Female sex

Hepatic dysfunction

Hypokalemia

Hypomagnesemia

Hypothyroidism

Left ventricular dysfunction or ventricular arrhythmias

Methadone

Solifenacin

Tetrabenazine

Thyroid abnormalities

TCAs, maprotiline, trazodone

Valbenazine

Vardenafil

Note.   SSRI=selective serotonin reuptake inhibitor; TCA=tricyclic antidepressant.
[a]Both agents have been withdrawn from the U.S. market; noted for historical purposes.

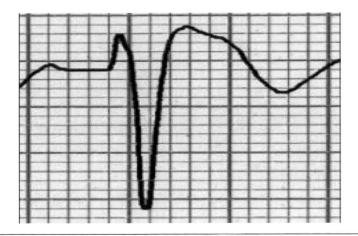

FIGURE 7–1. Brugada pattern on electrocardiogram.

Sudden cardiac death due to an arrhythmia is a particular concern in a number of clinical contexts. All antipsychotics, both FGAs and SGAs, may carry an increased (approximately twofold), dose-related risk for sudden cardiac death due to presumptive ventricular arrhythmias (Ray et al. 2009). Additionally, anticonvulsant drugs that block sodium channels (e.g., carbamazepine, gabapentin) have been linked with an approximately three- to sixfold increased risk for sudden cardiac death in epilepsy patients (Bardai et al. 2015). During treatment with antipsychotics, Glassman and Bigger (2001) identified 10–15 events per 10,000 patient years, also noting an approximate twofold increased risk for sudden death during antipsychotic therapy as compared to the general population. In addition, case reports exist of sudden death among children <age 14 after exposure to TCAs, particularly desipramine, often in the absence of a preexisting history of cardiac arrhythmia. Although TCAs are currently seldom used in children, appropriate precautions before their initiation in pediatric populations should involve a baseline ECG and identification of any underlying heart disease.

Antipsychotics

For many decades, antipsychotics have been known to have the potential for prolonging the time for ventricular repolarization (i.e., the QT interval on an ECG, corrected for heart rate [QTc*]), with an associated potential for causing TdP.

When Pfizer sought its indications for ziprasidone from the FDA, a comparative study was conducted to evaluate QTc prolongation with ziprasidone relative to several other conventional antipsychotics or SGAs, in the presence or absence of CYP inhibitors (see Glassman and Bigger 2001). Importantly, this is the sole study that provides direct comparative data across several antipsychotics (ziprasidone, risperidone, olanzapine, quetiapine, thioridazine [■], and haloperidol) under controlled conditions. Phenothiazines (including thioridazine [■] and mesoridazine [■]) are often considered to pose the greatest risk among antipsychotics for QTc prolongation. Antipsychotic-associated QTc prolongation may in general be a dose-related phenomenon (Reilly et al. 2000).

Table 7–3 provides a summary of information from both that Pfizer-sponsored study and from available FDA registration trial data of QTc effects with FGAs and SGAs, although absolute differences cannot easily be construed about relative QTc effects across agents due to between-subject differences in baseline risk factors for QTc duration. One must also consider that the paucity of head-to-head comparisons among antipsychotics makes it difficult to draw robust inferences about the "relative" safety of one agent over another with respect to the risk for repolarization abnormalities (although a meta-analysis of seven SGAs in schizophrenia concluded that aripiprazole appears to have the lowest overall risk for QTc prolongation [Chung and Chua 2011]).

The relationship between QTc prolongation and TdP is complex, impacted by multiple factors, and often patient-specific and context-dependent. For example, the clinical significance of a medication-associated QTc increase by 10 msec is likely different if a baseline QTc rises from 490 to 500 msec than from 380 to 390, or in a patient whose baseline QTc is in the higher versus lower range of normal. Importantly, the biological "propensity" of any single individual for QT prolongation and TdP is a key moderator of overall cardiac risk when deciding on the safety versus benefits of a medication that has the potential to prolong the QT interval. This point is illustrated by the example of database reports linking short-term use of azithromycin with sudden cardiac death, prompting an FDA warning about its use in patients with pre-existing or concomitant risk factors for QT prolongation (e.g., those described in Table 7-3) (https://www.fda.gov/drugs/drugsafety/ucm341822.htm).

The aforementioned Pfizer comparative study of antipsychotic effects on QTc intervals identified marked QTc prolongation with thioridazine, prompting imposition of a boxed warning (■) with thioridazine (see Table 1–6 in Chapter 1, "The Psychiatrist as Physician") and a physician notification letter warning of the risk for QTc prolongation and TdP. Mesoridazine received a similar boxed warning (■) shortly thereafter. The FDA traditionally categorizes increasing degrees of clinically meaningful risk associated with QTc prolongation from baseline as follows: ≤5 msec as "probably no concern," 6–10 msec as "increasing concern,"

11–20 msec as "uncertain concern," and >20 msec as "definite concern" (see also U.S. Food and Drug Administration 2005).

Generally, in patients with elevated QTc (i.e., ≥450 msec in men and ≥470 msec in women) and psychotic features, it is advisable to minimize or avoid exposure to all antipsychotics unless the perceived benefit outweighs the potential risk. In such patients, cautious observation with serial ECG monitoring may be warranted, as well as the elimination or correction of other potential causes of QTc prolongation (see Table 7–3). QTc intervals ≥500 msec pose a substantial hazard for developing potentially fatal ventricular arrhythmias (notably, TdP) and generally signal the need to eliminate antipsychotic drugs. In some instances, however, the clinical necessity of antipsychotic medication for patients with significant baseline QTc prolongation may warrant recommendations for cardiovascular implantable electronic devices such as permanent pacemakers, implantable cardioverter defibrillators, and cardiac resynchronization therapy devices (for further discussion of the psychiatrist's role in collaborative decision making alongside cardiologists in psychiatric patients at risk for TdP, see Brojmohun et al. 2013).

From a practical standpoint, it is often useful to compare current ECGs to prior ECGs in order to determine whether suspected abnormalities represent interval changes. New findings may warrant drug cessation or consultation with a cardiologist, whereas stable features may pose lesser concern for iatrogenic risks. Clinicians also should be mindful of cumulative risk factors for arrhythmias in a given patient, such as electrolyte abnormalities, hypothyroidism, advanced age, effects of alcohol, and the synergistic arrhythmogenic potential of concomitant drugs (e.g., fluoroquinolone antibiotics, anticholinergics, and other drugs noted in Table 7–3).

Some authors recommend that because of the potential for sudden cardiac death with all antipsychotics, clinicians should determine, before initiating an antipsychotic, whether a patient has had syncope, has relatives with known congenital QT prolongation syndrome, or has relatives who experienced sudden death at an early age, and should obtain a baseline ECG in older adults or those with a history of known cardiac disease (Glassman and Bigger 2001). The American Heart Association (AHA) also advises obtaining a baseline ECG (mainly to assure the absence of QT prolongation) before beginning a TCA or phenothiazine in children or adolescents (Gutgesell et al. 1999), with repeat assessment after steady-state dosing is achieved. Adult women generally may have a greater risk than men for developing TdP from medications that prolong QTc.

A summary of recommendations to aid decision making about antipsychotic use in the context of QTc prolongation is provided in Table 7–4.

TABLE 7–4.   Recommendations for the practitioner regarding the use of antipsychotics in patients with cardiac disease and/or risk factors for QTc prolongation

- Measure baseline QTc; serial QTc monitoring as clinically appropriate (e.g., after dosage increases or addition of other medications that can prolong QTc or inhibit CYP450 2D6).

- Avoid low-potency FGAs , IV haloperidol, ziprasidone, and possibly iloperidone.

- Favor atypical antipsychotics with low risk for QTc prolongation (e.g., aripiprazole, lurasidone).

- For IV haloperidol in hospital settings: obtain baseline and at least daily QTc, Mg^+, K^+, and PO_4^-, and continuous ECG monitoring for those with baseline QTc > 500 msec, significant risk factors, or high-dose requirements (e.g., total dose > 2 mg/day).

- If QTc increases to > 500 msec during treatment: check and replete K^+, Mg^+, PO_4^-; review overall medication regimen to identify other agents that may increase QTc; consider holding antipsychotic until QTc falls < 500 msec; consider alternative agents (e.g., nonantipsychotic drugs for agitation, such as divalproex or benzodiazepines).

Note. ECG = electrocardiographic; FGA = first-generation antipsychotic; IV = intravenous.

Antidepressants

TCAs may be arrhythmogenic by virtue of their anticholinergic and quinidine-like effects. Orthostatic hypotension may result from α_1-adrenergic blockade with tertiary amine TCAs (e.g., amitriptyline, imipramine). SSRIs generally lack effects on cardiac conduction with the apparent exception of citalopram and its enantiomer escitalopram; in August 2011, the FDA issued an alert that dosages of citalopram > 40 mg/day may prolong QT intervals and advised against the use of citalopram in patients with congenital long QT syndrome or other conditions associated with risk of QT prolongation, if possible. The maximum recommended dose of citalopram was changed to 20 mg/day for patients older than 60 years. Specifically, the FDA noted dose-related QTc increases with citalopram of 8.5, 12.6, and 18.5 msec at respective doses of 20, 30, and 40 mg/day, while escitalopram-related QTc increases were 4.5, 6.6, and 10.7 msec at respective doses of 10, 20, and 30 mg/day (http://www.fda.gov/Drugs/DrugSafety/ucm297391.htm). Accordingly, caution is recommended when using citalopram and possibly escitalopram in patients with other risk factors for QT prolongation (see Table 7–3). Citalopram also has been associated with significantly greater QT prolongation in overdoses as compared with changes seen in fluoxetine, fluvoxamine, paroxetine, or sertraline (Isbister et al. 2004). It is advisable to obtain a baseline ECG in patients taking ≥40 mg/day of citalopram and in those with risk factors for prolonged QTc.

In 2013, the FDA revised the package insert language for fluoxetine, stating that it should be used with caution in patients with congenital long QT syndrome, a previous history of QT prolongation, a family history of long QT syndrome or sudden cardiac death, and other conditions that predispose to QT prolongation, including CYP450 2D6 inhibitors or PM genotypes.

MAOIs lack anticholinergic adverse effects but may cause orthostatic hypotension, bradycardia, and shortened PR and QTc intervals on ECG (McGrath et al. 1987).

Stimulants

Psychostimulants, as well as atomoxetine, can mildly raise heart rate and blood pressure, but there is no compelling evidence that they in-crease QTc. There are rare reports in the literature of PVCs or ventricular or supraventricular tachycardias, as well as ST elevation and MI in overdose. Controversy remains about the necessity of routine ECG screening before the initiation of stimulant therapy (e.g., for attention-deficit/hyperactivity disorder). Stimulants can slightly raise heart rate and blood pressure, but the risk for sudden cardiac death from stimulants appears to be no higher than the background rate seen in the general population. Nonetheless, an AHA Scientific Statement suggests that in children and adolescents, it is "reasonable" to obtain a prestimulant ECG to identify underlying risk factors for sudden cardiac death, such as hypertrophic cardiomyopathies, long QT syndrome, and preexcitation or reentrant arrhythmias such as Wolff-Parkinson-White syndrome (Vetter et al. 2008). No similar AHA recommendation exists regarding baseline ECG screening in adults. More important than whether or not one obtains an ECG is the process by which a clinician evaluates cardiovascular risk before starting any sympathomimetic agent. An appropriate history would include assessment of the following:

- A history of fainting or dizziness
- Chest pain or shortness of breath on exertion
- Palpitations

- Hypertension
- History of heart murmur or known arrhythmia
- Current medications
- Family history of unexplained or sudden death before age 35
- Family history of cardiac arrhythmias

Decisions to obtain a baseline ECG or consultation with a cardiologist before stimulant initiation in adults are usually best determined in case-by-case fashion depending on an individual's history and suspected cardiac risk factors.

Other Cardiac Disturbances

Cardiomyopathies have been reported to occur during treatment with clozapine and risperidone. Myocarditis may occur with clozapine (■), and pericarditis is a rare adverse effect of gabapentin.

Cerebrovascular Accidents

General Recommendations

Elderly patients with underlying cerebrovascular or cardiovascular disease may be at greater risk for cerebrovascular events from use of SGAs, although causal links remain controversial. Clinicians should recognize the presence of baseline vascular disease when formulating risk-benefit treatment decisions.

Four controlled treatment studies of risperidone for dementia-related psychosis from 1999 to 2003 identified a significantly increased risk for transient ischemic attacks or cerebrovascular accidents with risperidone (4%) compared with placebo (2%) (Wooltorton 2002), prompting a subsequent FDA public health advisory linking the use of SGAs with an increased risk for cerebrovascular accidents. Subsequent case-control studies that failed to replicate these observations have pointed to possible confounding factors, such as vascular dementia, hypertension, and other noniatrogenic risk factors for transient ischemic attacks or cerebrovascular accidents that may have been overrepresented among antipsychotic recipients. At the same time, because SGAs demonstrate low efficacy but high dropout rates in dementia-related psychosis, enthusiasm for their use is modest. The absence of highly effective remedies for dementia-related psychosis requires thoughtful risk-benefit analyses when considering treatments, in addition to close monitoring for adverse neurological or cardiovascular changes.

Edema

General Recommendations

Clinicians should be aware of psychotropic drugs that may be associated with peripheral edema and assure the absence of other etiologies (i.e., cardiogenic factors, hepatic dysfunction, lymphatic obstruction, nephrotic syndrome, hypothyroidism) by history taking, physical examination, and appropriate laboratory measures (i.e., thyroid-stimulating hormone, serum protein, liver enzymes, urinalysis). After determining the absence of other noniatrogenic causes, diuresis may be advisable as an initial step in management.

Peripheral edema has a wide differential diagnosis that can include many drug-induced etiologies. It may result from a number of drug classes, including vasodilators (e.g., β-blockers and α_1-adrenergic receptor antagonists), calcium channel blockers, NSAIDs, estrogen-containing compounds, and thiazolidinediones. The mechanisms by which some psychotropic agents may cause peripheral edema are not well understood, although it is thought that extravasation from capillary beds in the lower extremities may result from vasodilation caused by α_1-blocking drugs, such as antipsychotics. Edema caused by some GABAergic anticonvulsants (e.g., divalproex, gabapentin, tiagabine) has been hypothesized to result from direct GABAergic effects on peripheral vascular resistance.

Case reports of lithium-associated peripheral edema date to the early 1970s and are thought to reflect redistribution of sodium from the intracellular to the extracellular compartment (water follows sodium) or alterations in renal tubular absorption of sodium. The phenomenon does not appear related to serum lithium levels or dosing toxicity and may variably resolve either spontaneously, via dosage reductions, or through coadministration of a potassium-sparing diuretic such as amiloride at a dosage of 5 mg bid.

Manufacturers' package insert information identifies peripheral edema as an uncommon side effect associated with olanzapine (3%) and divalproex (1%–5%), in the latter often arising during long-term therapy. In FDA registration trials of pimavanserin for psychosis associated with Parkinson's disease, peripheral edema was more common with active drug (7%) than with placebo (2%). Edema has also been reported in postmarketing studies during treatment with quetiapine, ziprasidone, risperidone, gabapentin, escitalopram, trazodone, and mirtazapine. Case reports also have described peripheral edema arising during cotherapy with divalproex plus risperidone or divalproex plus quetiapine.

The evaluation of peripheral edema involves the following considerations, which can greatly facilitate communication exchange and collaboration with primary care physicians when appropriate.

- *Is the edema unilateral or bilateral?* Unilateral edema in a lower extremity suggests an etiology that is less likely pharmacological than structural-anatomical (e.g., deep venous thrombosis, pelvic malignancies, lymphedema) or infectious (e.g., cellulitis).
- *Is there a suggestion of cardiopulmonary (rather than medication-induced) origin?* Edema caused by congestive heart failure or pulmonary hypertension will typically present with physical examination findings involving the lungs (e.g., wheezing or rales), heart (e.g., presence of an S_3 gallop), head and neck (e.g., jugular venous distension), or abdomen (e.g., hepatomegaly in right-sided heart failure). The presence of jugular venous distension suggests either a cardiac or pulmonary origin or the possibility of acute renal failure.
- *Is the onset acute or chronic?* Edema caused by medications typically has a relatively acute onset in close proximity to the initiation of a suspected causal medication. By contrast, chronic lower-extremity edema in adults over age 50 is most often caused by venous insufficiency.
- *Are electrolyte abnormalities present?* Hyponatremia may lead to peripheral edema due to fluid overload (e.g., water intoxication from polydipsia).
- *Is an eating disorder present?* Rebound fluid retention can occur from alternating patterns of dehydration, vomiting, and laxative or diuretic abuse.
- *Are serum protein and albumin normal?* Peripheral edema that is likely related to medications typically involves normal serum protein levels. Other medical etiologies of peripheral edema with normal serum protein levels include severe hypothyroidism, lymphedema, and angioedema (see the section "Allergic Reactions and Angioedema" in Chapter 20, "Systemic Reactions"). The presence of low serum protein and albumin raises the suspicion of hepatic or renal disease or of severe malnutrition.
- *Is proteinuria present?* Low serum protein or albumin levels with proteinuria point to nephrotic syndrome.
- *Are liver enzymes normal?* In the absence of proteinuria, abnormal liver enzymes suggest primary hepatic disease (e.g., cirrhosis).

Table 7–5 summarizes key points for psychiatrists in the assessment and management of peripheral edema.

TABLE 7–5. Key points in the management of drug-induced peripheral edema

- Determine the timing, onset, location, and extent of edema. Clarify if patient has a history of trauma, surgery, or predisposing medical conditions (e.g., past malignancy or liver disease) that may indicate etiologies other than drug-induced edema.

- By physical examination, determine location of edema (lower extremities [ankle or pretibial], upper extremities, sacral regions when recumbent), bilaterality, and degree of pitting. The presence of ulcerations or warmth may suggest cellulitis. Determine normal bilateral pedal and popliteal pulses. Palpable calf cords or tenderness, calf warmth, or pain on dorsiflexion may suggest deep venous thrombosis. Affirm normal cardiac and breath sounds by auscultation, and the absence of jugular venous distension. Physical examination may also help to assure the absence of ascites or hepatomegaly.

- Ensure that serum protein, liver enzymes, and electrolytes are normal; determine the absence of proteinuria (by urinalysis).

- Consider diuresing normokalemic and normonatremic patients with a brief (e.g., 5-day) course of furosemide or spironolactone.

- Track progress of diuresis by measuring baseline and daily weights.

- Obtain primary medical consultation if edema persists or if drug discontinuation and diuresis fail to resolve the problem, or when indicated when laboratory abnormalities or physical examination findings suggest a noniatrogenic underlying process.

If the absence of other medical etiologies has been established, the clinician can treat drug-induced edema—often a benign phenomenon—either conservatively (i.e., by leg elevation or compression stockings) or with the short-term use of a diuretic. Pitting pretibial edema caused by antipsychotics or anticonvulsants may respond to a brief (e.g., 3- to 5-day) course of furosemide 10–40 mg/day or spironolactone 50–100 mg/day [maximum 100 mg qid]). Generally, monitoring serum potassium levels is unnecessary in a normokalemic individual who begins a short course of furosemide, although this may be warranted during longer-term therapy. Thiazide diuretics, such as hydrochlorothiazide 25 mg/day, also may be used but tend to produce a less robust diuresis than does furosemide.

In the case of lithium-associated peripheral edema, the potassium-sparing diuretic amiloride (e.g., 5 mg bid) is preferred to diuretics that act on the distal convoluted tubule, such as hydrochlorothiazide, because amiloride is less likely to raise serum lithium levels. Loop-acting diuretics (e.g., furosemide) also have not been shown to increase serum lithium levels (Jefferson and Kalin 1979). If electing to diurese peripheral edema with a thiazide diuretic, the clinician might choose to reduce a standing lithium dosage or to monitor serum lithium levels more closely depending on the existing lithium dosage and the duration of diuretic therapy.

Referral to a primary care doctor should occur when causes other than drug-induced edema are suspected, laboratory abnormalities or physical examination findings suggest causes other than drug-induced bilateral edema, or edema persists despite diuresis.

The clinician should keep in mind that cessation of a likely causal agent typically leads to resolution of drug-induced edema, and the decision to discontinue a presumed offending agent (rather than manage the side effect of edema) depends on the persistence of the problem, recurrence after response to acute treatment of the edema, and availability of viable alternative primary psychotropic compounds.

Hypertension

General Recommendations

Patients who receive psychotropic drugs that can alter blood pressure should have their blood pressure monitored on a regular basis by the prescriber. Sympathomimetic (e.g., noradrenergic) agents reported to cause hypertension should not be administered in patients with unstable hypertension. Present recommendations are *not* to use sublingual or oral nifedipine for probable drug-induced hypertensive crises, but rather to obtain blood pressure measurements for suspected hypertension-induced signs (e.g., headache) and to seek medical attention as appropriate.

Catecholaminergic agents, including psychostimulants and noradrenergic agents (e.g., SNRIs, TCAs, atomoxetine, and bupropion), carry the risk of raising blood pressure and increasing heart rate via their sympathomimetic effects. In premarketing studies of venlafaxine XR (across dosages from 75 to 375 mg/day), sustained hypertension (defined as a diastolic blood pressure >90 mm Hg and ≥10 mm Hg above baseline, on three consecutive occasions) occurred in 3% of patients with major depression, with incidence rates of <1% in patients with anxiety disorders (i.e., panic disorder, generalized anxiety disorder, or social anxiety disorder). Incidence rates of sustained diastolic hypertension rose proportionally with increasing dosages, reaching 13% at dosages >300 mg/day. Among patients treated with venlafaxine XR across diagnoses in FDA registration trials, 1% of patients had a ≥20 mm Hg rise in systolic blood pressure (manufacturer's package insert, Wyeth Pharmaceuticals). The manufacturer of venlafaxine advises against initiating therapy in patients with poorly controlled preexisting hypertension, and either decreasing the dosage or discontinuing therapy in patients with new-onset hypertension arising during treatment with venlafaxine.

Rates of sustained diastolic hypertension with desvenlafaxine (0.7%–1.3%) or venlafaxine XR (0.5%–3%) are lower than the dose-related rates seen with venlafaxine IR (3%–13%). The SNRI duloxetine was associated with trivial changes in diastolic blood pressure (<1 mm Hg) across its indications at dosages ≤120 mg/day. The time course for developing hypertension that is likely attributable to an SNRI has not been identified from clinical trials, but hypertension may be dose dependent and more likely to arise sooner rather than later after treatment initiation. In normotensive patients who are stably dosed on an SNRI but who later develop elevated blood pressure, investigation and treatment of other causes of hypertension may be warranted before it is advisable or necessary to discontinue a long-standing SNRI.

As reported in manufacturers' prescribing information, the incidence of hypertension with bupropion is <1%, which is no different from the incidence with placebo. In FDA registration trials, hypertension occurred in only 1% of subjects taking mirtazapine, despite its noradrenergic properties, and hypertension occurred less frequently than in subjects taking TCAs (Watanabe et al. 2010).

Hypertensive crises are of well-known concern during pharmacotherapy with MAOIs. The calcium channel blocker nifedipine, and the nonselective α-adrenergic antagonist phentolamine, are traditionally the antihypertensive agents used in monitored settings to manage MAOI-associated hypertension. A contentious literature has emerged on the pros and cons of instructing MAOI recipients to carry 10-mg nifedipine capsules to swallow, bite and swallow, or place sublingually in the event of developing a headache that could be a manifestation of a hypertensive crisis. A 1996 review challenged the safety and efficacy of this practice, citing an increased risk for adverse cardiovascular or cerebrovascular consequences — with little evidence of benefit — from the practice of routinely instructing patients to take nifedipine capsules outside of a monitored setting if headaches occur during MAOI therapy (Grossman et al. 1996). Beta-blockers, with the exception of labetolol (which also blocks α-adrenergic receptors), are generally not advisable for treating MAOI-associated hypertensive crises because their blockade of β_2-adrenergic receptors allows unopposed α_1-adrenergic vasoconstriction, potentially making hypertension worse.

Another issue regarding cardiovascular safety with MAOIs involves the question about the necessity of discontinuing their use before surgery (or electroconvulsive therapy) in which general anesthesia is used. The manufacturers of tranylcypromine, phenelzine, isocarboxazid, and transdermal selegiline caution against the use of MAOIs during surgery that involves general anesthesia and recommend discontinuing an MAOI at least 10 days before undergoing elective surgery with general anesthesia. However, contemporary studies report no differences in blood pressure and heart rate attributable to the continued use of MAOIs during surgery involving general anesthesia, and most experts believe that discontinuing MAOIs preoperatively is not routinely necessary (El-Ganzouri et al. 1985). Nevertheless, cardiovascular safety may be jeopardized by the use of injectable sympathomimetic vasoconstrictors such as epinephrine during surgical procedures in patients taking MAOIs.

Finally, intravenous administration of ketamine exerts a CNS sympathomimetic effect and has been reported to increase systolic blood pressure by about 10–20 mm Hg transiently (up to 4 hours) in about one-third of patients during infusions for treatment of major depression.

Myocarditis and Cardiomyopathy

General Recommendations

Clinicians should recognize that myocarditis is a rare adverse effect with clozapine and should be alert to its presenting signs (e.g., fever, chest pain, shortness of breath), particularly during the first 1–2 months after treatment initiation. ECG and measurement of serum troponin or creatine kinase-MB and CRP should be obtained, along with consultation from a cardiologist in the setting of laboratory abnormalities. Clozapine should be discontinued and not reintroduced when myocarditis occurs.

Clozapine carries a known, rare risk for myocarditis (■), which arises through poorly understood mechanisms that may include clozapine-induced release of inflammatory cytokines, hypercatecholaminemia, and type I IgE–mediated acute hypersensitivity reactions (Merrill et al. 2006). Rapid clozapine titration also has been a factor implicated in case reports of myocarditis. Eosinophilia appears not to be a useful parameter in diagnosing clozapine-induced myocarditis, although elevated CRP (>100 mg/dL) has been reported even when troponin levels are normal. The majority of cases become manifest within the first 4–8 weeks of treatment initiation, and patients can present with a variety of signs and symptoms, including fever, chest pain, shortness of breath, tachycardia, and leukocytosis. Importantly, 20% of individuals may develop a benign and transient fever during clozapine initiation, making it important for clinicians to pay close attention to other systemic features that could signal the presence of myocarditis, NMS, or other correlates of fever during clozapine therapy — particularly given the rarity of myocarditis (with a reported incidence of 0.015%–0.188%) (Merrill et al. 2006). In their systematic review of the phenomenon, Merrill et al. (2006) advised that for clozapine recipients who develop chest pain, fever, dyspnea, or flulike symptoms, clinicians should consider obtaining an ECG (observing for T-wave changes or ST segment elevation) and serum troponin or creatine kinase-MB. Consultation with a cardiologist is advisable in the presence of abnormal parameters.

Management of clozapine-induced myocarditis hinges on discontinuation of clozapine, as well as the possible use of β-blockers (e.g., metoprolol), ACE inhibitors, and diuretics; the role of corticosteroids appears more controversial (Merrill et al. 2006). Also rarely, clozapine use has been associated with development of pericarditis, dilated cardiomyopathy, or congestive heart failure — the last-mentioned manifested by exertional dyspnea, orthopnea, dizziness, and fatigue; management involves drug cessation and serial echocardiographic monitoring.

Rechallenge with clozapine after resolution of myocarditis is highly controversial. Most authorities discourage even its contemplation, and there exist only a handful of case reports in the literature describing successful rechallenge. Manu and colleagues (2012) identified only four such cases, three of which involved successful rechallenge (ranging from 2–104 weeks after initial clozapine discontinuation) with serial troponins (e.g., three times per week) and frequent ECGs. Those authors concluded that insufficient safety data exist to justify reexposure to clozapine after myocarditis.

Case reports also have described myocarditis occurring during treatment with quetiapine, potentially as a drug hypersensitivity reaction associated with eosinophilia, leukopenia, and thrombocytopenia.

Orthostatic Hypotension

General Recommendations

Clinicians should be aware of drugs that can cause orthostatic hypotension, typically resulting from α_1-adrenergic blockade.

Orthostatic hypotension may not necessarily be dose related and may represent a persistent phenomenon during continued administration of a causal agent. Blood pressure and heart rate should be measured while the patient is sitting and standing, several minutes apart, to evaluate the presence and extent of autonomic changes. Increased oral hydration and salt intake may not reliably counteract pharmacological orthostatic hypotension, but avoiding dehydration may help to diminish exacerbation of the phenomenon. Patients should be advised to get up slowly from sitting or supine positions. Treatment with fludrocortisone, the vasoconstrictor midodrine, or the parasympathomimetic agent pyridostigmine may sometimes be appropriate antihypotensives. Significant orthostatic hypotension, particularly in patients with low resting blood pressure or cardiac disease, may warrant cessation of the causal agent.

Orthostatic hypotension may be associated with a wide range of psychotropic agents that cause vasodilation by blocking peripheral vascular α_1-adrenoreceptors. These agents include TCAs, MAOIs (e.g., tranylcypromine at dosages >30 mg/day), mirtazapine, atomoxetine, duloxetine, venlafaxine, desvenlafaxine, and SGAs, as well as cannabinoids. Antihypertensive α_1-blocking drugs such as prazosin (used sometimes to counteract nightmares; see the section "Nightmares and Vivid Dreams" in Chapter 19, "Sleep Disturbances") and terazosin (used sometimes to counteract hyperhidrosis; see the section "Hyperhidrosis" in Chapter 8, "Dermatological System") may cause orthostatic hypotension and syncope, particularly after a first dose. Patients who report dizziness upon standing or sitting after rising from a supine position should be examined for postural hypotension and tachycardia. Clinicians should consider other nonpharmacological etiologies when relevant, such as dehydration, prolonged bed rest, dysautonomias, anemia, and Parkinson's disease. The use of nonpsychotropic vasodilators or diuretics also may play contributing roles. The differential diagnosis of orthostatic hypotension also includes vasovagal syncope, as might occur when sudden-onset light-headedness includes visual, auditory, and other sensory abnormalities. Conservative management of pharmacologically induced orthostatic hypotension involves counseling patients to rise slowly from seated or supine positions, avoid dehydration, and assure the safe use of any concomitant drugs that may further cause anticholinergic, vasodilatory, arrhythmogenic, or extrapyramidal adverse effects.

Occasionally, orthostatic hypotension warrants pharmacological treatment. Use of antihypotensive drugs generally has been confined to the treatment of dysautonomias or cardiovascular dysregulation in critical care settings, and none has formally been studied to counteract iatrogenic orthostatic hypotension. The α_1 agonist midodrine (dosed typically at 5 mg three times daily, $t_{1/2}$=~3–4 hours) is a generally safe and well-tolerated vasopressor in people without significant heart or kidney disease, posing few side effects of its own (headache, flushing, dry mouth). Fludrocortisone, a synthetic mineralocorticoid and plasma volume expander, is dosed initially at 0.1–0.2 mg/day (with a usual maximum of 0.4–0.6 mg/day); patients must be monitored for hypokalemia and supine hypertension (the latter especially when fludrocortisone is added to midodrine). Finally, the cholinesterase inhibitor pyridostigmine (dosed initially as 30 mg twice daily and increased to a maximum of 60 mg three times daily [or as a 180 mg/day slow-release tablet]) yields a modest pressor effect by enhancing ganglionic neuro-transmission through the baroreflex pathway; its effect can be safely amplified by combining it with low-dose (e.g., 5 mg/day) midodrine.

8

Dermatological System

Alopecia

General Recommendations

Mineral supplements (e.g., zinc and selenium), oral biotin, or topical minoxidil may be worth attempting for the treatment of alopecia, but scalp hair loss attributable to psychotropic medications may be difficult if not impossible to counteract except through cessation of the suspected causal agent.

Diffuse scalp hair loss (*telogen effluvium*) has been reported in conjunction with several psychotropic medications, perhaps most notably with divalproex (incidence from 12% to 24%), lithium (incidence up to 10%), and carbamazepine (incidence up to 6%) (McKinney et al. 1996), and more rarely with fluoxetine, sertraline, venlafaxine, fluvoxamine, topiramate, amphetamine, methylphenidate, dopamine agonists, perphenazine, TCAs, olanzapine, risperidone, and mirtazapine. Reports also exist of hair loss occurring with one SSRI but not another in the same

The symbol ■ is used in this chapter to indicate that the FDA has issued a boxed warning for a prescription medication that may cause serious adverse effects.

145

patient. A World Health Organization database for international drug monitoring also identified a total of 337 cases of suspected lamotrigine-associated alopecia through April 1, 2009, occurring most often in women age <40 years and often resolving after drug cessation (Tengstrand et al. 2010).

Hair loss has been reported as a relatively rare adverse effect of a number of nonpsychotropic medications, including isotretinoin, allopurinol, androgens (testosterone formulations), anticoagulants, β-blockers, calcium channel blockers, colchicine, efavirenz, ergot alkaloids (migraine prophylaxis), NSAIDs, oral contraceptives, propylthiouracil, and ribavirin. A number of medical causes of alopecia warrant investigation before assuming that hair loss is an adverse effect of a suspected psychotropic agent. These include hypothyroidism, autoimmune diseases such as systemic lupus erythematosus or rheumatoid arthritis, vitiligo, and ulcerative colitis. Chemical damage caused by permanent curls or other caustic cosmetic products may cause hair loss in some individuals. Patchy areas of hair loss or hair loss in nonscalp areas might prompt clinicians to consider the possible presence of trichotillomania. Sudden physical or emotional stresses can be associated with hair loss over a period of weeks to months.

Alopecia from divalproex has been suggested to arise from interference with absorption of dietary zinc and selenium, for which supplementation (25–50 mg/day of zinc and 100–200 μg/day of selenium) is sometimes recommended. Case reports also suggest the possible efficacy of oral biotin 10,000 μg/day. However, in clinical practice, the efficacy of this strategy may not be robust. Cessation of divalproex generally halts the problem. The extended-release formulation of divalproex has been suggested by some to minimize the potential for alopecia (as reflected in a 7% incidence of alopecia during trials of Depakote ER for migraine headache, as compared with 13%–24% with Depakote DR for complex partial seizures), possibly via more distal absorption of the drug with lesser likelihood to interfere with gastrointestinal absorption of dietary minerals. Dosage reductions generally have not been shown to reverse drug-associated alopecia, although comparative studies of high- versus low-dose divalproex for complex partial seizures demonstrated more frequent alopecia among high-dose (24%) than low-dose (13%) recipients. Other clinicians advocate the use of topical minoxidil as a potential remedy; this option is likely safe, although it has not been systematically studied for this purpose.

Hyperhidrosis

General Recommendations

For sweating induced by SSRIs, SNRIs, or TCAs, clonidine 0.1 mg/day or terazosin 1–2 mg/day may be more effective than anticholinergic remedies such as benztropine 1 mg/day. Preliminary data also support the use of oxybutynin 5 mg qd–tid.

Excessive sweating (hyperhidrosis) occurs in up to 20% of individuals who take antidepressants, both as a daytime phenomenon or as night sweats, and may be dose related. It does not appear to dissipate during prolonged treatment but does remit when the causal antidepressant is stopped. Mechanisms thought to account for this phenomenon include dysregulation of cholinergically innervated sweat glands and dysregulation of the hypothalamic thermoregulatory center, mediated by prodopaminergic tone with reciprocal downregulation of serotonergic tone. Consequently, the most frequently employed strategies to counteract antidepressant-induced hyperhidrosis include anticholinergic agents, such as benztropine dosed at 1 mg/day (although its apparent benefit may be transient), and antiadrenergic agents, such as the α_2-adrenergic agonist clonidine (0.1 mg/day) or the α_1-adrenergic antagonist terazosin (1–2 mg/day), with visible efficacy within 3–4 weeks. The likelihood of sedation from either of the latter two agents would favor their use in a single nighttime dose. Other anticholinergic drugs that may be of value to counteract iatrogenic hyperhidrosis include glycopyrrolate 1 mg qd or bid or oxybutynin 5–10 mg qd–tid. Case reports also identify benefit with adjunctive mirtazapine (up to 60 mg/day) or the serotonin-blocking drug cyproheptadine 4 mg qd or bid, without reversing antidepressant efficacy.

Adjunctive aripiprazole 10 mg/day, but not ziprasidone, has been reported to alleviate daytime hyperhidrosis caused by fluoxetine or duloxetine, with a mechanism hypothesized to involve both its serotonin type 2A (5-HT_{2A}) antagonism and its dopaminergic partial agonism as modulating the hypothalamic thermoregulatory center (Lu et al. 2008).

Photosensitivity

General Recommendations

Clinicians should counsel patients about the potential for sun exposure to cause burnlike or hyperpigmentation reactions to antipsychotics (mainly FGAs) and less often to TCAs. Adequate prophylactic use of sunscreen is essential when patients are outdoors during warmer months. Photosensitivity reactions should be treated by use of conservative interventions (e.g., aloe lotions) and avoidance of further sun exposure until the resolution of signs and symptoms.

Phototoxic (i.e., nonimmune-mediated) sunburn-like reactions have long been recognized after sun exposure in patients taking FGAs (particularly chlorpromazine, occurring in up to 25% of patients, typically with dosages ≥400 mg/day) (Harth and Rapoport 1996). Case reports of phototoxic reactions also exist with some SGAs, including risperidone and clozapine. Photosensitivity-induced hyperpigmentation has been described as a relatively rare phenomenon in patients taking TCAs.

Adequate prevention of phototoxic reactions involves counseling patients who take antipsychotic medications to minimize sun exposure and make use of full skin protection from ultraviolet A and B (UVA, UVB) wavelengths. Typical treatment for photosensitivity reactions should include avoidance of further sun exposure and application of cool, wet dressings and emollient (e.g., aloe-based) lotions. Topical corticosteroids, NSAIDs, and oral antipruritic (e.g., antihistamine) agents are also sometimes helpful. Oral corticosteroids are more rarely indicated in the setting of more severe or persistent phototoxic reactions that do not remit with more conservative management.

Pruritus

General Recommendations

Evaluation of acute pruritus should include a general medical assessment with awareness of the most common dermatological and systemic conditions other than drug rashes that may be causal.

Generalized pruritus in the absence of a visible skin rash can occur with a variety of psychotropic agents, although the differential diagnosis of pruritus with respect to underlying medical etiologies is considerable. The sheer presence or absence of pruritus conveys little information about the nature of a suspected drug rash, other than that certain distinct types of rashes are usually pruritic (notably, atopic or allergic contact dermatitis, psoriasis, and seborrheic dermatitis); whether or not a rash is pruritic does not help to determine if it is likely drug related. Pruritic drug reactions may be allergic and usually are morbilliform or urticarial (see definitions in Table 8–1).

TABLE 8–1. Descriptive terminology in assessing skin rashes

Term	Description
Blanching	Transient white discoloration of a skin lesion that occurs with pressure
Bullous	Fluid-filled blisters greater than 5 mm in diameter
Confluent	Lesions that intermingle, often with ill-defined borders
Exanthematous (synonymous with *maculopapular*)	Meaning "eruptive"; skin eruptions or rashes
Exfoliative (also *desquamative*)	Peeling or shedding of skin in flakes or scales
Lichenified	Skin that has become thickened and leatherlike
Maculopapular (synonymous with *exanthematous*)	*Macular:* flat and circumscribed (typically <1 cm in diameter); *papular:* solid and elevated above the surrounding skin
Morbilliform	Rash that is measles-like in appearance
Pruritic	Itchy rash
Pustular	Visible collections of pus
Raised	Rash that rises above skin level
Red	Rash that indicates an inflammatory process
Ulcerative	Inflamed areas with loss of surrounding tissue, often surrounded by red, swollen, and tender skin
Urticarial	A wheal-and-flare reaction, often allergic in origin (hives), involving red, raised, pruritic, bumpy skin lesions
Weepy	Lesions that exude a liquid, often in very small droplets

The evaluation of patients who complain of itching should include assessment for the presence of skin lesions, which potentially could be self-inflicted from scratching or skin picking. Psychiatrists, in particular, should be alert to phenomena such as delusional parasitosis or somatoform pain disorders that involve complaints about unusual skin sensations. Skin picking that can cause excoriated lesions (dermatillomania) is less likely to be iatrogenic than to be a manifestation of underlying conditions such as impulse control disorders, body dysmorphic disorder, and obsessive-compulsive or other anxiety disorders.

Drugs known to cause pruritus include opiates, aspirin, NSAIDs, and drugs that may cause hepatotoxicity. Clinicians should consider whether an allergic, pruritic contact dermatitis is caused by environmental exposure (e.g., to cosmetics, detergents, rosins, epoxy resins). Psychotropic drugs (other than opiates or synthetic opiates such as tramadol) rarely cause pruritus apart from idiosyncratic hypersensitivity reactions. In fact, some SSRIs have been reported to improve pruritus associated with lymphoma, uremia, cholestasis, and opiate use. Similarly, some antipsychotics with antihistamine effects (notably, promethazine begun at a dosage of 25 mg/day) are often referred to as antiallergic neuroleptics for the treatment of pruritus.

Nonsedating antihistamines such as loratadine or cetirizine are generally safe interventions for nonspecific pruritus. Sedating antihistamines such as hydroxyzine (25–100 mg at bedtime) or doxepin (10–25 mg at bedtime) may be especially useful not only to counteract the degranulation of mast cells in suspected allergic reactions but also for their anxiolytic properties. Pruritus also may be managed with the use of hypoallergenic, nonalcohol-based skin lubricants; menthol-camphor-based topical agents (e.g., Sarna lotion); or Aveeno oatmeal bath treatments.

Skin Rashes

General Recommendations

Any drug can cause a skin rash, either from an allergic or a hypersensitivity reaction. Rashes should be evaluated to determine their location, appearance, and probable association with a suspected causal agent. Drugs suspected of causing a serious drug rash should be immediately discontinued, and appropriate dermatological evaluation should be obtained.

General Evaluation

Psychiatrists may feel ill equipped to evaluate potential medication-related skin rashes and to incorporate into their practice a working knowledge of the nature and characteristics of common skin rashes caused by psychotropic drugs. Although seeking formal consultation from a dermatologist for certain types of rashes is often helpful, psychiatrists can and should be familiar with the language used to describe the appearance of skin rashes, perform an initial assessment, and form an impression about likely associations with prescribed psychotropic medications on the basis of time course and appearance.

Upon discovering a skin rash, practitioners should obtain a basic patient history that identifies where the rash appears to be, when it began, what current medications are being taken (and whether doses or adherence have deviated from prescribed recommendations), and whether other novel environmental exposures (including concomitant medications, botanicals, animals, insect bites, or skin care products) may be contributing factors. One should also consider whether there has occurred a recent change in formulation or preparation of an existing medication within a treatment regimen, because rashes could reflect reactions to excipients rather than active drug ingredients (e.g., in a new generic formulation of an existing drug).

Allergic drug rashes usually arise within several days to a few weeks after beginning a medication. True allergic reactions are type I (immediate) hypersensitivity reactions mediated by IgE antibodies. These reactions require prior exposure to an allergen that sensitizes mast cells and basophils, which, upon reexposure, degranulate and cause the release of histamine, leukotrienes, and prostaglandins that cause an inflammatory reaction. Drug rashes are highly unlikely to arise for the first time after many months (or years) of stable exposure. A further consideration involves the potential for an allergic reaction to the vehicle coating the active drug (rather than the drug itself). If a rash occurs, the clinician should consider whether it is a possible idiosyncratic reaction in the aftermath of renewing an existing prescription, changing the formulation (e.g., from extended to immediate release), or substituting a generic for a branded product formulation.

A next step involves describing the appearance and location of a rash. Appropriate terminology for describing the appearance of suspected drug rashes is presented in Table 8–1, and common types of skin rashes are described in Table 8–2.

The most commonly encountered true drug rashes appear on the trunk and are exanthematous or morbilliform in appearance. Attention should be paid to whether the area is flat or raised, bumpy, red, and weepy or dry. An urticarial wheal-and-flare rash should be identified as a probable allergic reaction, and the patient should be assessed for other potentially serious manifestations of impending anaphylaxis, such as laryngeal constriction or shortness of breath. Rashes that occur in a dermatomal (often linear) distribution not crossing the midline are suggestive of varicella or herpes zoster (shingles); zoster classically manifests with painful pruritic or tingling vesicular lesions but may also be nonraised or pruritic. Antiviral drugs such as oral acyclovir tend to be most effective when begun within

TABLE 8–2.   Common skin rashes

Rash	Description	Likely drug associations	Common treatments
Acne (as caused or exacerbated by medications)	Red papules and pustules	Lithium may cause or exacerbate	Oral or topical antibiotics; benzoyl peroxide cream or lotion; tretinoin (Retin-A)
Acne rosacea	Red (inflammatory) diffuse facial rash	None	Oral or topical antibiotics to help reduce episodes
Atopic dermatitis (a type of eczema)	Scaly, itchy, red areas commonly affecting the face, neck, elbows, inner knees, and ankles; may burn or itch	None	Topical hydrocortisone, betamethasone, or fluticasone creams or ointments commonly recommended
Bacterial rashes (e.g., impetigo, caused by local staphylococcal infection)	Red, itchy, patchy skin areas that become pustular	None	Topical antibiotics often ineffective; may require oral antibiotics

TABLE 8–2. Common skin rashes (*continued*)

Rash	Description	Likely drug associations	Common treatments
Contact dermatitis	Skin irritation usually caused within 12–24 hours of *reexposure* to a specific allergen, following an *initial* exposure (sensitization); represents a type IV (delayed-type hypersensitivity [non–antibody-mediated]) reaction; typically manifests as papular, vesicular, scaly lesions	None	Medium- to high-strength topical steroid ointments
Fungal rashes (e.g., candida)	Scaly, exfoliative appearance, or may appear within skin folds (e.g., under the breast, inner groin) as red, flat, and tender to touch; may have small pustular edges	None	Antifungal topical creams (e.g., clotrimazole 1% or terbinafine 1%)
Hives or urticaria	Raised, itchy, wheal-and-flare reaction; may blanch; usually but not necessarily an allergic reaction; represents a type I (IgE-mediated) hypersensitivity reaction	Any drug	Antihistamines

TABLE 8–2.   **Common skin rashes** *(continued)*

Rash	Description	Likely drug associations	Common treatments
Psoriasis	Heritable condition involving red or pink, dry, flaky, patchy, or raised skin areas, usually nonpruritic; commonly affecting knees, elbows, and scalp	Lithium often may exacerbate; less commonly (case reports) associated with carbamazepine, divalproex, fluoxetine, paroxetine	Topical corticosteroids, vitamin D creams (e.g., calcipotriene), topical retinoids, inositol, salicylic acid, coal tar, ultraviolet light, or psoralen plus ultraviolet A (UVA) light (PUVA)
Purpura	Red or purple nonblanching discolorations <1 cm in diameter caused by bleeding under the skin, commonly resulting from infection, vasculitis, coagulopathies, or platelet disorders	Carbamazepine; otherwise unlikely except with other drugs that cause immunologically mediated thrombocytopenia	Discontinuation of suspected causal agents and treatment of underlying vascular, platelet, or coagulation disorders
Seborrhea	Red, itchy, exfoliative rash that affects skin areas containing sebaceous glands (scalp, face, and trunk)	Divalproex (incidence 1%–5%)	Medicated shampoos, topical antifungal agents (e.g., ketoconazole, clotrimazole), or topical steroids

TABLE 8–2. Common skin rashes *(continued)*

Rash	Description	Likely drug associations	Common treatments
Stevens-Johnson syndrome[a]	Systemic condition and dermatological emergency that usually involves blistering, burnlike lesions on oral and other mucocutaneous tissues, accompanied by fever, fatigue, and pharyngitis	May be caused by bupropion, carbamazepine, chlorpromazine, divalproex, lamotrigine, venlafaxine	Cessation of causal agent; systemic steroids sometimes administered early in the course of illness; monitoring of electrolytes; avoidance of suprainfections or sepsis
Viral rashes (e.g., shingles caused by varicella or herpes zoster)	Variable appearance and characteristics; shingles follows dermatomal distributions; postviral exanthematous rashes may involve diffuse tiny red bumps that may or may not be pruritic	None	Treatment of underlying disease process
Xerosis (dry skin)	Dry, dull, flaky skin with visible fine lines	None	Nonprescription emollients (e.g., Lubriderm or Eucerin cream or lotion)

Note. IgE=immunoglobulin E.
[a]Stevens-Johnson syndrome is considered a milder variant of toxic epidermal necrolysis.

48–72 hours after symptom onset and continued until crusting has occurred. Purpuritic (i.e., nonblanching red or purple skin discolorations) nodular or ulcerative rashes that are accompanied by systemic symptoms (e.g., fever, fatigue, weakness or numbness, myalgias or arthralgias) may suggest a vasculitis or infectious process rather than a typical drug reaction. While most vasculitides have idiopathic, infectious, or inflammatory etiologies, a handful of medications have been described in connection with their development, including sulfonamide (and other) antibiotics, NSAIDs, coumadin, and thiazide diuretics.

Common topical steroids that are sometimes used to treat rashes such as contact dermatitis are summarized in Table 8–3, grouped by relative strength.

Lithium-associated psoriasis has been reported to improve with the use of 4–6 g/day of omega-3 fatty acids or inositol 3–6 g/day. Case reports have indicated that atopic dermatitis and nondrug-induced psoriasis are responsive to treatment with bupropion.

Clinicians sometimes wonder whether a history of a drug rash with a particular medication class may help to predict the likelihood of the patient's developing a future rash with a drug that has not previously been taken (e.g., due to cross-sensitivity). For example, a history of rashes with other anticonvulsants has been shown to confer a 3-fold increased risk for developing a nonserious rash with lamotrigine (Hirsch et al. 2006), although a history of prior anticonvulsant-associated rashes appears less predictive for developing a rash with lamotrigine than with other anticonvulsants (Alvestad et al. 2008). According to the manufacturer of lamotrigine, a history of rash with penicillin or sulfa antibiotics increases the risk for nonserious rashes with lamotrigine.

Serious Rashes and DRESS Syndrome

Serious rashes require immediate evaluation and determination of the presence of an allergic reaction that could progress to anaphylaxis, a nonallergic systemic hypersensitivity reaction for which a suspected causal agent should be promptly discontinued, or an altogether unrelated phenomenon that may require independent medical management (e.g., poison ivy, shingles). The time course for developing a rash represents one element of its evaluation, because rashes that occur many months or years after drug initiation are unlikely to be iatrogenic. Serious rashes have been recognized in particular with lamotrigine and with carbamazepine—both of which carry boxed warnings in their manufacturers' product information materials regarding the potential for developing a serious rash. Additionally, a relatively small number of pediatric patients receiving the

TABLE 8–3. Topical steroids grouped from highest strength (Group I) to lowest strength (Group VII)

Group I	Group II	Group III	Group IV	Group V	Group VI	Group VII
Betamethasone dipropionate 0.25% (Diprolene)	Amcinonide 0.05% (Cyclocort)	Betamethasone dipropionate 0.05% (Diprosone)	Fluocinolone acetonide 0.01%–0.2% (Synalar, Synemol, Fluonid)	Desonide 0.05% (Tridesilon, DesOwen ointment)	Desonide 0.05% (DesOwen cream, lotion)	Hydrocortisone 1% (nonprescription) Hydrocortisone 2.5% (nonprescription)
Clobetasol propionate 0.05% (Temovate)	Desoximetasone 0.25% (Topicort)	Fluticasone propionate 0.005% (Cutivate)	Flurandrenolide 0.05% (Cordran)	Fluocinolone acetonide 0.025% (Synalar, Synemol cream)	Fluocinolone acetonide 0.01% (Capex shampoo, Derma-Smoothe/FS)	
Diflorasone diacetate 0.05% (Psorcon)	Fluocinonide 0.05% (Lidex)	Mometasone furoate 0.1% (Elocon ointment)	Hydrocortisone butyrate 0.1% (Locoid)	Fluticasone propionate 0.05% (Cutivate cream)	Prednicarbate 0.05% (Dermatop cream, ointment)	
Halobetasol propionate 0.05% (Ultravate)	Halcinonide 0.05% (Halog)	Triamcinolone acetonide 0.5% (Kenalog, Aristocort C cream)	Hydrocortisone valerate 0.2% (Westcort)	Hydrocortisone valerate 0.2% (Westcort cream)	Triamcinolone acetonide 0.025% (Aristocort A cream, Kenalog lotion)	
			Mometasone furoate 0.1% (Elocon cream, lotion)	Triamcinolone acetonide 0.1% (Kenalog, Aristocort R cream, lotion)		
			Triamcinolone acetonide 0.1% (Kenalog, Aristocort R ointment)			

wakefulness-promoting agent modafinil for attention-deficit disorder (ADD) developed serious rashes, which prevented the FDA from granting approval of modafinil for children and adolescents with ADD.

The DRESS syndrome (Drug Rash [or Reaction] with Eosinophilia and Systemic Symptoms) is an example of a hypersensitivity syndrome (for further discussion, see Chapter 20, "Systemic Reactions") in which systemic symptoms (e.g., fever, lymphadenopathy, inflammation) arise in conjunction with a morbilliform or maculopapular rash, usually arising 2–8 weeks after drug exposure. DRESS syndrome has been linked with several anticonvulsants as well as a number of other agents, as described below.

Carbamazepine

The incidence of either Stevens-Johnson syndrome or toxic epidermal necrolysis during treatment with carbamazepine (■) has been reported by the manufacturer as 1 per 500,000 patients. Notably, individuals of Han Chinese ancestry have been shown to carry an increased risk for developing carbamazepine-induced Stevens-Johnson syndrome or toxic epidermal necrolysis in association with the *HLA-B*1502* allele, which may represent a risk allele for which the FDA has recommended genotyping among Han Chinese Asians. With carbamazepine, as with lamotrigine, the risk for developing a serious skin rash is highest in the first few months of treatment.

Lamotrigine

Serious, life-threatening rashes — including Stevens-Johnson syndrome and toxic epidermal necrolysis — were observed in early studies of lamotrigine dosed aggressively for pediatric epilepsy. Subsequent studies identified that the risk for serious rashes with lamotrigine (■) appears highest when the dose escalation schedule occurs faster than recommended by the manufacturer (the recommendation is 25 mg/day for 2 weeks, followed by 50 mg/day for 2 weeks, then 100 mg/day for 1 week, then 200 mg/day; when combined with divalproex, dose escalation should occur at half this rate [i.e., 12.5 mg/day for 2 weeks, followed by 25 mg/day for 2 weeks, then 50 mg/day for 1 week, then 100 mg/day]). Divalproex delays phase II metabolism (glucuronidation) of lamotrigine, effectively increasing its levels and bioavailability. Risks of serious rashes also are higher when lamotrigine is coadministered with divalproex (particularly if the aforementioned dosing adjustment is not made) or when lamotrigine is used in children and adolescents. The risk for significant rashes appears to be highest during weeks 2–8 of treatment. Serious rashes typically involve blistering or burnlike lesions on soft, mucocutaneous tissues (as found in the oral cavity, nares, or conjunctivae) or skin exfoliation on the palms of the hands and soles of the feet. Systemic involvement often occurs, in which case patients may experience fever, malaise, lymphadenopathy, muscle pain, or facial edema. Serious rashes must be contrasted with benign rashes, which may occur on the extremities or trunk and are more often exanthematous (maculopapular), nonblanching, and nonpruritic.

The mechanism by which lamotrigine can cause serious rashes as part of a hypersensitivity syndrome is not well understood. Unlike delayed-type hypersensitivity reactions, the DRESS syndrome does not require prior exposure to the drug because the rash does not occur from a reactivation of sensitized mast cells and basophils.

Some authors have suggested undertaking dermatological precautions to minimize the risk for developing false-positive rashes that could be misattributed to lamotrigine rather than other more likely causes. Such precautions include avoiding exposure to other new medications or foods, cosmetics, deodorants, detergents, fabric softeners, sunburn, and environmental antigens such as poison ivy or poison oak. The potential for a rash to develop may also be diminished by avoiding the introduction of lamotrigine for 2 weeks following a prior rash, viral syndrome, or vaccination. Efforts such as these may lower the incidence of nonserious rash to about 5%.

Evidence suggests that patients taking lamotrigine who develop a nonserious rash that resolves after drug cessation may safely be rechallenged with lamotrigine, without recurrence of rash, by using a conservative dosing titration schedule (e.g., 5 mg every other day for 14 days, then increased every 14 days by 5 mg/day until reaching 25 mg/day, and thereafter following the manufacturer's usual recommended dosing schedule) (Aiken and Orr 2010; Lorberg et al. 2009).

Serious rashes thought to result from use of lamotrigine warrant prompt drug cessation and evaluation by a dermatologist. Steroids are sometimes indicated for the treatment of Stevens-Johnson syndrome during early phases of the rash but are sometimes controversial because they may also delay recovery.

Modafinil

During randomized placebo-controlled trials of modafinil for the treatment of ADD in 933 children and adolescents, 12 cases of severe cutaneous reactions (possible erythema multiforme or Stevens-Johnson syndrome, with one case identified as being definite) were identified

(Cephalon 2006). Subsequently, the FDA issued a "nonapprovable" letter regarding the pursuit by the manufacturer Cephalon of an ADD indication for modafinil in children and adolescents. The manufacturer ceased further efforts to obtain such an indication and did not conduct additional safety studies in children and adolescents with ADD. The risk of a serious dermatological reaction with modafinil in pediatric populations has been reported to be approximately 0.8%, with a median time to discontinuation (due to rash) of 13 days in clinical trials (manufacturer's product information). Although rare, rash warrants consideration during off-label treatment in pediatric patients.

Ziprasidone
In 2014, the FDA issued a warning linking ziprasidone with DRESS syndrome based on six reported cases to the agency in which symptoms developed within 11–30 days after drug initiation. Ziprasidone should be stopped immediately if a DRESS reaction is suspected.

9

Ear, Nose, and Throat

Bruxism

General Recommendations

Benzodiazepines such as clonazepam probably offer the most reliable and immediate relief for iatrogenic bruxism. Other potential pharmacological remedies may include buspirone, gabapentin, low-dose aripiprazole, propranolol, cyclobenzaprine, trazodone, divalproex, topiramate, metoclopramine, and hydroxyzine. Acrylic dental guards are considered the optimal strategy for long-term management. In severe or persistent cases, injection of botulinum toxin into the masseter muscle may provide symptomatic relief.

Bruxism is an involuntary grinding and gnashing of the teeth that may occur during sleep and in some instances may be considered a form of akathisia. Nocturnal bruxism is considered a type of non–rapid eye movement parasomnia and may be caused by a number of psychotropic agents, including SSRIs, SNRIs, buspirone, antipsychotics, atomoxetine, and dopaminergic compounds such as amphetamine or dopamine agonists used to treat Parkinson's disease. Among serotonergic antidepressants, reported incidence rates range from 14% to 24% and may be associated with older age and female sex (Uca et al. 2015). Several authors have suggested that at least in the case of SSRIs, iatrogenic bruxism may arise via inhibition of dopaminergic pathways controlling masticatory muscle activity. The persistence of bruxism over time may lead to erosion of dental enamel and potential tooth fractures or receding gums. Patient-specific risk factors include female sex, older age, smoking, stress (pertinent more for bruxing when the patient is awake than when he or she is asleep), and genetic vulnerabilities.

The clinical trial literature on pharmacotherapies for bruxism addresses bruxism in its primary (idiopathic) occurrence much more extensively than bruxism as a phenomenon secondary to medications or other etiologies, and therefore it is often necessary to extrapolate from idiopathic cases when treating its iatrogenic occurrence. No standard pharmacological treatment exists for bruxism, although acrylic dental guards ("appliance therapy") worn at night are usually considered the optimal intervention for persistent bruxism. Dosage reductions have been anecdotally reported as having potential benefit in SSRI-induced bruxism. Data from preliminary controlled trials suggest that in unmedicated, psychiatrically healthy sleep bruxers, benzodiazepines (notably, clonazepam 1 mg) may reduce bruxism and improve associated measures of sleep quality (Saletu et al. 2010). Anecdotal observations also support the possible value of cyclobenzaprine dosed from 2.5 to 10 mg at bedtime, trazodone 150–200 mg/night, divalproex 500 mg/night, hydroxyzine 10–25 mg/night, topiramate 25–100 mg/day, or metoclopramide 10–15 mg/night, all yielding improvement within 2–10 days following initiation. In a small double-blind crossover study, L-dopa 100 mg (dosed 1 hour before bedtime and again 4 hours later) has been shown to be better than placebo to reduce the frequency of noniatrogenic bruxing (Lobbezoo et al. 1997). Aripiprazole has been reported both to cause bruxism and to treat it when the bruxism is induced by SSRIs. Botulinum toxin injections into the masseter muscles also have been described as a novel periodontal procedure that can significantly reduce the number of bruxism events and consequent myofacial pain over time in individuals with persistent bruxism. There have also been anecdotal observations of preexisting bruxism *improving* after the initiation of SSRIs.

Case reports identify potential improvement in medication-induced bruxism with several other described agents, all yielding benefit within 2–7 days (Table 9–1).

Dysarthria

General Recommendations

Slow, slurred speech may be a consequence of psychotropic drugs, usually reflecting toxicity. Clinicians should be alert to the possible neurotoxic effects and the dosages of all medications and illicit substances being taken by a patient with dysarthric speech, as

TABLE 9–1. Medication-induced bruxism improved with other agents

Bruxism induced by	Improvement shown with
Antipsychotic-induced akathisia	Propranolol, 60–160 mg/day in three divided doses (Amir et al. 1997)
SSRI (sertraline) or venlafaxine	Buspirone, 10 mg bid or tid; potentially exerting an antibruxing effect via postsynaptic dopaminergic effect (Bostwick and Jaffee 1999; Jaffee and Bostwick 2000)
Venlafaxine	Gabapentin, 300 mg/day (Brown and Hong 1999)

Note. bid=twice daily; tid=three times daily; SSRI=selective serotonin re-uptake inhibitor.

well as consider and evaluate other pertinent noniatrogenic (e.g., neurological) etiologies. Nondevelopmental stuttering may rarely occur as a possible dose-related consequence of antipsychotic pharmacotherapy. Lack of improvement from dosage reductions may require discontinuation of a suspected causal agent.

Dysarthria involves impaired pronunciation of speech. When dysarthria is thought to result from psychotropic drugs, it usually reflects excessive dosing or toxicity, particularly during the use of benzodiazepines or other sedative-hypnotics and opiate analgesics, as well as lithium, divalproex, buspirone, antipsychotics, TCAs, and rarely, SSRIs. Dysarthria accompanied by difficulty clearing oral secretions may suggest possible laryngeal dystonia during antipsychotic therapy. The evaluation of dysarthria should include pertinent history taking; an assessment of the motor branch of the trigeminal nerve (V), facial nerve (VII), glossopharyngeal nerve (IX), vagus nerve (X), and hypoglossal nerve (XII) (see Table 9–2); and assessment of overall motor strength and deep tendon reflexes, in order to rule out upper motor neuron disease (e.g., strokes, basal ganglia deficits).

Nondevelopmental stuttering is a rare, possibly dose-dependent adverse drug event that has been identified in a handful of case reports with risperidone, olanzapine, clozapine, and FGAs. An equal number of cases have been reported that describe treatment of developmental (i.e., noniatrogenic) stuttering with SGAs, including risperidone, olanza-

TABLE 9–2.   Evaluation of cranial nerves that control speech and phonation

Cranial nerve	Evaluation
V Trigeminal nerve, motor branch	Assess jaw strength by palpating the temporal and masseter muscles as the patient clenches and moves the jaw.
VII Facial nerve	Ask the patient to raise the eyebrows, frown, resist opening the eyes while shut, smile (showing teeth), and puff out both cheeks.
IX Glossopharyngeal nerve	Observe the symmetry of palatal rise and fall; assess gag reflex (afferent limb).
X Vagus nerve	Assess gag reflex (efferent limb).
XII Hypoglossal nerve	As the patient protrudes and moves the tongue in various directions, inspect it for asymmetries, fasciculations, and deviation from the midline.

pine, and aripiprazole. The mechanisms by which antipsychotics could either cause or treat stuttering are not well understood, although preliminary functional imaging studies suggest that developmental stuttering may be related to increased hyperdopaminergic tone in the striatum. However, early suspicions that antipsychotic-induced stuttering could represent an extrapyramidal symptom were unsustained when adjunctive benztropine failed to demonstrate efficacy in its treatment. From a practical clinical standpoint, if new-onset stuttering does not improve via reducing the dosage of the suspected causal agent, drug discontinuation is likely warranted. Further neurological or otolaryngological evaluation is advisable if problems persist despite drug cessation.

Dysgeusia

General Recommendations

Abnormal taste sensation in the absence of other neurological adverse effects likely represents a benign phenomenon for which no intervention is medically necessary. A suspected causal medication may be eliminated if the problem persists, jeopardizes adherence, or otherwise remains objectionable to the patient. Drug cessation may be necessary.

Dysgeusia refers to an impaired sense of taste. It has rarely been identified as a manifestation of clinical depression. Iatrogenic dysgeusia can result from a number of psychotropic agents, including topiramate, carbamazepine, and lithium. In addition to being a side effect of nonpsychotropic medications (e.g., anti-inflammatory drugs, antineoplastic agents, allopurinol), dysgeusia can occur with numerous primary medical conditions, including oropharyngeal infections, vitamin or mineral (e.g., zinc) deficiencies, malignancies, Sjögren's syndrome, and smoking. Although no systematic studies have examined pharmacological antidotes for iatrogenic dysgeusia, the case report literature suggests possible value for sertraline to improve idiopathic primary dysgeusia (Mizoguchi et al. 2012).

Oral Lesions

General Recommendations

New oral lesions that arise within the first few days or weeks after starting any new medication should be evaluated for their possible association with a drug, as well as alternative (noniatrogenic) explanations. Particular attention should be paid to blistering lesions on oral mucosal tissue and any associated systemic features (e.g., fever, lymphadenopathy) that could be suggestive of serious dermatological reactions; the expected time course for such drug hypersensitivity reactions to occur is usually within the first 2 months of treatment initiation.

Oral ulcers can have many etiologies. They may be aphthous ulcers (canker sores), typically 3–10 mm in diameter, arising from a variety of causes, including physical trauma, stress, and immune deficiencies, among others. Aphthous lesions seldom persist beyond 1–2 weeks, typically remit spontaneously, and likely do not represent iatrogenic phenomena. Ulcerative tongue lesions can sometimes arise as part of a viral syndrome or reflect a chronic inflammatory process, the presence of autoimmune disease, or other immunocompromised states. They may be common phenomena in individuals with HIV. Persistent lesions sometimes warrant brush biopsies by an otolaryngologist or oral surgeon to evaluate the possibility of an oropharyngeal malignancy. Visually, malignancies usually do not appear synchronously as multiple lesions.

Inspection of the oral cavity should include assessment for the presence of thrush. Among patients taking psychotropic agents, rare cases of nonspecific oral ulcerations or mucositis have been reported in connection with carbamazepine, lithium, fluoxetine, and meprobamate. Among patients taking common nonpsychotropic drugs, oral lesions may rarely occur from the use of NSAIDs, β-blockers, thiazide diuretics, spironolactone, ACE inhibitors, and certain antibiotics. Of primary concern when evaluating oral lesions in the aftermath of starting a psychotropic drug is the recognition of blistering oropharyngeal lesions that may occur as part of the clinical presentation of a systemic rash, such as Stevens-Johnson syndrome or toxic epidermal necrolysis (see the section "Serious Rashes" in Chapter 8, "Dermatological System").

Symptomatic management of benign but painful oral ulcerative lesions can often be achieved by rinsing with oral solutions of viscous lidocaine with diphenhydramine and elixir antacids.

Sialorrhea

General Recommendations

If dosage reductions prove unhelpful for sialorrhea, the most compelling data support the use of glycopyrrolate 1 mg bid, biperiden 2 mg qd or bid, or metoclopramide 10–30 mg/day. Alternative strategies include atropine sulfate 1% ophthalmic solution 1–2 drops administered sublingually qhs or 2–3 times/day, or ipratropium bromide 0.03% nasal spray, 2 sprays administered sublingually qhs, potentially increased up to 3 times/day as needed.

Excessive drooling (*sialorrhea*) is a medically benign but often distressing side effect associated with several psychotropic agents, most notably clozapine (arising in about 30%–80% of clozapine-treated patients with schizophrenia), as well as risperidone, olanzapine, and quetiapine. Hypersalivation from clozapine appears to be a paradoxical phenomenon, in light of clozapine's antimuscarinic-anticholinergic and α_2-adrenergic antagonistic effects. Hypersalivation has been described in the absence of extrapyramidal symptoms and thus is unlikely a manifestation of parkinsonism. It also does not appear to be dose dependent in the case of clozapine, although a dose relationship may exist in cases associated with risperidone or quetiapine. Several mechanisms have been proposed to account for antipsychotic-induced hypersalivation, including postsynaptic α-adrenergic blockade at salivary glands; increased saliva production via M_4-muscarinic cholinergic receptor stimulation; decreased nocturnal pharyngeal peristalsis; and blockade of receptors at pharyngeal muscles that regulate swallowing. In addition, as noted in Chapter 2 ("Pharmacokinetics, Pharmacodynamics, and Pharmacogenomics"), preliminary pharmacogenetic studies suggest that a genetic variant of the dopamine D_4 receptor may contribute to the development of clozapine-induced sialorrhea.

Antimuscarinic anticholinergic agents represent the most extensively studied pharmacological class to counteract clozapine- or risperidone-induced sialorrhea, with varying efficacy. Significant improvement has been demonstrated from randomized data examining both oral glycopyrrolate (1 mg bid) and biperiden (2 mg qd or bid), with more robust effects seen with glycopyrrolate for clozapine-induced sialorrhea (Liang et al. 2010). Glycopyrrolate, as a peripherally acting agent, is significantly less likely than biperiden to impair cognitive function. Case reports also suggest possible value with oxybutinin 5 mg once or twice daily. Inasmuch as anticholinergic agents as a class carry the risk of cognitive dulling and sedation, their use becomes a further consideration that must be balanced against the potential for relief from hypersalivation.

A variety of other anticholinergic compounds have been used, with most having shown potential value from small proof-of-concept studies, often followed by lack of separation from placebo in larger randomized trials. These agents include the antimuscarinic-anticholinergic spray ipratropium bromide (favorable data from case reports, but negative findings from placebo-controlled trials) and the selective M_4-muscarinic receptor antagonist pirenzepine (significant reductions in hypersalivation from baseline in open-trial data reported at a dose of 50 mg/day or 25–100 mg/day, but negative data from an 8-week placebo-controlled trial begun at 25 mg/day and increased by 25 mg/week to a target dose of 100 mg/day [Bai et al. 2001]). Open data with trihexyphenidyl (mean dose=10.7 mg/day) have shown about a 50% reduction in hypersalivation, although no randomized controlled trials have as yet been reported for this use. The anticholinergic agent benztropine — popularly used to counteract parkinsonian adverse effects of antipsychotics, and known to cause dry mouth — has received little if any study for the intended purpose of counteracting hypersalivation.

A placebo-controlled trial using the D_2 antagonist metoclopramide dosed 10–30 mg/day found that sialorrhea fully or near-fully resolved in two-thirds of afflicted patients taking clozapine (Kreinin et al. 2016).

A number of case reports over the past two decades have described the local application of 1–2 drops of sublingual ophthalmic atropine sulfate 1% solution (initially qhs and then qam or bid) as an apparently effective and well-tolerated novel strategy (provided it is properly administered).

Similarly, ipratropium bromide 0.03% nasal spray can sometimes be used successfully to treat clozapine-associated sialorrhea, beginning with 2 sprays administered sublingually qhs and then increased as needed up to three times daily.

Open case reports have also described benefits from the α_2-adrenergic agonist clonidine (orally dosed from 0.05 to 0.1 mg/day) or a clonidine patch (0.1 mg/week), although randomized controlled trials have not been reported.

Stomatodynia (Burning Mouth Syndrome)

General Recommendations

Stomatodynia is rarely associated with psychotropic medicines. Topical clonazepam has been reported as being among the more successful interventions, although referral to an otolaryngologist may be necessary to clarify etiology and address therapeutic management.

Burning mouth syndrome involves a painful burning sensation of the tongue or oral mucous membranes that, in the absence of any visible physical or laboratory abnormalities, has been associated with the presence of major depressive disorder or generalized anxiety disorder. It is especially common in postmenopausal women and is rare in men, and it may be either constant or intermittent. It has no known pathophysiology or structural etiology, although conditions such as mucosal diseases, nutritional deficiencies (notably, deficiencies of vitamins B_1, B_2, B_6, or B_{12}; niacin; iron; folate; or zinc), oral thrush, non–insulin-dependent diabetes mellitus, xerostomia, or cranial nerve injuries should be ruled out when considering differential diagnosis. Some authors regard stomatodynia as a type of somatoform pain disorder. It may derive from depression or an anxiety disorder, rather than being a true pharmacodynamic consequence of treatment.

Psychotropic medications associated with burning mouth syndrome are quite rare and limited to case reports with some SSRIs (notably, fluoxetine or sertraline), venlafaxine, and clonazepam. A small number of nonpsychotropic medications, particularly ACE inhibitors such as lisinopril or enalapril, have been reported to cause burning mouth syndrome. The otolaryngological literature describes the use of TCAs and gabapentin as potentially beneficial for treating stomatodynia, as well as topical clonazepam (i.e., patients suck a 1-mg clonazepam tablet bid or tid near the pain site for several minutes, then spit).

Tinnitus

General Recommendations

Tinnitus is a rare, medically benign adverse effect without a clear antidote other than drug cessation if the symptom produces significant distress.

A small number of psychotropic drugs, including bupropion, buspirone, sertraline, and venlafaxine, have been suggested in case reports or premarketing studies to cause tinnitus. In addition, tinnitus can occur as part of withdrawal phenomena from SNRIs such as venlafaxine or short-half-life SSRIs such as sertraline. Divalproex has been reported both to cause tinnitus (Hori et al. 2003; Reeves et al. 2000) and to treat it (Menkes and Larson 1998). Tinnitus has not been observed to be dose related and often occurs in the first few weeks or months after drug initiation. Risk factors remain unidentified.

Primary (i.e., non-iatrogenic) tinnitus has been suggested in open trials to be responsive to carbamazepine, alprazolam, clonazepam, fluoxetine, duloxetine, ginkgo biloba, or melatonin, whereas randomized trials with paroxetine and with trazodone produced negative findings in treating idiopathic tinnitus in nondepressed subjects. A 4-week study of ondansetron 4–16 mg/day was superior to placebo in reducing the severity of idiopathic tinnitus (Taslimi et al. 2013). A 3-month randomized trial of intratympanic dexamethasone in combination with melatonin 3 mg nightly produced significant improvement for idiopathic tinnitus (Albu and Chirles 2014). Mirtazapine 7.5 mg/day has been reported to counteract tinnitus induced by sertraline, but there are no published open trials or systematic studies of any pharmacotherapies that specifically ameliorate tinnitus caused by psychotropic agents. Cessation of the likely causal agent typically eliminates the problem if tinnitus causes substantial distress.

Xerostomia

General Recommendations

Dry mouth is one of the most common side effects of numerous psychotropic drugs and is not necessarily dose related. It is usually of no medical consequence unless its chronic persistence leads to dental complications. Dry mouth that is of mild severity may attenuate with time or can sometimes be ameliorated by sugarless gum or glycerin-based oral lubrication solutions. Oral remedies may also include cevimeline 30 mg/day, pilocarpine 2.5–10 mg one to three times per day, and bethanechol 25 mg three times per day. Severe persistent dry mouth may necessitate drug discontinuation.

Xerostomia, or dry mouth, may result from a variety of psychotropic medications, most often from anticholinergic drugs and lithium, although dry mouth is identified as a more common adverse effect than seen with placebo in controlled trials of most classes of psychotropic compounds, regardless of an absence of known anticholinergic effects or other anticholinergic manifestations (e.g., constipation). It is often unrelated to drug dose (see Table 1–5 in Chapter 1, "The Psychiatrist as Physician"), although empirically, dosage reductions may sometimes lessen severity. Xerostomia differs from sheer thirst (as often occurs with lithium, which, as a salt, may stimulate the need for increased fluid intake).

Sugarless gums that contain aspartame, mannitol, sorbitol, or xylitol may help to stimulate saliva production. A number of nonprescription glycerin-based aerosolized sprays or gels may serve as oral moisturizers, including the glycerate polymer Biotene Oral Balance Gel, carboxymethyl cellulose or hydroxyethyl cellulose solutions (e.g., Oralube saliva substitute, Salivart Oral Moisturizer, Xero-Lube Artificial Saliva), and the water-glycerin solution Plax. Procholinergic or parasympathomimetic drugs are sometimes used to counteract the antimuscarinic effects of medications thought to cause xerostomia. These include bethanechol 25 mg three times per day, oral pilocarpine 2.5–10 mg one to three times per day (Masters 2005), and cevimeline 30 mg/day (typically used in Sjögren's syndrome or xerostomia after head and neck antineoplastic radiation therapy). Notably, in our experience, a single 10-mg dose of pilocarpine can cause profuse sweating, rhinorrhea, and diarrhea; therefore, the prudent action may be to initiate dosing at 2.5 or 5 mg to assure tolerability. Salivary stimulants versus saliva substitutes appear similar with respect to patient preference for their effects on xerostomia.

10

Electrolyte Abnormalities

Hyponatremia and SIADH

General Recommendations

Hyponatremia, with or without syndrome of inappropriate antidiuretic hormone secretion (SIADH), is a relatively rare complication of treatment with virtually all antidepressants, some anticonvulsants (notably, oxcarbazepine and carbamazepine), and many antipsychotics. In the absence of a known noniatrogenic cause for hyponatremia, psychotropic medications may need to be withheld pending determination of the etiology. Some authors advocate changing to an alternative psychotropic agent with a different pharmacological profile and closely monitoring serum sodium levels. Fluid restriction is usually the first-line treatment for mild psychotropically induced hyponatremia. Adjunctive demeclocycline or lithium sometimes may also help to reduce the risk of a recurrence of hyponatremia during continued therapy with a psychotropic drug suspected of contributing to SIADH or hyponatremia.

Hypotonic hyponatremia (often defined as a serum sodium level <130 or 135 mmol/L, depending on the study) has been reported in association with numerous psychotropic agents, including bupropion, carbamazepine, divalproex, lithium, lamotrigine, MAOIs, oxcarbazepine, SSRIs, SNRIs (including duloxetine and venlafaxine), mirtazapine, tertiary amine TCAs, other norepinephrine reuptake inhibitors such as reboxetine, and most FGAs and SGAs. Hyponatremia that has been observed to occur during treatment with an SSRI (citalopram) has been shown to recur after substitution with an SNRI (duloxetine). The mechanism(s) by which antidepressants can cause increased release of hypothalamic antidiuretic hormone (ADH), causing water retention and serum hypo-osmolarity, are not well understood. SIADH may be three times more likely among patients taking SSRIs than among patients taking other antidepressants (Movig et al. 2002). A review of relative risks for SIADH among antidepressants suggests that mirtazapine and tricyclics may be less likely than other antidepressants to cause SIADH (De Picker et al. 2014). Case reports also exist of antipsychotic-associated hyponatremia leading to NMS (Spigset and Hedenmalm 1995).

Known patient-specific risk factors for psychotropic-induced hyponatremia include the following (Spigset and Hedenmalm 1995):

- Increasing age (especially >65 years)
- Female sex
- Smoking (because nicotine increases antidiuretic hormone [ADH] secretion)

Mechanisms by which psychotropic drugs may cause SIADH are not well understood, although one proposal is that SSRIs may cause release of ADH or renal responsiveness to ADH. However, as noted earlier, nonserotonergic drugs such as bupropion also can cause SIADH, although in our experience bupropion often may be a reasonable and relatively low-risk alternative to SSRIs or SNRIs. SIADH has been reported to occur anywhere from 2 days to many months after the initiation of a causal psychotropic agent; typically it occurs during the first few weeks of treatment with an antidepressant but may have a more variable time of onset during therapy with other psychotropic agents. Many nonpsychotropic agents also may cause hyponatremia or SIADH; these drugs include, among others, diuretics (e.g., amiloride and thiazide diuretics), antineoplastic drugs (e.g., vinca alkaloids), and the fibrate clofibrate.

The formal diagnosis of SIADH entails the presence of hypotonic hyponatremia plus lower serum osmolality (usually ~240–275 mOsm/kg) than urine osmolality (usually >100–200 mOsm/kg), as well as increased urine sodium (>30 mEq/L). Patients are typically euvolemic and have normal hepatic, renal, cardiac, thyroid, and adrenal function. (Importantly, hyponatremia with *high* serum osmolality points to other medical etiologies than SIADH, such as hyperglycemia or hyperosmolar hyperglycemic nonketotic coma.) Hyponatremia may manifest without symptoms or may involve nonspecific features such as weakness, lethargy, headache, and weight gain. Neuropsychiatric signs (e.g., confusion, seizures) may occur when serum sodium levels fall below ~120 mmol/L. The differential diagnosis of noniatrogenic hyponatremia is vast, as summarized in Table 10–1.

Laboratory assessment of hyponatremia includes measurement of urine electrolytes and osmolality. A diagnosis of SIADH is supported by *concentrated urine* (i.e., elevation of both urine Na$^+$ [>20 mmol/L] and urine osmolality [>100 mmol/L]), whereas *dilute urine* (i.e., urine Na$^+$ <20 mmol/L and urine osmolality <100 mmol/L) more likely suggests psychogenic polydipsia.

In mild euvolemic hyponatremia caused by psychotropic agents, elimination of the suspected causal agent in addition to fluid restriction to about 1 L/day is usually the preferred first-line intervention and often leads to resolution of the abnormality. This intervention may require at least temporarily withholding most classes of major psychotropic drugs or, if necessary, choosing an alternative pharmacotherapy that involves a novel mechanism from that of the suspected causal agent. Most authorities caution against rapid correction of low serum sodium levels (e.g., via aggressive infusion of hypertonic saline) because of the risk for inducing central pontine myelinolysis. Severe acute hyponatremia should be gradually corrected in a medical setting via intravenous infusion of sodium chloride solution, usually no faster than an initial rate of 1–2 mmol/L per hour.

The tetracycline antibiotic demeclocycline is sometimes used in the treatment of hyponatremia because of its ability to inhibit the renal effects of ADH. For instances in which continued therapy with a suspected causal psychotropic agent is deemed clinically necessary, adjunctive demeclocycline initially dosed at 900–1,200 mg/day may be advisable (Spigset and Hedenmalm 1995). Polyuria typically occurs within 1–2 weeks, and the dosage may then be gradually reduced, usually to 300–900 mg/day, in order to maintain normal serum sodium levels. Notably, lithium also inhibits the renal effects of ADH and is sometimes recommended as an alternative strategy in the management of hyponatremia.

In medical patients with SIADH who are taking an antidepressant, psychiatrists are often asked to render an opinion on the likelihood that the antidepressant is a causal factor, along with recommendations about continuing versus stopping an existing antidepressant and advice about the choice and timing of starting an alternative antidepressant. Generally speaking, one is obliged to stop existing antidepressants unless

TABLE 10–1.   Medical (noniatrogenic) causes of syndrome of inappropriate antidiuretic hormone secretion

Acute intermittent porphyria	Hypothyroidism
Asthma	Malignancies
Brain abscess	Meningitis
COPD	Multiple sclerosis
Cirrhosis	Pneumonia
Congestive heart failure	Pneumothorax
Cystic fibrosis	Psychogenic polydipsia
Delirium tremens	Stroke
Empyema	Subarachnoid or subdural
Encephalitis	hemorrhage
Guillain-Barré syndrome	Thiazide diuretics[a]
Head trauma	Tuberculosis
Hydrocephalus	

Note.   COPD=chronic obstructive pulmonary disease.
[a]Hypokalemia and renal insufficiency typically present.

another known etiology exists. In the ideal, until serum sodium normalizes, one would not initiate another agent that could potentially also cause hyponatremia. However, in our experience, if ongoing antidepressant pharmacotherapy is indicated, it is reasonable to favor the initiation of either mirtazapine or bupropion, or sometimes a tricyclic or possibly a psychostimulant, when the risk–benefit ratio demands uninterrupted antidepressant therapy.

Metabolic Acidosis and Alkalosis

General Recommendations

A very limited number of psychotropic medications are associated, although rarely, with metabolic acidosis or alkalosis. Most notably, renal tubular acidosis can be induced by topiramate and lithium; toxicity is associated with TCA overdose; and hypokalemic hyperglycemic nonketotic acidosis can occur during treatment with SGAs. Mild acidosis may involve no presenting signs, but more severe acid-based derangements can involve an array of physical symptoms. Diagnosis is made by laboratory assessment, including arterial blood gas sampling. Treatment involves discontinuation of a presumptive causal agent, followed by supportive medical management.

Disorders of acid-base chemistry may manifest with metabolic acidosis or alkalosis, and may be either acute or chronic. When resulting from psychotropic medications, mild acidosis may be asymptomatic; or when more severe, it may manifest with variable symptoms that can include nausea, vomiting, malaise, headache, chest or abdominal pain, muscle or bone pain, and hyperpnea (long, deep breaths).

The anion gap represents the concentration of unmeasured ions in serum, as determined by calculating the sum of routinely measured cations (i.e., $[Na^+] + [K^+]$) minus routinely measured anions (i.e., $[Cl^-] + [HCO_3^-]$). A normal anion gap is usually 8–12 mEq/L. Causes of an increased anion gap are summarized in the mnemonic MUDPILES: **M**ethanol, **U**remia, **D**iabetic ketoacidosis, **P**ropylene glycol, **I**soniazid, **L**actic acidosis, **E**thylene glycol, **S**alicylates.

A normal anion gap acidosis may be caused by carbonic anhydrase inhibitors (e.g., topiramate), spironolactone, hyperparathyroidism, ammonium chloride, Addison's disease, diarrhea, hyperchloremia, organic solvents, diarrhea, or excess saline.

Hyperchloremic metabolic acidosis, without an anion gap, has been reported with the use of topiramate, due to renal bicarbonate loss resulting from carbonic anhydrase inhibition by topiramate. Acidosis may manifest clinically with dyspnea and confusion or other acute mental status changes, alongside laboratory values reflecting a rising serum chloride level with diminishing serum bicarbonate. This rare phenomenon has been reported to occur at any point during topiramate treatment and warrants consideration and evaluation of a basic metabolic laboratory panel in any patient receiving topiramate who develops acute mental status changes. Existing case reports suggest that the process generally ceases upon discontinuation of topiramate.

Other acid-base disturbances that can develop with specific psychotropic drugs include renal tubular acidosis caused by lithium and respiratory alkalosis resulting from TCA overdoses. Hypokalemic ketoacidosis may occur in association with sudden dramatic rises in blood glucose levels (e.g., as seen in hyperosmolar hyperglycemic nonketotic coma), a rare but potential risk associated with most if not all SGAs.

Lactic acidosis also can be a complication of treatment with the oral hypoglycemic agent metformin, usually when given at higher dosages. Patients taking metformin for possible reversal of psychotropic-induced weight gain (see Chapter 15, "Metabolic Dysregulation and Weight Gain," and Table 15–6) should be cautioned to pay attention to the development of sore muscles, which could indicate the presence of lactic acidosis.

11

Endocrinopathies

Bone Demineralization and Osteoporosis

General Recommendations

There is a small increased potential risk for osteoporosis during treatment with carbamazepine or SSRIs. Older adults or other patients who have an increased risk for osteoporosis may warrant periodic monitoring of bone mineral density during treatment with anticonvulsants or SSRIs, and consideration may be given to alternative pharmacotherapies when feasible.

Certain anticonvulsant drugs, particularly those that induce liver enzymes (e.g., carbamazepine), are known to decrease bone mineral density. In nongeriatric adults with epilepsy, long-term use of divalproex has been linked with an increased risk for osteoporosis or osteopenia in some studies but not others. Some investigators have suggested that drugs that inhibit histone deacetylase (e.g., divalproex) may have value in promoting osteoblast maturation, thereby mitigating a risk for bone demineralization. To date, no published reports have linked osteoporosis or osteopenia with gabapentin, lamotrigine, oxcarbazepine, topiramate, levetiracetam, or tiagabine.

Separately, SSRIs have been shown to reduce bone mineral density in hip and lumbar spinal joints by approximately 4%–6% in older adult men and women, presumably due to inhibition of serotonin sites in osteoblasts and osteoclasts. One prospective population-based study of 7,983 individuals found a 2.35-fold increased risk for nonvertebral fractures among SSRI recipients among individuals ≥age 55 (Ziere et al. 2008). Whether these observations pose a broad, clinically meaningful risk for fractures in older adults remains the subject of controversy, and at present no formal recommendation has been made either to perform bone densitometry studies on patients before and during treatment with SSRIs or to refrain from using SSRIs in osteoporotic patients for whom no other safety concerns exist regarding their use. Furthermore, depression itself has been suggested to induce bone loss via hypothalamic-pituitary-adrenocortical axis hyperactivity (Schweiger et al. 2000).

Of note, the use of hypermetabolic thyroid hormone as a psychotropic intervention (e.g., as may occur in rapid-cycling bipolar disorder) poses a potential risk for hastening bone demineralization. Some authorities advise periodic bone mineral densitometry testing in patients who continue high-dose thyroid hormone as a long-term therapy.

Hyperprolactinemia, Galactorrhea, and Gynecomastia

General Recommendations

Symptomatic hyperprolactinemia warrants either changing from a prolactin-elevating to a within-class prolactin-sparing drug or augmentation with a dopamine agonist such as bromocriptine or amantadine. Adjunctive aripiprazole also has preliminarily been shown to counteract hyperprolactinemia caused by other antipsychotics. Clinically asymptomatic hyperprolactinemia poses a long-term risk for osteoporosis and infertility and merits either periodic laboratory monitoring (if current benefits outweigh potential risks) or intervening by a medication change or augmentation with a dopamine agonist.

Antipsychotic-induced blockade of dopamine D_2 receptors on mammotropic cells of the anterior pituitary can cause release of prolactin. Hyperprolactinemia is a well-known consequence of virtually all FGAs and several SGAs (notably, risperidone and paliperidone), as described in Table 11–1. The clinician must bear in mind that hyperprolactinemia can result from other medications, including calcium channel blockers, TCAs, the sleep aid ramelteon, opiates, and histamine H_2 antagonists. Psychotropic agents other than antipsychotics have also been reported, although more rarely, to cause hyperprolactinemia and consequent gynecomastia with galactorrhea; these include venlafaxine, fluoxetine, paroxetine, diazepam (in the case of diazepam, possibly secondary to estrogen elevation), and methamphetamine. Hyperprolactinemia from some serotonergic antidepressants may arise via indirect GABAergic modulation of tuberoinfundibular dopaminergic projections (Emiliano and Fudge 2004). Among the SSRIs, the risk for hyperprolactinemia may be especially low with sertraline (Sagud et al. 2002). Rarely, carbamazepine and divalproex also have been implicated as causes of hyperprolactinemia.

Hyperprolactinemia also can result from a wide range of primary medical conditions, including pituitary tumors, macroprolactinomas, polycystic ovary syndrome, pregnancy, sarcoidosis, adrenal insufficiency, and hypothyroidism, as well as from decreased elimination due to renal or hepatic failure. Serum prolactin elevations due to antipsychotics or other psychotropic medications typically rise no higher than 100 mg/dL, although serum levels exceeding 200 mg/dL (usually otherwise suggestive of prolactinomas) have rarely been reported with use of risperidone (Melmed et al. 2011). A clinical practice guideline of The Endocrine Society advises against treating asymptomatic drug-induced hyperprolactinemia (Melmed et al. 2011). Limited patient-specific risk factors for the development of hyperprolactinemia during antipsychotic treatment have been identified and include female sex, possibly premenopausal > postmenopausal reproductive status, and antipsychotic dosage.

Reported rates of hyperprolactinemia with SGAs in controlled trials are summarized in Table 11–1.

Some SGAs, including aripiprazole and asenapine, have been reported in clinical trials to significantly *lower* serum prolactin levels from baseline. However, it is often a matter of speculation as to whether reductions in prolactin occur via an active normalizing effect of a newly introduced agent, or rather, the diminution of hyperprolactinemia after simply discontinuing a previous prolactin-elevating drug. SGAs appear less prone to elevate serum prolactin if they minimally interfere with tuberoinfundibular dopamine transmission and have "loose" D_2 binding affinities (i.e., high dissociation constants), as seen with quetiapine and clozapine. On the other hand, lurasidone demonstrates minimal prolactin elevation despite its low D_2 dissociation constant. It has been suggested that differences in prolactin elevation among SGAs may reflect their differential blood-brain disposition, with greater likelihood for hyperprolactinemia among agents with higher pituitary than striatal D_2 occupancy (Kapur et al. 2002).

Risk for hyperprolactinemia with a given agent may also vary on the basis of patients' clinical characteristics. For example, in studies that controlled for risperidone dosage, episode number, or illness duration,

TABLE 11–1.   Incidence rates of hyperprolactinemia with second-generation antipsychotics

| Agent | Changes from baseline in serum prolactin levels | | SMD (95% CI)[a] |
	Acute trials	Long-term trials	
Clozapine	*Schizophrenia:* No appreciable changes (Hamner 2002).	*Schizophrenia:* No appreciable changes (Hamner 2002).	Not available.
Cariprazine	*Schizophrenia:* –13.4 to –14.1 mg/dL.	*Schizophrenia:* –18.3 mg/dL (48-week open-label flexible-dose studies).	No data.
Aripiprazole	*Bipolar disorder:* –12.7-mg/dL (significantly greater than with placebo: –7.2 mg/dL) (Keck et al. 2003); –12.6-mg/dL (significantly greater than with placebo: –7.8 mg/dL) (Sachs et al. 2006b). *Schizophrenia:* –56.5% (Marder et al. 2003).	*Schizophrenia:* –34.2 mg/dL over 26 weeks in a multisite randomized industry-supported trial in schizophrenia (Hanssens et al. 2008).	–0.22 (–0.46, 0.03)

TABLE 11–1. Incidence rates of hyperprolactinemia with second-generation antipsychotics (*continued*)

| Agent | Changes from baseline in serum prolactin levels | | SMD (95% CI)[a] |
	Acute trials	Long-term trials	
Quetiapine	*Bipolar disorder*: 84-day placebo-controlled monotherapy trial, −15.3±40.9 mg/dL (no different from placebo) (Adler et al. 2007). *Schizophrenia*: In 6-week placebo-controlled monotherapy (comparison with paliperidone)[b] trial, −8.9±20.6 mg/dL (Canuso et al. 2009).	*Schizophrenia*: −10.6 mg/dL over 9.2-month median exposure in CATIE (Lieberman et al. 2005).	−0.05 (−0.23, 0.13)
Asenapine	*Bipolar disorder*: +4.9 mg/dL over 3 weeks. *Schizophrenia*: −6.5 mg/dL over 6 weeks (manufacturer's package insert, Merck Pharmaceuticals).	*Schizophrenia*: −26.9 mg/dL over 52 weeks.	0.12 (−0.12, 0.37)

TABLE 11–1. Incidence rates of hyperprolactinemia with second-generation antipsychotics *(continued)*

Agent	Changes from baseline in serum prolactin levels		SMD (95% CI)[a]
	Acute trials	Long-term trials	
Olanzapine	*Pooled FDA registration trial data across adult indications:* +30% increase from baseline over 12 weeks (cf. 10.5% of placebo-treated patients). *Adolescents with schizophrenia or bipolar disorder:* Serum prolactin elevations observed in 47% (cf. 7% with placebo) (manufacturer's package insert, Eli Lilly and Company).	–8.1 mg/dL over 9.2-month median exposure in CATIE (Lieberman et al. 2005).	0.14 (0.00, 0.28)
Iloperidone	*Schizophrenia:* FDA registration trials reported a mean serum prolactin change of +2.6 mg/dL over 4 weeks, with elevated prolactin levels seen in 26% of iloperidone recipients. A pooled analysis of 6-week acute phase trials demonstrated significant reductions from baseline in serum prolactin levels (ranging from –23.1 to –38.0 mg/dL) (Weiden et al. 2008).	Unavailable.	0.21 (–0.09, 0.51)

TABLE 11–1. Incidence rates of hyperprolactinemia with second-generation antipsychotics *(continued)*

Agent	Changes from baseline in serum prolactin levels		
	Acute trials	Long-term trials	SMD (95% CI)[a]
Brexpiprazole	*Schizophrenia:* Pooled findings from three acute trials identified mean serum prolactin changes ranging from –1.31 to 3.42 mg/dL (females) and –2.16 to –0.47 mg/dL (males) (Correll et al. 2016). *Major depressive disorder:* 2 mg/day adjunctive therapy over 6 weeks: +8.3 mg/dL (females), +2.2 mg/dL (males) (Thase et al. 2015a); 1 or 3 mg/day adjunctive therapy over 6 weeks: 0 patients taking 1 mg/day and 0.4% of those taking 3 mg/day had serum prolactin levels >3 times the upper limit of normal (Thase et al. 2015b).	No data.	No data.

TABLE 11–1. Incidence rates of hyperprolactinemia with second-generation antipsychotics (*continued*)

Agent	Acute trials	Changes from baseline in serum prolactin levels	
		Long-term trials	SMD (95% CI)[a]
Ziprasidone	Transient elevation from baseline that normalizes in healthy volunteers or across studies in psychotic disorders (Hamner 2002).	−5.6 mg/dL over 9.2 month median exposure in CATIE (Lieberman et al. 2005).	0.25 (0.01, 0.49)
Lurasidone	*Schizophrenia:* −1.1 mg/dL (dose dependent; +0.3 ng/mL with 40 mg/day; +1.1 mg/dL with 80 mg/day; +3.3 mg/dL with 120 mg/day; manufacturer's package insert, Sunovion Pharmaceuticals).	−1.9 mg/dL at 24 weeks; −5.4 mg/dL at 36 weeks; −3.3 mg/dL at 52 weeks (from schizophrenia open-label extension phase studies by manufacturer).	0.34 (0.11, 0.57)

TABLE 11–1. Incidence rates of hyperprolactinemia with second-generation antipsychotics (*continued*)

Agent	Changes from baseline in serum prolactin levels		
	Acute trials	Long-term trials	SMD (95% CI)[a]
Risperidone	*Schizophrenia:* Up to 66% of women and 45% of men demonstrated significant elevations in serum prolactin from baseline (Kinon et al. 2003). *Across diagnoses in children and adolescents:* In FDA registration trials, up to 87% had dose-dependent serum prolactin elevations (manufacturer's package insert, Janssen Pharmaceutica).	+13.8 mg/dL over 9.2-month median exposure in CATIE (Lieberman et al. 2005).	1.23 (1.06, 1.40)
Paliperidone	*Schizophrenia:* 6-week placebo-controlled monotherapy (comparison with quetiapine)[b] trial +38.4±42.8 mg/dL (Canuso et al. 2009).	No data.	1.30 (1.08, 1.51)

Note. CATIE=Clinical Antipsychotic Trials of Intervention Effectiveness; FDA=U.S. Food and Drug Administration; SD=standard deviation; SMD=standardized mean difference.
[a]Reported SMDs and 95% confidence intervals based on meta-analysis findings from Leucht et al. 2013.
[b]Industry trial sponsored by Ortho-McNeil Janssen Scientific Affairs, Johnson & Johnson Pharmaceutical Research and Development, and Janssen-Cilag.

serum prolactin levels were significantly higher among risperidone-treated patients with paranoid versus disorganized schizophrenia or schizoaffective disorder—possibly reflecting differences in basal dopaminergic tone among subtypes of psychotic disorders. The clinician does not routinely measure serum prolactin levels in patients taking antipsychotics without a clinical reason to do so. For example, because hyperprolactinemia is expectable with FGAs, its documentation may help to affirm treatment adherence. In patients who develop gynecological disturbances (e.g., amenorrhea, oligomenorrhea, gynecomastia, galactorrhea), measurement of serum prolactin can help clarify etiology.

No authoritative recommendation indicates whether or when iatrogenic hyperprolactinemia requires intervention. Persistent hyperprolactinemia can lead to osteoporosis, infertility, and hypogonadism in men. Some authors advise favoring prolactin-sparing SGAs in patients with existing osteoporosis, or in women with breast cancer or a history of breast cancer, inasmuch as prolactin may be trophic to some breast tumors (such that aripiprazole may be the preferred agent) (Citrome 2008).

In symptomatic patients with antipsychotic-induced hyperprolactinemia, most authorities favor changing from a prolactin-elevating antipsychotic (e.g., risperidone, paliperidone) to a prolactin-sparing antipsychotic (e.g., cariprazine, aripiprazole, quetiapine; see Table 11–1) as the first-line intervention. Alternatively, the cautious use of adjunctive dopamine agonists (e.g., bromocriptine 2.5–10 mg/day, amantadine 100–300 mg/day, pramipexole ≤1 mg/day, pergolide 0.05–0.1 mg/day, or ropinirole 0.75–3 mg/day) may effectively suppress antipsychotic-induced hyperprolactinemia, although the clinician must observe for rare but possible exacerbations of psychosis or mania. Adjunctive low-dose aripiprazole (3 mg/day) has also been described in open trials as an effective strategy to normalize hyperprolactinemia induced by risperidone or paliperidone and in a randomized placebo-controlled study (dosed at 15–30 mg/day) to counteract haloperidol-induced prolactin elevation (Shim et al. 2007), with no adverse effect on psychopathology.

Gynecomastia occurs from a hypertrophic effect of prolactin on mammary tissue. Although gynecomastia is not medically significant, it can be a distressing side effect for men or women. Long-standing high prolactin exposure to mammary tissue may cause a pharmacologically irreversible hypertrophy that may be remediable only by surgical procedures (e.g., liposuction, breast reduction). Treatment with dopamine agonists has not shown reductions in hypertrophic mammary tissue caused by elevated prolactin levels.

Several apparently safe herbal remedies have been reported to counteract antipsychotic-induced hyperprolactinemia, although their mechanisms of action are not well defined. The herb *Peony-glycyrrhiza decoction* dosed at 45 g/day significantly reduced risperidone-induced hyperprolactinemia over 4 weeks, with magnitude comparable to that seen with bromocriptine 5 mg/day; other herbal remedies with open or preliminary randomized controlled data to reduce antipsychotic-induced hyperprolactinemia without exacerbating psychiatric symptoms include *Shakuyaku-kanzo-to, Zhuang Yang* capsule, and *Tongdatang* serial recipe (reviewed by Hasani-Ranjbar et al. [2010]).

Menstrual Disturbances and Polycystic Ovary Syndrome

General Recommendations

New-onset menstrual disturbances should be evaluated for changes related to medications that may elevate serum prolactin or otherwise interfere with the menstrual cycle. In women of childbearing potential, menstrual cycles should be monitored during treatment with divalproex due to a potential increased risk for polycystic ovary syndrome (PCOS).

A number of psychotropic agents can cause menstrual irregularities through a variety of mechanisms. Irregular menstruation caused by hyperprolactinemia (e.g., secondary to antipsychotic medications) is readily diagnosed by measurement of serum prolactin levels.

PCOS was defined by the National Institutes of Health as the presence of hyperandrogenism with oligomenorrhea (Zawadzki and Dunaif 1992). Documented anatomical evidence of subcapsular ovarian cysts (known as polycystic ovaries) is not considered necessary for the diagnosis of PCOS, although it is often present.

Concerns that divalproex might contribute to PCOS arose following a large observational study of 238 women with epilepsy, in whom the use of divalproex was associated with a higher prevalence of irregular menses (45%) or anatomical evidence of polycystic ovaries (43%) than occurred during treatment with carbamazepine or other anticonvulsants (Isojärvi et al. 1993). Extensive subsequent debate ensued about parsing the effects of divalproex on the menstrual cycle relative to the potential unique contributions of epilepsy, obesity, and other factors. A later study specifically in women with bipolar disorder found a 7.5-fold increased relative risk for developing PCOS during divalproex treatment than during therapy with other anticonvulsants (Joffe et al. 2006). Collectively, these reproductive findings and the drug's teratogenic risks have prompted some authorities to advise against the use of divalproex among women of childbearing potential. Less extreme perspectives would favor monitoring the menstrual cycle of any woman of reproductive potential who receives divalproex, and further evaluation (i.e., measurement of serum androgen levels) would likely be warranted in the presence of clinical signs of a change in menstrual patterns. The treatment of PCOS involves the discontinuation of agents that may be causing it or the administration of oral contraceptives.

There is no absolute contraindication to prescribing divalproex in women with preexisting PCOS. In other words, no evidence indicates clinical worsening of existing PCOS after superimposition of divalproex, although most practitioners would likely be reluctant to risk further disruption of the hypothalamic-pituitary-gonadal steroid axis by prescribing divalproex.

Table 11–2 provides recommendations for monitoring reproductive safety in women who take divalproex during reproductive years.

Parathyroid Abnormalities

General Recommendations

Noniatrogenic causes of hypercalcemia in conjunction with hyperparathyroidism should be investigated medically. Iatrogenic hyperparathyroidism may result from lithium and thiazide diuretics. Lithium discontinuation may not necessarily reverse secondary hyperparathyroidism. Imaging studies to discern hyperplasia from multiglandular pathology should occur in conjunction with endocrinological consultation. Parathyroidectomy or use of calcimimetics may be necessary to restore calcium homeostasis.

Hypercalcemia in conjunction with both hyperplastic and multiglandular hyperparathyroidism has been reported to occur in about 10%–25% of patients taking lithium, more commonly (4:1 ratio) in women than in men (Albert et al. 2013; Meehan et al. 2015; Shapiro and Davis 2015). Lithium can cause a shift in the inhibitory set point for parathyroid hormone secretion to a higher serum calcium concentration, while antagonizing the calcium sensing receptor (CaSR) located on the surface of parathyroid cells, which results in an increase in the threshold levels of extracellular calcium required to suppress PTH release from the parathyroid gland, leading to increased serum PTH. Lithium also can inhibit renal excretion of calcium, causing hypercalcemia with inappropriately low-normal urinary calcium excretion, measurable by 24-hour urine collection. (By con-

TABLE 11–2. **Reproductive safety considerations during divalproex therapy in premenopausal women**

1. Discuss possibility of reproductive and endocrinological side effects with female patients before beginning divalproex treatment.

2. Measure baseline body weight and body mass index, and follow both at each visit; evaluate weight gain.

3. Obtain baseline information about menstrual cycle and assess for menstrual irregularities at each visit.

4. Consider obtaining baseline and subsequent information about ovarian structure (by ultrasound) and serum sex hormone concentrations, including the following:

   • Pregnancy test

   • Lutenizing hormone (LH)/follicle stimulating hormone (FSH) ratio (if >2–3 may be consistent with polycystic ovary syndrome [PCOS])

   • Morning, fasting 17-hydroxyprogesterone during follicular phases of menstrual cycle (values >200 ng/dL may suggest 21-hydroxylase deficiency due to late-onset congenital adrenal hyperplasia)

   • Dehydroepiandrosterone (DHEA; usually normal or slightly elevated in PCOS; values >800 µg/dL may suggest possible androgen-secreting adrenal tumor)

   • Prolactin (usually normal or only mildly elevated in PCOS; marked elevation in the absence of dopamine-blocking drugs may suggest pituitary hyperprolactinoma)

   • Total testosterone (may be normal [<150 ng/dL] in PCOS; higher levels may reflect an androgen-secreting ovarian or adrenal tumor)

5. Obtain baseline and annual serum lipid profiles.

6. Evaluate at baseline signs of androgen excess (e.g., hirsutism, alopecia, acne) and follow up at each visit.

7. Refer to a reproductive endocrinologist if abnormalities in the laboratory values described above are accompanied by two or more of the following symptoms: hirsutism, menstrual disturbances, obesity, alopecia, or infertility; consider discontinuing divalproex if a thorough risk-benefit analysis demonstrates unfavorable risk.

8. Counsel patient on nutrition and weight management strategies.

TABLE 11–2.   Reproductive safety considerations during divalproex therapy in premenopausal women (continued)

---

9. For women <age 20 years:

  • Divalproex is not contraindicated, but use with caution and follow the recommendations listed above.

  • Consider pretreatment workup consisting of serum testosterone level and pelvic ultrasound, and consider repeating annually.

  • Consider changing to a different mood stabilizer if clinical symptoms of hyperandrogenism or PCOS appear.

Source.   Adapted from Ernst CL, Goldberg JF: "The Reproductive Safety Profile of Mood Stabilizers, Atypical Antipsychotics, and Broad-Spectrum Psychotropics." *Journal of Clinical Psychiatry* 63 (suppl 4):42–55, 2002.

trast, primary hyperparathyroidism typically causes both hypercalcemia and hypercalciuria.) Duration of lithium exposure may be a predisposing risk factor. We recommend periodic monitoring of serum calcium and PTH in patients taking lithium.

Exacerbations of preexisting hyperparathyroidism, as well as multiglandular disease, have both been implicated in the pathogenesis of lithium-induced hyperparathyroidism (Szalat et al. 2009). Cessation of lithium does not necessarily lead to normalization of parathyroid function. The calcimimetic drug cinacalcet is sometimes used to treat secondary hyperparathyroidism (via activating the CaSR, in turn downregulating PTH release), usually for instances in which parathyroidectomy is either not indicated or unsuccessful.

Thyroid Abnormalities

General Recommendations

Lithium, carbamazepine, and quetiapine all may infrequently cause secondary hypothyroidism. Baseline measurement of thyroid function tests should include measurement of antithyroid antibodies when serum thyroid-stimulating hormone (TSH) is elevated. Repletion typically involves supplemental L-thyroxine (T_4), usually begun at 0.025 mg/day, followed by reassessment of thyroid function tests after 6 weeks, with increases by 0.025 mg every 3–6 weeks until TSH levels normalize.

Subclinical hypothyroidism may manifest as a consequence of lithium use in 5%–35% of individuals receiving lithium, particularly women

(Kraszewska et al. 2016), and usually within the first 6–18 months of treatment. The duration of exposure appears not to contribute to risk (Kraszewska et al. 2016). The condition is thought to result from several effects of lithium, including antagonism of TSH, reduced deiodination of peripheral T_4 to triiodothyronine (T_3), and interference with cyclic adenosine monophosphate–mediated production of thyroid hormone within the thyroid gland. More rarely, lithium may also cause hyperthyroidism due to thyroiditis or Graves' disease (Lazarus 2009). Some studies suggest that lithium-associated hypothyroidism may be more common among individuals who have circulating thyroid antibodies. Typically, in patients with an elevated serum TSH level, the clinician measures antiperoxidase and antithyroglobulin to determine whether autoimmune thyroiditis is present. Note that in contrast to goiter, thyroid nodules are generally not thought to result from treatment with lithium.

No firm consensus exists on when supplemental thyroid hormone should be added to the regimen of patients with an elevated serum TSH level who are taking lithium. Some authorities advocate more frequent monitoring of serum TSH levels (e.g., every 3 months) in the setting of biochemical hypothyroidism, without adding exogenous thyroid hormone unless serum TSH levels exceed 10 mU/L or clinical manifestations emerge. Others advise a lower threshold for adding supplemental thyroid hormone *whenever* serum TSH levels rise above the upper limit of a laboratory's reference range, particularly in the setting of affective symptoms. T_4 is usually preferred over T_3 to produce steadier hormone levels, even though T_3 may exert more potent psychotropic (e.g., antidepressant) effects.

Supplementation of thyroid hormone for lithium-induced hypothyroidism usually begins with the addition of 0.025 mg/day of T_4, followed by a reassessment of thyroid function tests after 6 weeks, and iterative increases of T_4 by 0.025 mg/day until TSH levels have normalized. High-dose exogenous thyroid hormone—as is sometimes used to achieve suprametabolic levels of free T_4 in rapid-cycling bipolar disorder—requires clinicians to recognize the potential for developing arrhythmias (notably, atrial fibrillation) and promoting bone demineralization and osteoporosis (sometimes prompting a need for obtaining periodic bone mineral densitometry assessments).

Carbamazepine also hastens the metabolism of T_4 and T_3 and may produce secondary hypothyroidism. In addition, a handful of case reports have described hypothyroidism induced by quetiapine, usually in patients with a history of past thyroid abnormalities (Kelly and Conley 2005), and potentially subject to spontaneous resolution (Kontaxakis et al. 2009). Proposed mechanisms include competitive metabolism of thyroid hormones and quetiapine by uridine diphosphate–glucuronosyltrans-ferase (Kelly and Conley 2005) or possibly an autoimmune-mediated process, although the rarity of this phenomenon does not appear to warrant routine monitoring of thyroid function during quetiapine treatment.

12

Gastrointestinal System

Diarrhea, Hypermotility, and Constipation

General Recommendations

Loose stools may occur during initiation of treatment with serotonergic antidepressants or as part of discontinuation syndromes upon abrupt cessation of these drugs. Loose stools are usually self-limited phenomena that can be managed conservatively (e.g., via oral replenishment of fluid losses and over-the-counter remedies such as loperamide or bismuth subsalicylate).

Serotonergic antidepressants may cause gastrointestinal (GI) hypermotility, usually near treatment initiation. Symptoms are usually self-limited and resolve with time on the drug. As identified in manufacturers' product information materials, FDA registration trials of SSRIs across their indications collectively report incidence rates of diarrhea that are generally within the range of ~6%–20%, with the highest being vilazodone (28%).

The symbol ■ is used in this chapter to indicate that the FDA has issued a boxed warning for a prescription medication that may cause serious adverse effects.

Some SNRIs (e.g., duloxetine, desvenlafaxine) identify lower rates (~10%), while the lowest rates among antidepressants (>1%–2%, but no different from placebo) are described with bupropion XL, mirtazapine, and venlafaxine XL. Among mood-stabilizing agents, significant or persistent diarrhea with lithium or divalproex should be considered as a possible indicator of drug toxicity. Frank microscopic colitis also has been associated with paroxetine, sertraline, and carbamazepine, remediable by drug cessation (Beaugerie and Pardi 2005).

When necessary, conservative interventions to manage diarrhea symptoms include increasing dietary fiber (e.g., psyllium husk–containing products, such as Metamucil), use of aluminum hydroxide (e.g., Amphojel) products, cyproheptadine, or over-the-counter antidiarrheal medicines such as loperamide or bismuth subsalicylate. Oral probiotics (e.g., lactobacillus acidophilus) also represent popular nonprescription antidiarrheal remedies, but their potential efficacy for psychotropically induced GI hypermotility has not been formally studied. Severe or persistent diarrhea in the absence of other identified etiologies may warrant drug cessation.

Constipation is among the more common adverse effects associated with drugs that possess antimuscarinic anticholinergic properties (e.g., many SGAs, TCAs, benztropine, and some SSRIs [notably, paroxetine]). Anticholinergic antipsychotics (e.g., clozapine) may cause constipation in up to half of patients. Assessment should rule out the possibility of a functional bowel obstruction (e.g., failure to pass gas, distended abdomen with crampy abdominal pain, nausea/vomiting). Clozapine-induced gastrointestinal hypomotility is a rare and potentially lethal adverse effect associated with high doses or concomitant anticholinergic drugs that can cause bowel obstruction, megacolon, necrosis, and intraabdominal sepsis.

Similar incidence rates for constipation (ranging from ~3% to 16%) have been reported in manufacturers' product information materials from FDA registration trials involving SSRIs, SNRIs, bupropion, and mirtazapine. Clinicians obviously should, when possible, attempt to minimize the cumulative anticholinergic burden of an overall drug regimen. Short-term use of bulk-forming hydrophilic laxatives (e.g., methylcellulose, psyllium seed), stimulant laxatives (e.g., senna), or cathartic osmotic laxatives (e.g., lactulose) offer relatively conservative first-line interventions, while agents that stimulate peristalsis (e.g., metoclopramide or bethanechol) may offer additional mechanistically specific strategies to counteract anticholinergic-associated constipation.

Gastrointestinal Bleeding

General Recommendations

SSRIs, particularly in combination with NSAIDs or aspirin, may increase the risk for upper GI bleeding. In SSRI recipients with a history of peptic ulcer disease or upper GI bleeding, gastroprotective cotherapy (e.g., with a proton pump inhibitor) may be advisable.

SSRIs have been associated with an approximate 2-fold increased risk for upper GI bleeding, with a crude incidence rate of 1 in 8,000 SSRI prescriptions (Andrade et al. 2010). Mechanisms thought to account for this phenomenon include decreased platelet aggregation due to inhibition of serotonin uptake from blood into platelets, as well as a direct effect causing increased gastric acid secretion (see further discussion in Chapter 14, "Hematological System," in the section on platelet aggregation disorders and bleeding risk). SSRIs (but not TCAs) have also been shown to increase the risk for peptic ulcer disease by 1.5-fold, with a 24% reduction in risk observed with concomitant proton pump inhibitors (e.g., omeprazole, lansoprazole, or pantoprazole) (Dall et al. 2010). Identified risk factors for upper GI bleeding during SSRI therapy include concomitant use of NSAIDS, aspirin, or antiplatelet drugs (conferring an 8- to 28-fold increased likelihood) or the presence of liver failure or cirrhosis (Andrade et al. 2010), while cotherapy with proton pump inhibitors among SSRI recipients as a group may reduce bleeding risk (Dall et al. 2009). No increased risk of lower GI bleeding during SSRI treatment has been reported.

Some authors advocate the coadministration of a proton pump inhibitor or other gastroprotective agent (e.g., H_2 histamine blocker) in SSRI recipients with a history of upper GI bleeding or peptic ulcer disease, although the low absolute risk for upper GI bleeding likely obviates the necessity of gastroprotective measures for most SSRI recipients. Some authors also advise the discontinuation of SSRIs before elective surgery in patients with a history of upper GI bleeding, although such decisions are usually made on a case-by-case basis depending on the nature of the surgery and the presence of other risk factors for increased bleeding.

Hepatic Impairment and Transaminitis

General Recommendations

Most psychotropic drugs require lower dosing in the setting of hepatic failure, but few absolute contraindications exist for use of these drugs in patients with hepatic dysfunction. Although many anticonvulsants and some antidepressants and SGAs can infrequently raise hepatic enzyme levels, routine laboratory monitoring is generally less useful or relevant than regular clinical monitoring for signs and symptoms suggestive of hepatotoxicity.

The evaluation of hepatic function involves assessment of liver enzymes (i.e., ALT and AST), as well as other enzymes (e.g., alkaline phosphatase) and synthetic proteins made by the liver (e.g., serum albumin, total protein, total bilirubin, prothrombin time). AST:ALT ratios of 2:1 or 3:1 often suggest alcohol-induced hepatotoxicity. The detection of recent heavy alcohol use can be aided by the measurement of serum carbohydrate-deficient transferrin, a highly specific but only moderately sensitive marker for drinking behavior. γ-Glutamyl transpeptidase (γGTP), another enzyme synthesized exclusively by the liver, is a nonspecific measure of liver dysfunction that is sometimes used as an indicator of even modest alcohol consumption or as a means to clarify hepatic- versus bone-based causes of an elevated serum alkaline phosphatase. An elevated γGTP level also may occur in congestive heart failure or other conditions that involve liver injury and by itself does not help to distinguish a cause for hepatic dysfunction.

Medication-induced hepatotoxicity often involves serum ALT > AST. In overweight individuals at risk for metabolic syndrome, mild transaminitis (in which ALT and AST levels usually do not exceed 4 times the upper limit of normal) may reflect nonalcoholic steatohepatitis, a hepatic inflammatory condition affecting 2%–5% of Americans (particularly middle-aged, overweight adults) that can lead to hepatocellular damage, fibrosis, and eventual cirrhosis. Importantly, 10%–25% of Americans have simple fatty liver without inflammation (nonalcoholic fatty liver disease), addressable by treating the underlying metabolic risk factors (particularly obesity and hyperlipidemia).

Many psychotropic drugs, including divalproex, carbamazepine, TCAs, SNRIs, and SGAs, can be associated with modest elevation of serum liver enzyme levels. For example, incidence rates of transaminitis with carbamazepine in epilepsy patients range from 5% to 15%, although fewer than 20 cases of significant liver impairment were reported over a 12-year period studied (Pellock and Willmore 1991). Frank hepatotoxicity has been reported in connection with the use of carbamazepine, divalproex (■), duloxetine, and nefazodone (■). Hepatic enzyme elevation may be caused by numerous nonpsychotropic medications, including acetaminophen, NSAIDs, statins, ACE inhibitors, omeprazole, allopurinol, certain antibiotics, and oral contraceptives, among others. There are no formal manufacturers' recommendations or guidelines on the indications for monitoring of liver enzymes, with the exceptions of divalproex and carbamazepine (see Table 1–2 in Chapter 1, "The Psychiatrist as Physician"), unless indicated based on the emergence of clinical signs (e.g., icteric sclerae or jaundice, changes in stool color).

Some authorities point out that regular, routine laboratory monitoring of liver enzymes or other parameters that reflect hepatic function (e.g., prothrombin time, partial thromboplastin time, protein levels) are often normal in anticonvulsant recipients who subsequently develop hepatotoxicity; more relevant to safety monitoring is the ability to recognize clinical signs of hepatic failure (e.g., nausea, vomiting, anorexia, lethargy, jaundice) (Pellock and Willmore 1991).

In general, most hepatically cleared drugs can be continued unless liver enzymes exceed 3 times the upper limit of normal. That generalization reflects one of three pillars that has come to be known as Hy's law (Reuben 2004), a principle relevant for gauging the likelihood of fatal drug-induced liver injury. Other components of this triad include total serum bilirubin >2 times the upper limit of normal, and absence of another etiology (e.g., alcoholic hepatitis, hepatic ischemia).

Preexisting liver disease (e.g., hepatitis, alcoholic liver disease) does not automatically contraindicate use of hepatically metabolized psychotropic drugs. Degrees of hepatic impairment are rated with the Child-Pugh classification scale (see Table 3–1 in Chapter 3, "Vulnerable Populations"), which takes into account total bilirubin, serum albumin, ascites, INR, and presence of hepatic encephalopathy. The extent to which hepatic dysfunction may alter drug clearance, and potentially necessitate hepatic dosing of psychotropic medications, is summarized in Table 12–1.

Hyperammonemia

General Recommendations

In patients with an acute mental status change who are taking divalproex or carbamazepine, serum ammonia level should be measured to determine the possible presence of hyperammonemia. If either of these agents is the suspected cause of hyperammonemia, discontinue the drug and consider administration of L-carnitine 1,000 mg twice daily and/or lactulose to hasten the elimination of serum ammonia. Asymptomatic hyperammonemia caused by divalproex or carbamazepine does not necessarily require intervention.

Laboratories vary in defining reference range upper limits for serum ammonia levels, although levels exceeding 70 µg/dL in adults are gen-

TABLE 12–1.   Dosing adjustments or precautions in the presence of hepatic failure

Agent	Comment
Anticonvulsants and lithium	
Carbamazepine	Caution is advised when used in patients with hepatic dysfunction.
Divalproex	Drug is contraindicated in the setting of significant hepatic dysfunction.
Gabapentin	Drug is not appreciably metabolized and is excreted unchanged; dosing adjustment in the setting of hepatic disease therefore is unnecessary.
Lamotrigine	Dosing should be reduced by 25%–50% in the setting of moderate or severe hepatic impairment, according to the manufacturer's package insert. Metabolized by Phase II glucuronidation.
Lithium	All preparations of lithium are renally excreted with no hepatic metabolism; no dosing adjustment is necessary in the setting of hepatic failure.
Oxcarbazepine	No dosing adjustment is necessary in patients with mild to moderate hepatic impairment; caution is advised when used in patients with severe hepatic dysfunction.
Topiramate	Dosing should be reduced and intervals between doses should be increased in the setting of hepatic dysfunction.
Antidepressants and related agents	
Atomoxetine	Initial dosing should be reduced by 50% in patients with moderate hepatic impairment and by 75% in those with severe hepatic impairment.
Bupropion	Caution is advised in the setting of mild to moderate hepatic impairment; in severe hepatic impairment, the manufacturer of bupropion XL advises dosages no higher than 150 mg every other day.

TABLE 12–1. Dosing adjustments or precautions in the presence of hepatic failure *(continued)*

Agent	Comment
Antidepressants and related agents *(continued)*	
Buspirone	Hepatic insufficiency may increase serum buspirone levels 13-fold. The manufacturer advises against using buspirone in individuals with severe hepatic dysfunction.
Mirtazapine	Oral clearance of mirtazapine is decreased by approximately 30% with hepatic insufficiency. Consequently, dosages should be reduced in patients with moderate or severe hepatic impairment.
Nefazodone	Plasma concentrations increase by ~25% in the setting of liver disease. Boxed warning (■) indicates that nefazodone should not be administered in patients with active liver disease or when liver enzymes exceed 3 times the upper limit of normal.
SNRIs	*Desvenlafaxine:* In mild to moderate impairment, dosing should be reduced by at least 50%. Desvenlafaxine should not be dosed >100 mg/day in the setting of hepatic impairment. *Duloxetine:* Administration is not recommended for patients with any hepatic insufficiency. *Levomilnacipran:* No dosing adjustment is necessary per the manufacturer in the setting of mild, moderate, or severe hepatic impairment. *Venlafaxine:* In mild to moderate impairment, dosing should be reduced by at least 50%.

TABLE 12–1.   Dosing adjustments or precautions in the presence of
               hepatic failure *(continued)*

Agent	Comment

Antidepressants and related agents *(continued)*

SSRIs
: *Citalopram:* Half-life approximately doubles in the setting of hepatic dysfunction; a dosage of 20 mg/day is recommended.
: *Escitalopram:* A dosage of 10 mg/day is recommended with hepatic impairment.
: *Fluoxetine:* Lower or less frequent doses are advised.
: *Fluvoxamine:* Plasma clearance is decreased by ~30%; low initial dosing is advised.
: *Paroxetine:* Plasma concentrations are increased approximately 2-fold; low initial dosing is advised.
: *Sertraline:* Plasma concentrations are increased approximately 3-fold; low initial dosing is advised.

Transdermal selegiline
: No dosing adjustment is necessary in patients with mild or moderate hepatic impairment.

Vilazodone
: No dosing adjustment is necessary in patients with mild or moderate hepatic impairment.

Vortioxetine
: The manufacturer recommends no need for dosing adjustments in the setting of mild, moderate, or severe hepatic impairment.

Sedative-hypnotics

Eszopiclone
: The manufacturer advises no need for dosing adjustment in the setting of mild to moderate hepatic impairment and a maximum dose of 2 mg/day in the setting of severe hepatic impairment.

Ramelteon
: The manufacturer notes that drug exposure increases 4-fold in the setting of mild hepatic impairment and >10-fold in patients with severe hepatic failure (for whom caution is advised if using ramelteon).

TABLE 12–1. Dosing adjustments or precautions in the presence of hepatic failure *(continued)*

Agent	Comment
Sedative-hypnotics *(continued)*	
Suvorexant	No dosing adjustment needed in mild or moderate hepatic impairment; the manufacturer advises against using suvorexant in patients with severe hepatic impairment.
Tasimelteon	The manufacturer advises no necessary dosing adjustments in the setting of mild to moderate hepatic impairment (Child-Pugh scores ≤ 9) but recommends against using tasimelteon in patients with severe hepatic impairment (Child-Pugh scores of 10–15).
Zolpidem	The manufacturer recommends maximum dosing of 5 mg/day in patients with mild to moderate hepatic impairment and discourages use of zolpidem in the setting of severe hepatic impairment.
SGAs	
Aripiprazole	No dosing adjustment is necessary in the setting of any hepatic impairment (Child-Pugh scores of 5–15).
Asenapine	Drug is not recommended for use in patients with hepatic failure. It is metabolized by Phase I oxidation (CYP1A2) and Phase II glucuronidation (UGT1A4).
Brexpiprazole	In moderate to severe hepatic impairment (Child-Pugh scores ≥ 7), the manufacturer's maximum recommended dose is 2 mg/day (major depressive disorder) or 3 mg/day (schizophrenia).
Cariprazine	The manufacturer advises no necessary dosing adjustments in patients with mild to moderate hepatic impairment (Child-Pugh scores of 5–9) but avoidance of cariprazine in the setting of severe hepatic impairment (Child-Pugh scores of 10–15).

TABLE 12–1.   Dosing adjustments or precautions in the presence of hepatic failure *(continued)*

Agent	Comment
SGAs *(continued)*	
Lurasidone	In moderate or severe hepatic impairment, maximum dosage recommended by the manufacturer is 40 mg/day.
Olanzapine	Mild hepatic impairment (Child-Pugh scores of 5–9) produces little effect on clearance of olanzapine.
Paliperidone	No dosing adjustments are necessary for mild to moderate hepatic impairment.
Quetiapine	The manufacturer advises that patients with hepatic impairment begin treatment at 25 mg/day, with daily increases of 25–50 mg/day based on clinical response and tolerability.
Risperidone	In the setting of hepatic impairment, dosage increases should be no higher than 0.5 mg twice daily, and increases above 1.5 mg twice daily should occur at least 1 week apart.
Ziprasidone	No dosing adjustments are necessary for mild to moderate hepatic impairment.

Note. CYP=cytochrome P450; SGA=second-generation antipsychotic; SNRI = selective norepinephrine-serotonin reuptake inhibitor; SSRI=selective serotonin reuptake inhibitor; XL=extended release.

erally thought to reflect clinically significant elevation. Hyperammonemia may be associated with hepatic encephalopathy and warrants consideration in the differential diagnosis of patients with an acute mental status change when hepatic disease (e.g., cirrhosis, hepatitis, alcohol withdrawal) may be present. Clinicians should be attentive to the presence of vomiting and asterixis or other focal neurological signs (e.g., hyperreflexia) when considering the possibility of hepatic encephalopathy.

In the early 1980s, case reports began to emerge describing asymptomatic hyperammonemia as well as hyperammonemic encephalopathy in both child and adult epilepsy patients taking divalproex. A prospective case series by Raja and Azzoni (2002) identified asymptomatic hyperammonemia (serum ammonia>97 µg/dL) with normal liver enzyme levels in 51% of adult psychiatric inpatient recipients of divalproex, ameliorated solely by divalproex dosage reductions. Divalproex-associated hyperammonemia may be clinically asymptomatic in about half of cases. Notably, no clear correlation has been demonstrated between asymptomatic hyperammonemia (or even valproate-related hyperammonemic encephalopathy) and serum valproate levels. The clinical significance of asymptomatic hyperammonemia due to divalproex is uncertain, although serum ammonia levels >127 μg/dL may be more likely associated with encephalopathy irrespective of serum valproate levels.

Hyperammonemia has also been reported as an idiosyncratic phenomenon in association with carbamazepine in the absence of laboratory indices of hepatic impairment, remedied by oral lactulose and the cessation of carbamazepine. Other possible causes of hyperammonemia include barbiturates, opiates, diuretics, and cigarette smoking, as well as hemolytic processes (e.g., GI bleeding), reduced ammonia clearance due to fulminant hepatic failure (e.g., following acetaminophen overdose), and inborn errors of metabolism in both children and adults. Excessive exercise or seizures can also increase direct ammonia production from skeletal muscle.

Numerous factors can predispose to the development of hyperammonemia among divalproex recipients, including severe alcoholism, high dietary nitrogen intake in the setting of low caloric intake, urea cycle disorders among pediatric patients, and combinations of anticonvulsant drugs among epilepsy patients. Hyperammonemia is thought to result from the effects of propionic acid (a metabolite of divalproex that inhibits carbamoyl phosphate synthetase, in turn impairing the conversion of ammonia to urea in the urea cycle). Additionally, divalproex may directly elevate serum ammonia levels by depleting body stores of carnitine, a quaternary ammonium compound synthesized from the essential amino acids methionine and lysine in the liver that is a necessary cofactor for β-oxidation of fatty acids. Measurement of serum carnitine levels is thought to be uninformative in estimating its bioavailability in the liver because it is stored mainly in muscle. The use of oral lactulose is generally reserved for hyperammonemic patients who manifest clinical signs of encephalopathy.

Case reports have suggested that supplemental dietary L-carnitine (1 g po bid) can reverse signs of lethargy and mental slowing in the setting of otherwise asymptomatic hyperammonemia during divalproex therapy. There is presently no consensus recommendation within the field as to the necessity for routinely monitoring serum ammonia levels in the absence of lethargy or other CNS features suggestive of encephalopathy, or in routine supplementation of oral L-carnitine in asymptomatic divalproex recipients. In our experience, given the relative rarity of symptomatic hyperammonemia and the dubious clinical significance of its asymptomatic presence, we concur with the manufacturer in not advocating routine measurement of serum ammonia levels during divalproex treatment, although it likely warrants evaluation in patients taking divalproex who develop acute mental status changes, for which treatment with supplemental L-carnitine (1 g bid) may be ameliorative.

Malabsorption Disorders

General Recommendations

Some anticonvulsants may interfere with absorption or metabolism of vitamin B_{12} and folic acid. Folic acid supplementation is commonly recommended during anticonvulsant therapy in pregnancy to minimize risk for neural tube defects. However, routine screening or repletion of these vitamins during anticonvulsant therapy in nonepileptic patients generally is not done in the absence of clinical signs of deficiency.

Low serum levels of vitamin B_{12} (cobalamin) and folic acid found in epileptic adults have been associated with a number of anticonvulsants, including carbamazepine, divalproex, gabapentin, oxcarbazepine, and topiramate (but not lamotrigine or zonisamide) (Kishi et al. 1997; Sander and Patsalos 1992). Impaired GI absorption has been proposed as one possible mechanism, although other plausible explanations for this phenomenon include impaired plasma binding, disrupted renal secretion, and (at least in the case of carbamazepine, oxcarbazepine, or topiramate) hastened metabolism via induction of CYP microenzymes (Linnebank et al. 2011). Because folic acid and vitamin B_{12} are necessary to convert homocysteine to methionine, deficient levels can elevate plasma homocysteine, in turn predisposing to vascular endothelial damage and cardiovascular or cerebrovascular disease. Clinically, low levels of vitamin B_{12} or folic acid may also cause megaloblastic anemia, neuropathy, cognitive deficits, and osteoporosis, among other metabolic or homeostatic disturbances. Low serum folic acid levels due to anticonvulsant exposure during pregnancy are well-recognized contributors to neural tube defects (see the section "Breast-Feeding and Teratogenicity" in Chapter 21, "Pregnancy and the Puerperium"). Although some authors advocate periodic laboratory monitoring of serum folic acid and vitamin B_{12} levels during therapy with most anticonvulsants in women (irrespective of pregnancy status) as well as men, with repletion (e.g., 1 mg/day of oral folic acid [Morrell 2002] or 1,000–2,000 µg/day of oral vitamin B_{12} [Kuzminski et al. 1998]), there is no formal recommendation by the American Epilepsy Society or the American Academy of Neurology either for routine serum monitoring or replacement therapy in asymptomatic anticonvulsant recipients.

Nausea and Gastrointestinal Upset

General Recommendations

Nausea often occurs as a transient side effect from serotonergic antidepressants that indiscriminately stimulate postsynaptic serotonin type 3 (5-HT_3) receptors, and may be minimized by co-administration with food or over-the-counter antiemetics such as bismuth subsalicylate or antihistamines. Prescription-strength antihistamine antiemetics, such as trimethobenzamide or promethazine, may be useful if significant nausea persists.

Serotonergic agents commonly cause nausea due to their undesirable affinity for 5-HT_3 receptors, resulting in the most frequent adverse effect associated with SSRIs. Accordingly, psychotropic agents that block postsynaptic 5-HT_3 receptors (notably, mirtazapine or olanzapine) have a lower likelihood for causing nausea than do drugs that nonselectively agonize this receptor and may in fact possess potent antiemetic properties. The novel serotonergic antidepressant vortioxetine was associated with an approximate 20%–30% incidence of dose-dependent, mild to moderate nausea, mainly in the first 2 weeks of exposure, during FDA registration trials; however, since this drug is a potent 5-HT_3 antagonist (Ki=~3.7 nM), the mechanism by which it may produce nausea is likely related to other receptors or transmitter systems (e.g., 5-HT_{1A} agonism). Consequently, anti-nausea drugs that exert their effects via 5-HT_3 antagonism (e.g., ondansetron, granisetron) would represent less compelling treatment options to remedy vortioxetine-associated nausea because vortioxetine already blocks 5-HT_3 receptors. Ondansetron has formally been studied to treat or prevent nausea and vomiting from emetogenic cancer chemotherapy, radiation therapy, or postoperative nausea and vomiting, although it is commonly used "off label" in emergency departments and other medical settings to treat nausea and vomiting from other etiologies, with comparable efficacy to prochlorperazine. Anti-nausea pharmacotherapies that are unrelated to 5-HT_3 binding might include trimethobenzamide, prochlorperazine, or metaclopramide.

Nausea and GI upset are usually transient phenomena with most psychotropic medications that cause them. Antipsychotic drugs generally do not cause nausea, and some in fact are commercially marketed as antiemetics (e.g., phenothiazines such as prochlorperazine, or the dopamine D_2 antagonist metoclopramide) — albeit with high risk for extrapyramidal side effects by virtue of their D_2 antagonistic effects, including in the chemoreceptor trigger zone. Patients' complaints of nausea should be evaluated not only from the standpoint of their acclimation to a new drug but also as possibly indicating erratic treatment adherence with frequent missed doses and withdrawal states. Anecdotally, compared with branded formulations, generic formulations of serotonergic antidepressants may be more likely to cause nausea and GI upset. Specifically, in the case of lithium, long-acting preparations that are absorbed more distally in the GI tract (e.g., Eskalith CR) or lithium citrate solution may be associated with less upper GI upset but potentially more lower GI symptoms (e.g., loose stools or diarrhea).

Adjunctive pharmacotherapies may sometimes be appropriate and useful to counteract transient nausea, although a more overriding concern is determining whether nausea represents a more serious adverse drug effect (e.g., pancreatitis from divalproex) or drug toxicity state (e.g., elevated lithium levels). In patients taking lithium, associated neurological signs (e.g., ataxia, tremor) or other GI symptoms (e.g., abdominal cramping) should alert the clinician to recognize nausea as a potential indicator of drug toxicity rather than merely a benign adverse effect remediable by symptomatic treatment. Antihistamines with antiemetic properties, such as trimethobenzamide (300 mg tid prn) or promethazine (12.5–25 mg bid prn), are perhaps the most reliable and safe pharmacological interventions for transient nausea. Antiemetic phenothiazines such as prochlorperazine or the D_2 antagonist/5-HT_3 antagonist metoclopramide also may be of value, although their potential for causing movement disorders due to their nigrostriatal antidopamine effects limits enthusiasm for their long-term use. (The FDA has approved use of metoclopramide for no longer than 4–12 weeks.)

Pancreatitis

General Recommendations

Patients who develop an acute abdomen require prompt evaluation. Patients taking divalproex, or less commonly, some SGAs (e.g., quetiapine, olanzapine, clozapine), should be assessed for iatrogenic pancreatitis through physical examination, measurement of serum lipase and amylase, and possible radiographic evaluation. In the setting of acute pancreatitis, the aforementioned drugs should be discontinued and not reintroduced.

Divalproex (both delayed- and extended-release formulations) may rarely be associated with the development of acute pancreatitis (■). The mechanism by which this may occur is not well understood. From 1979 to 2005, 90 cases were reported worldwide, although the true incidence may be underrecognized and underreported (Gerstner et al. 2007). Cases have been reported to occur during both recent and long-term treatment, up to 19 years after drug initiation (Taira et al. 2001). Routine screening of serum lipase or amylase levels in divalproex recipients is neither recommended nor clinically indicated in the absence of clinical signs that are suggestive of acute pancreatitis (i.e., development of an acute abdomen). Pancreatitis does not appear to be a class adverse effect among anticonvulsants, although rare case reports have been published that involved lamotrogine as part of DRESS syndrome (see section "Antiepileptic Hypersensitivity Reactions" in Chapter 20, "Systemic Reactions"), as well as carbamazepine, and levetiracetam. Gabapentin and pregabalin have also been described as viable treatments for pancreatitis-associated visceral pain.

Some SGAs (e.g., quetiapine, olanzapine, clozapine) have been associated with acute pancreatitis independent of hypertriglyceridemia or hyperglycemia, arising via poorly understood mechanisms. Rare case reports also exist of recurrent pancreatitis arising in connection with the use of mirtazapine.

Many nonpsychotropic drugs can also cause acute pancreatitis; these include estrogen, calcium, anticholinesterases, thiazide diuretics, pentamidine, ACE inhibitors, furosemide, tetracycline, metronidazole, isoniazid, rifampin, sulfonamides, cyclosporine, asparaginase, vinca alkaloids, and other antineoplastic drugs. Careful attention should be paid to other factors that may predispose patients to acute pancreatitis — notably, alcohol abuse or dependence (which often may be comorbid with conditions for which divalproex or an SGA may be used, such as bipolar disorder or impulsive aggression) — or hyperlipidemic states. Divalproex or the aforementioned SGAs should be discontinued and not reintroduced following identification and proper medical management of acute pancreatitis.

13

Genitourinary and Renal Systems

Dysuria and Urinary Retention

General Recommendations

Anticholinergic drugs or α_2-adrenergic blocking agents, as well as SNRIs and psychostimulants, may in rare cases cause urinary hesitancy or retention. Risk factors apart from preexisting benign prostatic hypertrophy have not been identified. Drugs suspected of causing urinary hesitancy or retention generally should be discontinued. Dysuria is an uncommon consequence of psychotropic agents that if not secondary to urinary hesitancy or retention, likely warrants independent urological evaluation. Symptomatic relief from urinary hesitancy or retention may occur from the temporary use of bethanechol (10–50 mg tid to qid), and dysuria may respond to the urinary tract analgesic phenazopyridine (200 mg tid with meals).

Anticholinergic agents can be associated with dysuria or urinary hesitancy, as well as urinary retention. Acute urinary retention also has been reported with SSRIs, SNRIs, and their combination (e.g., fluoxetine plus venlafaxine). Randomized controlled trials of duloxetine for major depression have collectively identified an incidence of 1% (20 of 2,097 subjects) encountering obstructive voiding symptoms, usually occurring

(>80% of cases) within the first 2 weeks of treatment initiation; no subjects developed urinary retention requiring catheterization (Viktrup et al. 2004). SNRI-associated urinary retention presumably arises due to α_2-adrenergic receptor antagonism, leading to contraction of the striated urethral sphincter. Amphetamine use has infrequently been associated with both urinary retention and incontinence. The risk for urinary hesitancy or urinary retention would presumably be higher in individuals with existing risk factors, such as benign prostatic hypertrophy, or in patients taking additional medications that may constrict bladder outflow. Urinary retention also has been reported as a rare adverse effect (~1% incidence) with the novel stimulant modafinil according to the manufacturer's product information.

The parasympathomimetic agent bethanechol is sometimes used to counteract urinary hesitancy. Typical adult dosing is 10–50 mg tid to qid. Pyridium is a urinary tract analgesic that is frequently used for the symptomatic relief of pain caused by irritation of the urinary tract mucosa. Adult dosing is typically 200 mg tid with meals.

Symptoms of burning when urinating, increased urinary frequency and urgency, hematuria, or pelvic discomfort leads most health care professionals to think of urinary tract infections, although it should be kept in mind that patients who have repeated exposures to ketamine incur a risk for ulcerative cystitis, thought to occur from damage to interstitial cells lining the bladder, as well as endothelial microvascular damage to the bladder and kidneys.

Enuresis and Urinary Incontinence

General Recommendations

Urinary incontinence may be a rare adverse effect with a number of antipsychotic, antidepressant, or anticonvulsant drugs. Enuresis is not clearly dose related, although it may be influenced in part if heavy sedation occurs. Reasonable pharmacological remedies for enuresis and urinary incontinence include adjunctive anticholinergic drugs (e.g., benztropine), ephedrine, intranasal desmopressin acetate (DDAVP; 10 μg in each nostril at bedtime), oxybutynin (5 mg bid to tid), or substitution of alternative pharmacotherapies for the presumptive offending agent.

Enuresis is a relatively infrequent adverse effect associated with clozapine and may respond to the anticholinergic drugs trihexyphenidyl (5 mg nightly) or benztropine (0.5–2 mg nightly). Urinary incontinence has been reported with risperidone (especially during co-therapy with SSRIs such as fluoxetine, which may increase serum risperidone levels), olanzapine, clozapine, gabapentin, SSRIs (including paroxetine and sertraline), and some SNRIs (e.g., venlafaxine). Diagnostic evaluation of enuresis with SGAs may require determining the absence of diabetes mellitus and nocturnal seizures or the presence of neurogenic bladder dysfunction. Ephedrine, up to 150 mg/day, has been reported as a potentially useful strategy to counteract olanzapine- or clozapine-induced urinary incontinence.

Drugs that may cause urinary retention (e.g., modafinil, anticholinergic drugs, and SNRIs such as duloxetine) may potentially counterbalance urinary incontinence if co-therapy is otherwise appropriate within an overall pharmacotherapy regimen. With respect to more traditional strategies for managing urinary incontinence, lack of efficacy was reported with the bladder-specific antimuscarinic agent tolterodine 2 mg bid in an adolescent female whose clozapine-induced enuresis was ultimately ameliorated by intranasal desmopressin (English et al. 2001). When used to counteract clozapine-induced enuresis, desmopressin nasal spray (typically dosed as 10 µg in each nostril at bedtime) may be associated with significant hyponatremia (Sarma et al. 2005). Oxybutynin, dosed at 5 mg bid or tid, also may be of value in the general management of iatrogenic enuresis. Persistent enuresis that is unresponsive to the pharmacological interventions recommended in this section and that does not eventually remit spontaneously may ultimately require replacement of the suspected causal agent with an alternative psychotropic medication.

Nephrotic Syndrome

General Recommendations

Symptoms of nephrotic syndrome (proteinuria, hypoalbuminemia, and peripheral edema) can have multiple etiologies and require careful evaluation. In rare cases, lithium may cause nephrotic syndrome, which is remediable by cessation of the drug.

Nephrotic syndrome arises from damage to the glomerular basement membrane (causing leakage of protein from filtered blood to urine), therefore manifesting with proteinuria (i.e., without hematuria [cf. nephritic syndrome]), as well as hypoalbuminemia, edema, and hyperlipidemia. Nephrotic syndrome can be a primary disorder or may be secondary to other medical conditions, such as diabetes mellitus, viral infections, amyloidosis, preeclampsia, or systemic lupus erythematosus. A handful of published cases have linked its occurrence with lithium therapy, although no risk factors for its development have been identified. Drug cessation, sometimes followed by corticosteroids, generally leads to resolution of symptoms.

Nephrotoxicity and Nephrogenic Diabetes Insipidus

General Recommendations

Lithium-associated polyuria or nephrogenic diabetes insipidus (NDI) can usually be effectively managed by the addition of amiloride 5 mg qd or bid, sometimes in combination with hydrochlorothiazide; periodic monitoring of serum potassium levels would be appropriate in cases of ongoing or long-term amiloride use. Once-daily lithium dosing may diminish the potential for developing long-term lithium-induced glomerulosclerosis.

During the course of lithium therapy, urinary frequency or quantity (i.e., polyuria) is common (evident in up to 70% of otherwise healthy individuals) and potentially seen more often in women and individuals with increased body weight (Kinahan et al. 2015). NDI is the most common adverse renal effect of lithium, occurring with an incidence of up to 40% (Grünfeld and Rossier 2009), and is a clinical diagnosis defined by the presence of polyuria, polydipsia, and a dilute urine with low urine electrolytes and osmolality, caused by impaired urinary concentrating ability. In contrast to diabetes mellitus, NDI involves an absence of glycosuria or hyperglycemia. A first step in identification involves obtaining a urinalysis to determine whether urine specific gravity is low, as well as measurements of urine electrolytes and osmolality. Serum sodium levels may be elevated due to hypovolemia caused by polyuria. Although some authorities believe that the development of NDI warrants cessation of lithium, others advise treating it with the potassium-sparing diuretic amiloride (typically dosed at 5 mg bid) (Finch et al. 2003), which has been shown to restore renal medullary osmolytes (i.e., concentrating ability). The thiazide diuretic hydrochlorothiazide can paradoxically improve NDI via decreasing distal tubular sodium reabsorption, leading to increased urinary sodium excretion, decreased extracellular fluid volume, and increased proximal tubular sodium and water reabsorption with resultant decreased urine volume. The combination of amiloride plus hydrochlorothiazide may together further increase urine osmolality and reduce urine volume. In addition, NSAIDs such as indomethacin also can reduce urinary free water loss and are sometimes used to help manage NDI. One must keep in mind that NSAIDs (especially indomethacin) can increase serum lithium levels with great variability across agents and across individuals, leading some experts to advise monitoring of serum lithium levels as often as every 4–5 days during long-term NSAID use until a new steady state is determined.

Lithium-associated nephrotoxicity has long been debated as a possible consequence of acute overdose, but whether it occurs at therapeutic dosages during long-term maintenance treatment has been more controversial. Before 2000, an extensive literature altogether challenged the nephrotoxicity of lithium, or the assertion that long-term lithium use caused changes in glomerular filtration rate (GFR) (Gitlin 1999; Schou 1988, 1997). Histopathological evidence from autopsy studies demonstrated unequivocal evidence of lithium-induced chronic tubulointerstitial nephrotoxicity (primarily affecting distal and collecting tubules) and segmental or global glomerulosclerosis (Markowitz et al. 2000), which challenged prior assumptions about the rarity (or even nonexistence) of structural kidney changes caused by lithium.

Reports in the literature have traditionally estimated the incidence of renal insufficiency as ranging from 4% (Gitlin 1993) to 20% (Lepkifiker et al. 2004), with variability based on the duration of exposure and the definition of renal insufficiency (e.g., loosely defined in some retrospective studies based on serum creatinine levels >1.5 mg/dL). Using a decision-analytic model based on 20 years of lithium exposure, Wernicke and colleagues (2012) estimated an approximate 14% risk of developing end-stage renal disease once chronic kidney disease (CKD), defined as a serum creatinine level ≥ 1.7 mg/dL, has developed. A cross-sectional report found that about half of bipolar patients taking lithium >20 years had at least some degree of reduced renal function (Bocchetta et al. 2015). On the other hand, other prospective long-term data dispute any increased risk for lithium to reduce GFR after age, baseline GFR, co-prescription of nephrotoxic drugs, and past episodes of lithium toxicity were controlled for (Clos et al. 2015). Thus, while some experts identify the duration of lithium exposure as a key factor in the risk for eventual chronic renal disease, it is important to recognize the potential impact of confounding factors on this relationship (Presne et al. 2003).

Although existing proprietary formulations of lithium carbonate advise administration in divided doses two or three times daily, it can be dosed all at once, given its 24-hour elimination half-life; moreover, once-daily lithium dosing has been suggested to pose a lesser risk than multiple daily doses for developing glomerulosclerosis or chronic kidney disease (Hetmar et al. 1991; Plenge et al. 1982). In fact, a large joint database study from the Massachusetts General Hospital and Brigham and Women's Hospital found that the most robust predictors of developing renal insufficiency while taking lithium were dosing more than once daily and having a maintenance serum lithium level that exceeds 0.6 mEq/L (Castro et al. 2016).

It is customary practice to monitor serum creatinine levels every 6 months for patients receiving long-term lithium therapy. Generally, if serum creatinine levels rise >25% from a patient's own previous level, or exceed 1.6 ng/mL, further investigation is warranted (Gitlin 1993). Creatinine clearance (CrCl), which is an approximation of the GFR, is a more specific measurement of renal function than serum creatinine. It reflects the flow rate of fluid undergoing filtration through the renal tubular system. Moreover, serum creatinine alone may be insensitive to milder degrees of renal insufficiency and can be normal even in the setting of substantially reduced GFR (Jefferson 2010). As noted in the section "Older Adults" in Chapter 3 ("Vulnerable Populations"), GFR typically diminishes by 10 mL/min for every decade after age 40 and is also dependent on weight. A normal GFR is approximately 97–137 mL/min for men and 88–128 mL/min for women.

CrCl can be estimated by the Cockcroft-Gault equation:

$$\text{CrCl} = \frac{(140 - \text{age}) \times \text{weight (in kg)} \times (0.85 \text{ if female})}{72 \times \text{serum creatinine}}$$

Use of estimating equations such as this one are considered the best overall indicator of kidney function (National Kidney Foundation 2002) but can be imprecise in early stages of chronic kidney disease and may sometimes underestimate true GFR (Jefferson 2010). Some authorities point out that the Cockcroft-Gault equation is inadequate because of its standardization to CrCl rather than true GFR. Newer, alternative methods of calculating GFR include the Modification of Diet in Renal Disease (MDRD) study equation and the Chronic Kidney Disease Epidemiology Collaboration equation (CKD-EPI). There also has been increasing interest in the measurement of serum cystatin C, a low-molecular-weight renally filtered protein that has a stronger and more linear relationship to true GFR than does creatinine. Patients who exercise heavily or lift weights also may have elevated levels of muscle creatine kinase, favoring the measurement of serum cystatin C over serum creatinine. When measured alone or in conjunction with creatinine, cystatin C–based eGFRs may provide more accurate estimates of true GFR and the potential for underlying kidney disease (Shlipak et al. 2013). Degrees of chronic kidney disease are classified by the National Kidney Foundation's (2002) Kidney Disease Outcomes Quality Initiative, as summarized in Table 13–1.

Clinicians also should consider other possible causes of age-related inappropriately diminished CrCl, such as medications (e.g., cimetidine, ACE inhibitors, and certain nephrotoxic antibiotics such as trimethoprim and cephalosporins).

Priapism

General Recommendations

Iatrogenic priapism is a rare phenomenon that may occur during treatment with trazodone, as well as several SGAs, SSRIs, psychostimulants, or bupropion. Priapism constitutes a medical and possible surgical emergency and requires urgent evaluation in an appropriate medical setting such as an emergency department.

Priapism is defined by the American Urological Association as an erection that occurs without sexual stimulation and lasts longer than 4 hours. As a type of compartment syndrome, it poses a medical (if not surgical) urological emergency and involves a specific management strategy as outlined in clinical guidelines published by the American Urological Association (Montague et al. 2003). Urologists differentiate between priapism that is ischemic (low-flow, painful) and nonischemic (high-flow, less common, and generally nonemergent, usually resulting from arterial steal or shunting of blood). Psychotropically induced priapism involves ischemic priapism. Nonischemic priapism may result from several primary medical conditions, including sickle cell anemia, hematological malignancies, thalassemia, and genital trauma.

By definition, ischemic priapism is not ameliorated by sexual intercourse or masturbation. Its proper evaluation and treatment should occur in an emergency department or similar medical setting. The American Urological Association advises urgent intracavernous injection of an α-adrenergic sympathomimetic agent, such as phenylephrine, with or without evacuation of blood in the corpus cavernosum, performed with local or regional anesthesia. If this treatment fails to alleviate priapism, a surgical shunting procedure may be necessary. Oral medications such as β_2-adrenergic agonists (e.g., terbutaline) or the oral α-adrenergic agonist pseudoephedrine, although sometimes used in nonischemic priapism, are not recommended for the treatment of ischemic priapism.

TABLE 13–1.   Classification of chronic kidney disease

Stage	Description	Glomerular filtration rate (GFR)
1	Kidney damage with no GFR increase	≥ 90 mL/min/1.73 m^2
2	Kidney damage with mild GFR decrease	60–89 mL/min/1.73 m^2
3	Moderately decreased GFR	30–59 mL/min/1.73 m^2
4	Severely decreased GFR	15–29 mL/min/1.73 m^2
5	Kidney failure	<15 mL/min/1.73 m^2 (or dialysis)

Source.   National Kidney Foundation 2002.

Priapism is an exceedingly rare but often-mentioned adverse effect associated with trazodone (incidence of approximately 1 in 6,000; reports include its occurrence after only a single dose; most reported cases occur within the first 28 days of its initiation). Less well recognized are rare cases of priapism associated with both FGAs and SGAs, possibly mediated by α_1-adrenergic blockade (Andersohn et al. 2010), including reports involving quetiapine, risperidone, ziprasidone, clozapine, and olanzapine. Rare cases of priapism also have been reported with atomoxetine, fluoxetine, fluvoxamine, citalopram, and bupropion. In 2013 the FDA issued a warning that methylphenidate products may cause priapism, based on reports of 15 such cases to the FDA Adverse Event Reporting System (FAERS) from 1997 through 2012; no such warning was applied to amphetamine products (https://www.fda.gov/Drugs/DrugSafety/ucm375796.htm). Case reports (and product manufacturers' warnings) also identify priapism as a risk associated with the use of PDE type 5 inhibitors such as sildenafil or vardenafil.

When using medications that may increase the risk for priapism, clinicians should recognize the presence of pretreatment baseline risk factors, such as the presence of blood dyscrasias (e.g., sickle cell disease, multiple myeloma, leukemia). Paradoxically, PDE type 5 inhibitors can also sometimes effectively treat recurrent ischemic priapism (also termed "stuttering priapism").

Cases of clitoral priapism that manifest with vulvar pain lasting from 24 to 60 hours have been described in connection with the use of trazodone, olanzapine, nefazodone, citalopram, and bupropion; this effect is managed with drug cessation and the administration of α-adrenergic agonists in analogous fashion to that of male priapism. Clinicians should consider a broad differential diagnosis for priapism, particularly in women with respect to vascular obstruction due to pelvic floor and bladder malignancies.

Renal Calculi

General Recommendations

A history of renal calculi is a relative contraindication to treatment with topiramate. Adequate hydration is imperative in all patients taking topiramate to minimize the risk of stone formation.

Calcium phosphate renal calculi are a known risk (approximately 1% incidence) in individuals taking topiramate, attributable to topiramate's inhibition of carbonic anhydrase in the kidney, which in turn can cause hypocitraturia, hypercalciuria, and acidified urine. Accordingly, a history of nephrolithiasis is a relative contraindication to the use of topiramate. Some practitioners advise increased oral water intake in patients taking topiramate, although it is not clear whether this precaution meaningfully counters the risk for developing renal calculi. Notably, individuals who follow a ketogenic diet (i.e., high-protein diet with avoidance of carbohydrates) may be independently predisposed to the development of renal calculi due to hypercalciuria, decreased urinary citrate excretion, and acidified urine; hence, the use of topiramate in conjunction with a ketogenic diet may warrant particular caution with respect to monitoring for nephrolithiasis (Paul et al. 2010).

Renal calculi (composed of calcium or urate salts) appear to be a rare phenomenon with zonisamide (15 cases reported from 1,296 clinical trial subjects [1.2% incidence] over an 8.7-year period; Wroe 2007). However, the manufacturer's product information identifies a 4% incidence rate during drug development for adult epilepsy, arising most often from 6 to 12 months after drug initiation but with new cases still occurring >1 year after beginning therapy. The manufacturer advises that patients drink 6–8 glasses of water daily to help prevent kidney stone formation.

Renal Insufficiency

General Recommendations

Random creatinine measurements are advisable semiannually with lithium; serum creatinine rises of >25% from a prior baseline may warrant collection of 24-hour urine for direct measurement of CrCl. No absolute value has been established for GFRs below which lithium or other renally cleared drugs should be discontinued, but progressive declines in renal function or the emergence of moderate to severe renal impairment signals the need for closer, more frequent renal monitoring, as well as renal dosing of many medications and their probable eventual discontinuation.

Most psychotropic drugs either are directly excreted renally or have active metabolites that are renally excreted. Hence, the presence of impaired renal clearance often requires reduced dosing depending on the magnitude of renal insufficiency, as described in Table 13–1. A 2012 review alongside recommendations by the European Renal Best Practice (ERBP) observed that in patients with CKD stages 3–5, marked reductions in drug clearance were observed for oral selegiline, venlafaxine, desvenlafaxine, milnacipran, bupropion, reboxetine, and tianeptine.

Table 13–2 summarizes manufacturers' recommendations for dosing adjustments of psychotropic medications in the setting of renal insufficiency.

Sexual Dysfunction

Impaired Arousal, Erectile Dysfunction, and Anorgasmia

General Recommendations

Lowest incident rates of antidepressant-associated sexual dysfunction have been reported in FDA registration trials with bupropion, desvenlafaxine, duloxetine, mirtazapine, nefazodone, selegiline transdermal system, vilazodone, and vortioxetine. SNRIs may be somewhat less likely than SSRIs to cause this phenomenon, although such differences have not been affirmed in comparative trials. Bupropion added to SSRIs has shown modest benefit to overcome existing iatrogenic sexual dysfunction. Adjunctive sildenafil 50–100 mg/day, up to 200 mg/day, appears to be the most effective pharmacological intervention to remedy sexual arousal that is diminished by serotonergic antidepressants in men or women. Other evidence-based antidotes to iatrogenic sexual dysfunction include adjunctive buspirone, testosterone, mirtazapine, and dehydroepiandrosterone (DHEA).

TABLE 13–2. Renal considerations for psychotropic agents

Agent	Recommendations
Atomoxetine	No dosing adjustment is necessary in the setting of renal insufficiency.
Buspirone	Patients with CrCl of 10–70 mL/min demonstrate an approximate 4-fold increase in serum drug levels. Dosages should be reduced accordingly.

Anticonvulsants and lithium

Agent	Recommendations
Carbamazepine	No dosing adjustment is necessary in the setting of renal insufficiency.
Divalproex	Renal failure is associated with an increased unbound fraction (and slightly reduced clearance) of free valproic acid. No dosage adjustment is necessary in the setting of renal failure.
Gabapentin	For CrCl of 30–60 mL/min, maximum dosage=300 mg bid; for CrCl of 15–30 mL/min, maximum dosage=300 mg/day; for CrCl <15 mL/min, maximum dosage=300 mg every other day.
Lamotrigine	Manufacturer's product information states that "reduced maintenance doses may be effective for patients with significant renal impairment" and that "Lamictal should be used with caution in these patients" because "there is inadequate experience in this population."
Lithium	In chronic kidney disease patients for whom alternatives to lithium may not be feasible, some authors advise the following: for GFR >50 mL/min, no dosing modification is necessary; for GFR=10–50 mL/min, administer 50%–75% of usual dose; for GFR <10 mL/min, administer 20%–50% of usual dose (Aronoff et al. 1999). In end-stage renal disease patients undergoing hemodialysis, administer a single dose of 200–600 mg after each hemodialysis session, guided by levels checked immediately before hemodialysis (Cohen et al. 2004).

TABLE 13–2.   Renal considerations for psychotropic agents *(continued)*

Agent	Recommendations
Anticonvulsants and lithium *(continued)*	
Oxcarbazepine	Dosing is halved when CrCl is <30 mL/min (in which case, dosing should be started at 150 mg bid).
Pregabalin	Dosing must be reduced in the presence of renal failure (for CrCl of 30–60 mL/min, maximum dosage=75–300 mg/day in 2–3 divided doses; for CrCl of 15–30 mL/min, maximum dosage= 25–150 mg/day given once or in 2 divided doses daily; for CrCl of <15 mL/min, maximum dosage=25–75 mg/day).
Topiramate	For CrCl of <70 mL/min, the usual dosage is halved and upward titration is done slowly.
Antidepressants	
Bupropion	ERBP advises against dosing >150 mg/day in CKD stages 3–5 (Nagler et al. 2012).
Citalopram	No dosing adjustment is necessary for individuals with mild to moderate renal impairment. Caution is advised for use in severe renal disease, although ERBP advises that no dosing adjustments are necessary in CKD stages 3–5 (Nagler et al. 2012).
Desvenlafaxine	Recommended dosage in the setting of moderate renal impairment is 50 mg/day; 50 mg every other day is advised in severe renal impairment; ERBP advises dosing of 25 mg/day with "careful increases" in CKD stage 3 and dosing no higher than 25 mg/day in CKD stages 4–5 (Nagler et al. 2012).
Duloxetine	Administration is not recommended for patients with end-stage renal disease or severe renal impairment (i.e., CrCl of <30 mL/min). ERBP recommends no dosing adjustment in CKD stage 3 but careful increases >40 mg/day in CKD stages 4–5 (Nagler et al. 2012).

TABLE 13–2.   Renal considerations for psychotropic agents *(continued)*

Agent	Recommendations
Antidepressants *(continued)*	
Escitalopram	No dosing adjustment is necessary for individuals with mild to moderate renal impairment. Dosages >10 mg/day should be done with caution in CKD stages 4–5 (Nagler et al. 2012).
Fluoxetine	No dosing adjustment is necessary in the setting of renal insufficiency.
Fluvoxamine	Low initial dosing is advised in the setting of mild to moderate renal impairment, although ERBP advises no dosing adjustments as being necessary in CKD stages 3–5 (Nagler et al. 2012).
Levomilnacipran	Maximum dosage is 40 mg/day in setting of moderate renal impairment (CKD stages 3–4) and 80 mg/day in severe renal impairment (CKD stage 5); not recommended in patients with ESRD.
MAOIs	Isocarboxazid, phenelzine, and tranylcypromine are not recommended in patients with clinically significant renal disease; however, the ERBP advises that in CKD stages 3–5, no dosing adjustment is necessary with isocarboxazid or phenelzine, but in CKD stages 4–5, tranylcypromine should be started at 30 mg/day and "increased carefully." Transdermal selegiline requires no dosing modification in the setting of renal insufficiency, although the ERBP advises oral selegiline dosing no greater than 5 mg/day in CKD stages 4–5.
Mirtazapine	Clearance of mirtazapine is reduced by ~30% in moderate renal insufficiency (CrCl of 11–39 mL/min) and by ~50% for CrCl ≤10 mL/min. The manufacturer advises caution when administering to patients with renal impairment. ERBP advises no dosing adjustment in CKD stage 3 but "careful increases" above 15 mg/day in CKD stages 4–5 (Nagler et al. 2012).

TABLE 13–2.   Renal considerations for psychotropic agents *(continued)*

Agent	Recommendations
Antidepressants *(continued)*	
Nefazodone	No dosing adjustment is necessary in the setting of renal insufficiency, although the ERBP advises caution if dosing >100 mg/day in CKD stages 3–5 (Nagler et al. 2012).
Paroxetine	Mean plasma concentrations increase approximately 4-fold in the setting of severe renal impairment (i.e., CrCl of <30 mL/min), and about 2-fold when CrCl is 30–60 mL/min. Dosage reductions and slowed titration schedules are therefore advised if dosing >10 mg/day occurs in CKD stages 3–5 (Nagler et al. 2012).
Sertraline	No dosing adjustment is necessary in the setting of renal insufficiency; however, the ERBP advises "careful increases" if dosing above 50 mg/day in CKD stage 4 and if dosing above 25 mg/day in CKD stage 5, with a reduced maximum dose (Nagler et al. 2012).
TCAs	In CKD stages 3–5, the ERBP advises no necessary dosing adjustments with doxepin, nortriptyline, and amitriptyline; for desipramine, no dosing adjustments are advised for CKD stages 3–4, while dosing initiation at 25 mg/day should be "increased carefully" in CKD stage 5; for clomipramine or imipramine, no dosing adjustment is recommended for CKD stage 3, but dose initiation should be 10 mg/day and the doasge "increased carefully" in CKD stages 4–5 (Nagler et al. 2012).
Venlafaxine	For CrCl of 10–70 mL/min, total daily dosing should be decreased by 25%–50%. ERBP advises no dosing adjustment in CKD stage 3 but dosing only from 37.5–112.5 mg/day in CKD stages 4–5 (Nagler et al. 2012).

TABLE 13–2. Renal considerations for psychotropic agents *(continued)*

Agent	Recommendations
Antidepressants *(continued)*	
Vilazodone	No dosing adjustment is necessary in the setting of renal insufficiency.
Vortioxetine	No dosing adjustment is necessary in the setting of renal insufficiency.
Benzodiazepines	Short-acting agents, and those with fewer active metabolites, such as oxazepam or lorazepam, are preferred over longer-acting agents (e.g., clonazepam or chlordiazepoxide) and those with many active metabolites (e.g., diazepam).
SGAs	
Aripiprazole	No significant pharmacokinetic differences in patients with significant renal failure (Mallikaarjun et al. 2008); renal dosing adjustments are likely unnecessary.
Asenapine	No dosing adjustment is necessary in the setting of renal impairment.
Brexpiprazole	For patients with CKD stages 3–5, the maximum recommended dosage is 2 mg/day in major depressive disorder and 3 mg/day in schizophrenia.
Cariprazine	No dosing adjustment is necessary in mild to moderate renal impairment (CrCl≥30 mL/min). Use is not recommended when CrCl<30 mL/min.
Lurasidone	For CrCl of 10–50 mL/min (i.e., moderate to severe renal impairment), the manufacturer recommends that daily dosage should not exceed 40 mg/day.
Olanzapine	No dosing adjustment is necessary in the setting of renal impairment.
Paliperidone	In mild impairment (CrCl of 50–80 mL/min), recommended dosage is 3–6 mg/day. In moderate to severe impairment (CrCl of 10–50 mL/min), recommended initial dosage is 1.5 mg/day and maximum dosage is 3 mg/day.

TABLE 13–2.   Renal considerations for psychotropic agents *(continued)*

Agent	Recommendations
SGAs *(continued)*	
Quetiapine	Plasma concentrations of quetiapine appear no different in the setting of renal insufficiency. Dosing adjustment is therefore not necessary in the setting of renal impairment.
Risperidone	The manufacturer advises an initial dosage not exceeding 0.5 mg bid in patients with renal impairment, with subsequent increases of no more than 0.5 mg bid; dosage increases above 1.5 mg bid should occur at least 1 week apart.
Ziprasidone	Dosing adjustment is not necessary in the setting of renal impairment.
Sedative-hypnotics	
Eszopiclone	Dosing adjustment is not necessary in the setting of renal impairment.
Suvorexant	Dosing adjustment is not necessary in the setting of renal impairment.
Zolpidem	Dosing adjustment is not necessary in the setting of renal impairment.
Other CNS agents	
Deutetrabenazine	No data, but because deutetrabenazine is renally excreted, usage in CKD stages 4–5 should likely be done with caution pending further studies.
Valbenazine	Dosing adjustment is not necessary in mild to moderate renal impairment (CrCl ≥ 30 mL/min); not recommended in CKD stages 4–5.

Note.   bid=twice daily; CKD=chronic kidney disease; CNS=central nervous system; CrCl=creatinine clearance; ERBP=European Renal Best Practice; ESRD=end-stage renal disease; GFR=glomerular filtration rate; MAOI= monoamine oxidase inhibitor; SGA=second-generation antipsychotic; TCA= tricyclic antidepressant.

Patient concerns about impaired sexual functioning resulting from psychotropic medications rank among the highest reasons for poor adherence to continued treatment with antidepressants and other (usually serotonergic or antidopaminergic) agents (Kennedy and Rizvi 2009; Serretti and Chiesa 2011). However, because patients tend not to spontaneously discuss sexual functioning, either as a possible drug side effect or illness symptom, clinicians need to proactively assess sexual function with an awareness of the relative adverse sexual effects of different psychotropic agents, as well as the distinct areas of human sexual responsivity affected by common medications. Indeed, although premarketing studies of many antidepressants identify relatively low rates of spontaneously reported sexual dysfunction, adverse sexual effects are often not proactively assessed in pivotal trials, and hence are underreported. Findings from studies in which patients were specifically asked about sexual dysfunction with SSRIs or other antidepressants suggest that incidence rates may be as high as 80% (Hu et al. 2014). Formal assessment ratings, such as the Arizona Sexual Experiences Scale (ASEX; McGahuey et al. 2000), the Changes in Sexual Functioning Questionnaire (CSFQ; Clayton et al. 1997), or the Psychotropic-Related Sexual Dysfunction Questionnaire (PRSexDQ; Montejo and Rico-Villademoros 2008) (see "Rating Scales for Measuring Adverse Drug Effects" in Appendix 3) may aid clinicians in detecting and monitoring sexual dysfunction during longitudinal treatment.

The human sexual response cycle is divided into three components, including interest (libido), excitation and arousal (i.e., erections in men and vaginal lubrication in women), and orgasm. Diminished interest in sex is a common adverse effect of serotonergic antidepressants, although even nonserotonergic antidepressants have been associated with an increased risk for delayed ejaculation in some studies. Men taking antidepressants appear significantly more likely than women to encounter impaired sexual desire and orgasm, whereas women may be more prone to impaired arousal (Clayton et al. 2006). SSRI treatment may be more likely to lead to remission of impaired sexual desire and arousal in depressed women, but not orgasmic dysfunction in depressed men.

Antidepressants

Serotonergic antidepressants may adversely affect all components of sexual functioning, as well as sexual satisfaction. Although it is often difficult to distinguish whether depression itself or antidepressants are the proximal cause of decreased libido and sexual dysfunction, antidepressants are often thought to be more prone to impair excitation and arousal (i.e., erectile dysfunction and delayed ejaculation in men, or impaired lubrication in women) and orgasm, whereas depression may more often impair libido than other phases of the sexual response cycle.

Agonism of serotonin type 2A (5-HT$_{2A}$) postsynaptic receptors is believed to contribute to impaired sexual functioning and, consequently, may be an unintended effect of serotonergic agents that fail to block or antagonize 5-HT$_{2A}$ receptors. Correspondingly, serotonergic agents that block postsynaptic 5-HT$_{2A}$ receptors may incur minimal sexual dysfunction, as has been demonstrated in preliminary open-label fashion with mirtazapine (Saiz-Ruiz et al. 2005) or adjunctive trazodone for SSRI-induced sexual dysfunction (Stryjer et al. 2009). Preliminary data suggest that adjunctive mirtazapine is superior to placebo for improving FGA-associated orgasmic dysfunction in schizophrenia (Terevnikov et al. 2017), but data are lacking on the use of adjunctive mirtazapine for SSRI- or SNRI-associated sexual dysfunction.

A prospective multicenter study comparing various SSRIs found that paroxetine caused significantly more orgasmic delay, ejaculation, or impotence than did fluoxetine, sertraline, or fluvoxamine (Montejo-González et al. 1997). These authors also found SSRI-induced sexual dysfunction to be a dose-related phenomenon. Similarly, paroxetine 20 mg/day was significantly more likely than citalopram 20 mg/day (Waldinger et al. 2001) or mirtazapine 30 mg/day (Waldinger et al. 2003) to delay orgasm and ejaculation in affectively healthy men with premature ejaculation. Another study of men with premature ejaculation, comparing paroxetine 20 mg/day, fluoxetine 20 mg/day, sertraline 50 mg/day, fluvoxamine 100 mg/day, and placebo, found that paroxetine caused the greatest delay in ejaculation and that fluvoxamine caused the least (Waldinger et al. 1998).

The novel serotonergic antidepressants vortioxetine and vilazodone appear to have relatively modest incident rates of prospectively measured sexual dysfunction in clinical trials of major depression. For ex-ample, a randomized 8-week comparison of vortioxetine (10–20 mg/day) or escitalopram (10–20 mg/day) among treated major depression patients who had developed sexual dysfunction while taking sertraline, paroxetine, or citalopram found a significantly greater improvement in overall sexual functioning, as well as in component domains (e.g., desire, arousal, orgasm), among those switched to vortioxetine than among those switched to escitalopram (Jacobson et al. 2015). Pooled analyses of seven randomized trials of vortioxetine for major depressive disorder or generalized anxiety disorder found no differences from placebo in ASEX scores at doses of 5 mg/day or 10 mg/day, but treatment-emergent sexual dysfunction was higher than with placebo at doses of 15 mg/day or 20 mg/day (Jacobson et al. 2016). Across dosages, ASEX scores were lower with vortioxetine than with duloxetine (which was studied as an active comparator).

Another prospective trial comparing paroxetine, sertraline, venlafaxine, and moclobemide found that men were more likely than women to encounter diminished sexual desire but that no gender differences emerged in arousal and orgasm (Kennedy et al. 2000). Overall rates of sexual dysfunction were lower with moclobemide or venlafaxine than with SSRIs. Other trials similarly suggest a lower incidence of sexual dysfunction with SNRIs (e.g., duloxetine, dosed at 40–120 mg/day) than with pure serotonergic reuptake inhibitors (e.g., paroxetine, dosed at 20 mg/day) (Delgado et al. 2005).

Antipsychotics

SGAs might be expected to incur relatively low rates of sexual dysfunction by virtue of their postsynaptic 5-HT_{2A} blockade, although agents that increase prolactin release can in turn induce sexual adverse effects. In patients with chronic schizophrenia, findings from the CATIE study found relatively similar rates of sexual dysfunction (19%–27%) across the FGAs and SGAs studied, without clear links to differences in reported changes in serum prolactin (Lieberman et al. 2005). In fact, even agents that showed *reductions* from baseline serum prolactin levels in CATIE (i.e., quetiapine and ziprasidone) had approximate 20% incidence rates of sexual dysfunction. Because of interindividual variability between changes in serum prolactin and the potential for sexual dysfunction, other endocrinological or physiological factors likely contribute to (or mediate) iatrogenic sexual dysfunction from SGAs.

A meta-analysis of reported incidence rates of sexual dysfunction with FGAs and SGAs ($N=7,975$ subjects) identified the following rank ordering of global sexual dysfunction (most dysfunction to least dysfunction): thioridazine > clozapine > haloperidol > risperidone > olanzapine > aripiprazole > perphenazine > ziprasidone > quetiapine. In addition, aripiprazole and ziprasidone caused the least degree of impaired sexual desire, whereas aripiprazole and quetiapine both caused the least degree of arousal dysfunction and orgasmic dysfunction (Serretti and Chiesa 2011).

Other Agents

Tables 13–3 through 13–6 summarize information regarding iatrogenic sexual dysfunction from randomized controlled trials with commonly used psychotropic medications: SGAs (Table 13–3), sedative-hypnotics

(Table 13–4), lithium and anticonvulsants (Table 13–5), and antidepressant and related noradrenergic or serotonergic agents (Table 13–6).

Case reports exist of divalproex-associated anorgasmia and decreased libido in men and women with bipolar disorder, migraine, or epilepsy; these effects are possibly dose related and are generally in the context of cotherapy with other medications. Dosage reductions have not reliably eliminated sexual side effects in reported cases, although drug cessation has. With respect to lithium, one study of 104 outpatients with bipolar disorder revealed an incidence of sexual dysfunction among 14% of those undergoing monotherapy but among 49% of those taking lithium plus a benzodiazepine (Ghadirian et al. 1992). A subsequent review identified only 13 publications examining lithium-associated sexual dysfunction, noting from preclinical studies that lithium can reduce testosterone levels and impair nitric oxide–mediated relaxation of corpus cavernosum musculature (Elnazer et al. 2015).

Controlled trials conducted outside of industry, for purposes other than label indications, often reveal higher rates of sexual dysfunction with antidepressants than identified in FDA registration trials. These include incidence rates for overall sexual dysfunction of 22% and 25% with bupropion IR and SR, respectively, over a variable duration from less than 1 week to more than 3 years (Clayton et al. 2002); 33% with duloxetine over 8 months (Clayton et al. 2007); and 49% with escitalopram over 8 months (Clayton et al. 2007).

Management

Strategies to manage anorgasmia or other sexual side effects of SSRIs — apart from switching altogether to alternative primary agents — focus mainly on the use of adjunctive pharmacotherapies, although the concept of "weekend holidays" from an SSRI (specifically, sertraline or paroxetine, but not fluoxetine) has been suggested to significantly improve sexual functioning (Rothschild 1995). The potential benefit of such a break must be weighed against the potential for SSRI-discontinuation withdrawal symptoms.

A wide range of pharmacotherapy strategies have been proposed on mechanistic grounds and studied empirically as intended remedies to counteract antidepressant-induced sexual dysfunction. Some capitalize on putative mechanisms of action (e.g., introducing blockade of 5-HT$_2$ receptors) or efforts to reverse antidepressant-induced increases in peripheral/genitourinary serotonergic tone (e.g., cyproheptadine) or to "override" serotonergic effects by introducing catecholaminergic agents (e.g., bupropion, stimulants). Others focus on the role of nitric oxide and PDE

TABLE 13–3. Incidence of sexual dysfunction in clinical trials of second-generation antipsychotics

Agent	Rates reported in FDA registration trials or randomized controlled studies
Aripiprazole	Libido either increased or decreased in <1% across FDA registration trials. Greater improvement from baseline in overall sexual functioning was seen with aripiprazole compared with olanzapine, risperidone, or quetiapine in a 26-week multisite open randomized industry-supported study (Schizophrenia Trial of Aripiprazole; Hanssens et al. 2008).
Asenapine	In all registration trials for bipolar mania or schizophrenia, both short- and long-term, incidence of sexual dysfunction was ≤1% (per manufacturer).
Brexpiprazole	NR
Cariprazine	NR
Iloperidone	In schizophrenia FDA registration trials, decreased libido and anorgasmia were reported in ≥1%; ejaculation failure occurred in 2% across dosages.
Lurasidone	NR
Olanzapine	Across indications, FDA registration trials reported decreased libido in ≤1%. In CATIE, sexual dysfunction was reported in 27% (Lieberman et al. 2005).
Paliperidone	NR
Pimavanserin	NR
Quetiapine	Across all indications, FDA registration trials reported decreased libido in 1%–2% and abnormal ejaculation in ≤1%. In CATIE, sexual dysfunction was reported in 20% (Lieberman et al. 2005).

TABLE 13–3.   Incidence of sexual dysfunction in clinical trials of second-generation antipsychotics *(continued)*

Agent	Rates reported in FDA registration trials or randomized controlled studies
Risperidone	Across indications, FDA registration trials and postmarketing reports identified impaired ejaculation in ≤1%, and decreased libido and anorgasmia in <1%. In CATIE, sexual dysfunction was reported in 27% (Lieberman et al. 2005).
Ziprasidone	In FDA registration trials for schizophrenia, impotence, anorgasmia, or abnormal ejaculation occurred in ≤1%. In CATIE, sexual dysfunction was reported in 19% (Lieberman et al. 2005). Incidence rates of sexual dysfunction in trials for bipolar disorder were not reported.

Note.   CATIE=Clinical Antipsychotic Trials of Intervention Effectiveness; FDA=U.S. Food and Drug Administration; NR=not reported.

inhibitors, such as sildenafil, vardenafil, or tadalafil. Inhibition of PDE prevents the catabolism of cyclic guanosine monophosphate, which in turn facilitates the relaxation of smooth muscle lining the corpus cavernosum. A related strategy involves using L-arginine, a precursor of nitric oxide, for a similar purpose.

PDE inhibitors were initially studied and adapted for the treatment of sexual dysfunction in men, although more recent studies have also demonstrated their value in SSRI-associated sexual dysfunction in women (see Table 13–7). Notably, however, adjunctive sildenafil in women appears better than placebo in helping to improve anorgasmia but not desire, arousal-sensation, arousal-lubrication, or orgasmic satisfaction (Nurnberg et al. 2008). By contrast, in men, all measured components of sexual functioning, including sexual desire, arousal, erectile function, ability to orgasm, and orgasmic satisfaction, have shown significant improvement with adjunctive sildenafil (Fava et al. 2006; Nurnberg et al. 2003).

PDE inhibitors represent the best studied and most robust strategy to counteract sexual dysfunction caused by serotonergic antidepressants. A 2013 Cochrane Review reported an overall 11.5-fold improvement in erectile function among men taking tadalafil (vs. placebo) caused by se-

TABLE 13–4. Incidence of sexual dysfunction in sedative-hypnotic clinical trials

Agent	Rates reported in FDA registration trials or randomized controlled studies
Benzodiazepines	In general, ≤1%–3% incidence of sexual dysfunction across agents
Eszopiclone	Decreased libido in <3% of patients taking 3 mg/day; no reports of erectile dysfunction or anorgasmia
Suvorexant	NR
Zaleplon	Decreased libido or impotence in <1%
Zolpidem	Decreased libido or impotence in <0.1%

Note. FDA=U.S. Food and Drug Administration; NR=not reported.

rotonergic antidepressants, while potential benefits in women appear more uncertain (Taylor et al. 2013). Prescribers must be aware of the potential of PDE inhibitors to cause modest decreases in blood pressure (e.g., sildenafil has been shown to lower blood pressure in healthy volunteers by about 9/6 mm Hg). The vasodilatory effects of sildenafil pose at least a theoretical risk for exacerbating underlying cardiovascular disease, although adverse hemodynamic effects in men with coronary artery disease have not been demonstrated, and use of sildenafil is not necessarily contraindicated in this population.

There have been rare reports of vision loss from sildenafil or vardenafil due to nonarteritic anterior ischemic optic neuropathy. The manufacturers of these drugs point out that most people who take them have underlying predispositions to visual problems (e.g., diabetic retinopathy), although risk factors for developing loss of vision with PDE inhibitors have not been described. Patients who begin a PDE inhibitor should be counseled to inform the prescriber if they notice any visual changes, and treatment should be discontinued unless alternative explanations are identified.

A number of other pharmacological approaches have been described and studied with more variable results, as summarized in Table 13–7. Also, with few exceptions, there has been little study of combination therapy approaches that use complementary and possible synergistic mechanisms to overcome impaired sexual functioning caused by psychotropic agents.

TABLE 13–5.   Incidence of sexual dysfunction in FDA registration trials of lithium and anticonvulsants

Agent	Impotence	Decreased libido	Delayed ejaculation	Anorgasmia
Carbamazepine	<5%	NR	NR	NR
Divalproex	NR	NR	NR	NR
Gabapentin	NR	≥1%	<1%	<1%
Lamotrigine	<1%	<1%	<1%	NR
Lithium	NR	NR	NR	NR
Oxcarbazepine	NR	NR	NR	NR
Topiramate	NR	1%–3%	NR	NR

Note.   FDA=U.S. Food and Drug Administration; NR=not reported.

Noteworthy from the findings presented in Table 13–7 is the failure in two studies (DeBattista et al. 2005; Masand et al. 2001) of adjunctive bupropion to reverse SSRI-induced sexual dysfunction with dosages of 150 mg/day, but the apparent benefit in other studies with dosages of 75–150 mg/day (Ashton and Rosen 1998) or 150 mg twice daily (Safarinejad 2010). A further corollary to these observations is that replacement (rather than augmentation) of purely serotonergic agents with catecholaminergic, nonindoleaminergic antidepressants (such as bupropion) or with antidepressants that selectively block 5-HT$_{2A}$ postsynaptic receptors (e.g., mirtazapine) may produce substantially less sexual dysfunction than seen with an SSRI. The incidence of sexual dysfunction with SNRIs (i.e., duloxetine, venlafaxine, desvenlafaxine) appears less than that seen with purely serotonergic agents.

In unmedicated men with erectile dysfunction (Lebret et al. 2002) or women with sexual arousal disorder (Meston and Worcel 2002), the combination of yohimbine (6 mg/day) with the nitric oxide precursor L-arginine glutamate (6 g/day) has shown benefits over placebo that may reflect synergistic effects (presynaptic α$_2$ blockade may both enhance genital nitric oxide release and reduce risk of hypotension from nitric oxide–related vasodilation, while nitric oxide donation may increase genital effects of yohimbine). However, this combination has not been studied specifically as a strategy to counteract sexual dysfunction induced by antidepressants or other psychotropics. Other possible viable strategies for noniatrogenic hypoactive sexual arousal in postmenopausal women include DHEA 300 mg/day.

TABLE 13–6. Incidence of sexual dysfunction in U.S. Food and Drug Administration registration trials of antidepressant and related noradrenergic or serotonergic agents[a]

Agent	Impotence	Decreased libido	Erectile dysfunction	Delayed ejaculation	Anorgasmia
Atomoxetine	NR	4%	9%	3%	≥2%
Bupropion	<1%	<1%	NR	<1%	NR
Buspirone	<0.1%	<1%	NR	<0.1%	NR
Citalopram	3%	3.8% (men), 1.3% (women)	NR	6.1%	1.1% (women)
Desvenlafaxine[b]	NR	4%–5%	3%–6%	1%–5%	0–3%
Duloxetine[c]	NR	NR	NR	NR	NR
Escitalopram	2%	6% (men), 3% (women)	NR	12%	3% (women)
Fluoxetine	NR	4%	NR	NR	NR
Fluvoxamine	2%	4%–8%	3%	11%	4%–5%
Levomilnacipran	NR	NR	6%	5%	NR
MAOIs other than transdermal selegiline: isocarboxazid, phenelzine, tranylcypromine	NR	NR	NR	NR	NR
Mirtazapine	<1%	≥1%	NR	≥1%	NR

TABLE 13–6. Incidence of sexual dysfunction in U.S. Food and Drug Administration registration trials of antidepressant and related noradrenergic or serotonergic agents[a] *(continued)*

Agent	Impotence	Decreased libido	Erectile dysfunction	Delayed ejaculation	Anorgasmia
Paroxetine	10%	7%–9%	NR	26%–27%	NR
Sertraline	NR	6%	NR	14%	NR
TCAs	NR	NR	NR	NR	NR
Transdermal selegiline	≤1%	≤1%	NR	≤1%	≤1%
Venlafaxine	NR	3%–8%	NR	8%–19%	NR
Vilazodone	NR	3%–5%	2%	2%	2%–4%
Vortioxetine[d]	NR	1.6% (men), 0.8% (women)	0.2%	0.5%	0.4% (men), 0.3% (women)

Note. FDA=U.S. Food and Drug Administration; MAOI=monoamine oxidase inhibitor; NR=not reported; TCA=tricyclic antidepressant.

[a]Reported incidence rates are based on spontaneous reports rather than on systematic assessments, unless otherwise noted.

[b]Adverse effects as reported with desvenlafaxine dosages of 50–100 mg/day for major depression.

[c]Adverse sexual effects with duloxetine were assessed in FDA trials using the Arizona Sexual Experiences Scale (McGahuey et al. 2000), which revealed significantly poorer scores versus placebo for global sexual function among men but not women and significantly greater difficulty reaching orgasm with duloxetine than placebo in men but not women. No significant drug-placebo differences were observed in sex drive; arousal; ability to achieve erections (men) or lubrication (women); orgasmic satisfaction; or ease of reaching orgasm (women).

[d]As reported from spontaneous reports of pooled trials of vortioxetine in major depressive disorder and generalized anxiety disorder (N=3,377) (Jacobson et al. 2016).

TABLE 13–7. Pharmacological strategies used to counteract drug-induced sexual dysfunction

Agent	Rationale	Positive data	Equivocal or negative data
Phosphodiesterase type 5 inhibitors (e.g., sildenafil, vardenafil, tadalafil)	Nitric oxide–mediated vasodilator	Case reports describe improvement or resolution of SSRI-associated ejaculatory delay with sildenafil 50–100 mg/day prn or higher (up to 200 mg/day; Seidman et al. 2003), including improvement of anorgasmia in women (Nurnberg et al. 2008). Significant improvement also identified from placebo-controlled data (Fava et al. 2006; Nurnberg et al. 2003), and in placebo-controlled trials of sildenafil (25–50 mg/day) to counteract antipsychotic-associated sexual dysfunction (Gopalakrishnan et al. 2006). Vardenafil (10 mg 30 minutes before sexual activity; Berigan 2004) and tadalafil (20 mg/day; Segraves et al. 2007) have been described in case reports and open trials as a strategy to counteract sexual dysfunction secondary to antidepressants.	None.

TABLE 13–7. Pharmacological strategies used to counteract drug-induced sexual dysfunction (*continued*)

Agent	Rationale	Positive data	Equivocal or negative data
Amantadine	Dopamine agonism	Case reports indicate favorable results when used to treat anorgasmia related to fluoxetine (Balogh et al. 1992; Balon 1996) or paroxetine (Shrivastava et al. 1995).	In women with sexual dysfunction secondary to fluoxetine, adjunctive amantadine (50–100 mg/day) was no different from placebo (Michelson et al. 2000).
Aripiprazole	Relatively prolactin sparing	Over 12–26 weeks, open-label add-on or substitution from another SGA significantly improved libido and overall sexual satisfaction in men and women ($N=27$), ejaculatory or erectile dysfunction in men, and menstrual dysfunction in women (Mir et al. 2008).	None.
Bethanechol	Procholinergic, may help counteract sexual dysfunction caused by anticholinergic drugs (e.g., TCAs or MAOIs)	Case reports used 10–50 mg/day (Gross 1982).	None.

TABLE 13–7. Pharmacological strategies used to counteract drug-induced sexual dysfunction (*continued*)		
Agent	Rationale	Positive data	Equivocal or negative data
Bupropion	Prodopaminergic and noradrenergic agent without known serotonergic effects	Outpatients (*N*=47) taking SSRIs received open-label bupropion 75–150 mg 1–2 hours before sexual activity, yielding improvement in 38%; a standing adjunctive dose of bupropion 75 mg tid for 2 weeks reversed sexual dysfunction in 66% of patients (Ashton and Rosen 1998). In a 12-week randomized comparison of bupropion SR 150 mg bid or placebo added to SSRIs in 234 remitted male depressed patients with SSRI-induced sexual dysfunction, significantly greater improvement occurred in overall sexual functioning (by ASEX) with bupropion than placebo (Safarinejad 2010). In 12-week randomized comparison of bupropion SR 150 mg bid or placebo added to SSRIs in 218 remitted female depressed patients with SSRI-induced sexual dysfunction, significantly greater improvement in desire and lubrication occurred with bupropion than placebo (Safarinejad 2011).	In 6-week randomized comparison of bupropion SR 150 mg/day or placebo (*N*=41) added to SSRIs in remitted depressed patients with SSRI-induced sexual dysfunction, no differences were found between drug and placebo on any measures of sexual functioning (DeBattista et al. 2005); identical findings in a similarly designed 3-week study with the same dosing (*N*=30) were reported by Masand et al. (2001).

TABLE 13–7. Pharmacological strategies used to counteract drug-induced sexual dysfunction (*continued*)

Agent	Rationale	Positive data	Equivocal or negative data
Buspirone	5-HT$_{1A}$ partial agonist	In 4-week comparison of placebo vs. flexibly dosed buspirone (20–60 mg/day; mean dose=49 mg/day) added to citalopram or paroxetine, greater improvement in sexual function occurred with buspirone (58%) than placebo (20%); results more pronounced in women than men (Landén et al. 1999).	Among women with sexual dysfunction secondary to fluoxetine, adjunctive buspirone (20–30 mg/day) was no different from placebo (Michelson et al. 2000).
Cyproheptadine	Serotonin antagonist	Case series data show improvement of delayed male ejaculation from fluoxetine, fluvoxamine, or clomipramine using adjunctive cyproheptadine (4–12 mg) 1–2 hours before sexual activity (Aizenberg et al. 1995).	None.

TABLE 13–7. Pharmacological strategies used to counteract drug-induced sexual dysfunction *(continued)*

Agent	Rationale	Positive data	Equivocal or negative data
Ginkgo biloba	Hypothesized effects on vasodilation and stimulation of prostaglandin synthesis	Favorable open-label data were reported in men and women (*N*=63) with dosages of 60–120 mg/day (Cohen and Bartlik 1998).	In 2-month comparison of *Gingko biloba* (*N*=19) or placebo (*N*=18), no significant differences were found (Kang et al. 2002). In 12-week trial of *Ginkgo biloba* 240 mg/day or placebo in 24 antidepressant-treated subjects, no significant differences were found (Wheatley 2004).
Maca root (*Lepidium meyenii*; a Peruvian plant)	Unknown	In 12-week double-blind, randomized comparison of 1.5 vs. 3.0 g/day of maca in 20 SSRI-treated outpatients with remitted major depression, improved libido and sexual functioning from baseline were seen with 3.0-g/day dosage (Dording et al. 2008).	

TABLE 13–7. Pharmacological strategies used to counteract drug-induced sexual dysfunction *(continued)*

Agent	Rationale	Positive data	Equivocal or negative data
Methylphenidate	Dopamine agonism may increase sexual function	Case reports (Roeloffs et al. 1996).	No significant differences were found between methylphenidate extended release (OROS) and placebo with respect to change in ASEX scores for sexual functioning over 4 weeks in patients with treatment-resistant major depression (Pae et al. 2009).
Mirtazapine	Postsynaptic 5-HT$_{2A}$ blockade may counteract 5-HT$_{2A}$ serotonergic stimulation	In depressed outpatients in remission with SSRIs receiving open-label adjunctive mirtazapine 15–30 mg/day (N=49), significant improvement was seen usually after 4 weeks (Ozmenler et al. 2008).	Improvement from baseline found with mirtazapine (N=36) but similar to placebo (N=39) over 1 month in premenopausal women receiving fluoxetine (Michelson et al. 2002).

TABLE 13–7. Pharmacological strategies used to counteract drug-induced sexual dysfunction *(continued)*

Agent	Rationale	Positive data	Equivocal or negative data
Saffron (*Crocus sativis* L.)	Reported to have aphrodisiac effects in animals and humans	Randomized 4-week comparison of 30 mg/day for fluoxetine-associated sexual dysfunction in women (*N*=34) demonstrated significant improvement in global sexual functioning, arousal, lubrication, and pain (Kashani et al. 2013).	
Testosterone (gel or transdermal)	Improves libido and arousal	Improved ejaculatory function in men (randomized 6-week placebo-controlled trial; Amiaz et al. 2011) or sexual satisfaction in women (randomized 12-week placebo-controlled trial; Fooladi et al. 2014).	
Trazodone	5-HT$_{2A}$ postsynaptic antagonism	Open-trial data using trazodone 50–100 mg/day added to SSRIs for 4 weeks led to improvement in desire, arousal, orgasm, and overall satisfaction in men and women (*N*=20) (Stryjer et al. 2009).	

TABLE 13–7. Pharmacological strategies used to counteract drug-induced sexual dysfunction *(continued)*

Agent	Rationale	Positive data	Equivocal or negative data
Yohimbine (+/− L-arginine glutamate)	Presynaptic α_2-adrenergic antagonism increases noradrenergic tone	In 2-week crossover study of yohimbine 6 mg/day+L-arginine glutamate 6 g/day vs. yohimbine 6 mg/day or placebo (N=45), combination therapy was found superior to placebo (Lebret et al. 2002). Five favorable outcomes were found in 6 open cases receiving yohimbine as needed for SSRI-induced sexual dysfunction (Hollander and McCarley 1992). Improved sexual function was found in 8 of 9 fluoxetine-treated outpatients given open-label yohimbine 5.4 mg tid (Jacobson 1992).	Improvement from baseline found with yohimbine (N=35) but similar to placebo (N=39) after 1 month among women with SSRI-induced sexual dysfunction (Michelson et al. 2002). May cause anxiety, tachycardia, and hypertension.

Note. 5-HT$_{1A}$=serotonin type 1A ; 5-HT$_{2A}$=serotonin type 2A ; ASEX=Arizona Sexual Experiences Scale; bid=twice daily; MAOI= monoamine oxidase inhibitor; OROS=osmotic-release oral system; prn=as needed; SGA=second-generation antipsychotic; SR=sustained release; SSRI=selective serotonin reuptake inhibitor; TCA=tricyclic antidepressant; tid=three times daily.

In addition to the findings from randomized trials summarized in Table 13–7, a handful of case reports and proof-of-concept open trials describe novel strategies to counteract antidepressant-induced sexual dysfunction. One such example, focusing on patients who developed sexual dysfunction after successful treatment for generalized anxiety disorder with an SSRI or SNRI, involved substituting the novel GABAergic anticonvulsant tiagabine for the original agent; the change yielded significant overall improvement in sexual function with sustained improvement in anxiety symptoms (Schwartz et al. 2007).

Drug-induced sexual dysfunction typically remits after cessation of the suspected causal agent. However, some case reports describe sexual dysfunction that may persist indefinitely after the discontinuation of citalopram, fluoxetine, or sertraline and that remains unimproved with a variety of dopamine agonists.

Sexual dysfunction due to antipsychotic medications has been attributed to likely effects of hyperprolactinemia, although the postsynaptic 5-HT$_{2A}$ blockade exerted by SGAs should, at least in theory, minimize sexual adverse effects. As noted in Table 13–7, adjunctive sildenafil has demonstrated value in improving erectile dysfunction and orgasmic satisfaction in men taking antipsychotics (Gopalakrishnan et al. 2006). Also, according to a Cochrane Database analysis, sildenafil constitutes the sole known effective adjunctive therapy to counteract antipsychotic-associated sexual dysfunction (Berner et al. 2007) apart from the use of adjunctive dopamine agonists.

Remarkably, only a small literature exists describing the use of dopamine agonists such as bromocriptine (dosed at 5–7.5 mg/day) to overcome sexual dysfunction caused by antipsychotics. Perhaps this dearth of studies results from concerns that dopamine agonism could potentially reverse the antipsychotic effects of dopamine D$_2$ antagonism or otherwise cause a direct psychotomimetic effect. Preliminary open-trial data suggest value for ropinirole (begun at 0.25 mg/day and increased to 2–4 mg/day, with a mean dose of about 2 mg/day to alleviate antidepressant-induced sexual dysfunction). Dopamine agonists such as bromocriptine, amantadine, pramipexole, or ropinirole could at least in theory diminish antipsychotic-associated sexual dysfunction via reduction of antipsychotic-induced hyperprolactinemia.

Retrograde Ejaculation

General Recommendations

Retrograde ejaculation may be caused by a select number of FGAs or SGAs. Dosage reductions, or if necessary, drug cessation typically ameliorates the complication.

The phenomenon of retrograde ejaculation has been reported with a limited number of antipsychotic agents, most notably thioridazine, risperidone, and clozapine. Some authors have suggested that retrograde ejaculation more likely occurs due to α_1-adrenergic antagonism than to other mechanisms (e.g., hyperprolactinemia) because of the lack of interference with arousal or the ability to attain or sustain erections. Short of altogether discontinuing the causal agent, the prescriber can try dosage reductions to resolve the side effect.

14

Hematological System

Myelosuppression: Agranulocytosis and Thrombocytopenia

General Recommendations

Clinicians should recognize the risk for agranulocytosis in patients taking carbamazepine or clozapine, and more infrequently in those taking other SGAs or mirtazapine. Drug discontinuation is necessary in the setting of neutropenia.

Myelosuppression refers broadly to the failure of bone marrow to produce blood cells (red cells [anemia], white cells [agranulocytosis], and platelets [thrombocytopenia]). *Aplastic anemia* refers to a more serious form of myelosuppression. *Neutropenia* refers to an abnormally low number of neutrophils, and the *absolute neutrophil count* (ANC) is calculated from the percentage of neutrophils plus the percentage of bands (immature neutrophils). The ANC is typically defined on the basis of severity gradations that indicate the risk for infection as being *mild* (1,000–1,500/mm^3), *moderate* (500–1,000/mm^3), or *severe* (<500/mm^3). A normal platelet

---

The symbol ■ is used in this chapter to indicate that the FDA has issued a boxed warning for a prescription medication that may cause serious adverse effects.

count is 150,000 to 450,000 cells/μL of blood; clinically significant thrombocytopenia with risk for bleeding, requiring emergency intervention, is generally identified by a platelet count <50,000 cells/μL of blood. Myelosuppression can occur as rare adverse effects associated with a select number of psychotropic agents, as described in the following subsections.

Carbamazepine

Benign, transient leukopenia is a common phenomenon during initial treatment with carbamazepine. In the original Veterans Administration Multicenter Antiepileptic Drug Trial, leukocyte counts <5,000/mm^3 were observed in approximately 30% of carbamazepine recipients during the first 6 months of treatment (Mattson et al. 1985). A pharmacoepidemiological study of 977 patients at McLean Hospital taking carbamazepine found a point prevalence of 2.1% (Tohen et al. 1995). Frank aplastic anemia is an exceedingly rare event with carbamazepine (■), with an estimated occurrence of 1 in 200,000 exposures. Thrombocytopenia from carbamazepine, potentially related to immunologically mediated platelet destruction, typically occurs in conjunction with other systemic signs (e.g., rash, liver enzyme elevation). Some authorities advise obtaining a complete blood count (CBC) at baseline, then weekly for 2 months, and then once every 3 months. The myelosuppressive effects of carbamazepine are thought to result from toxicity caused by its epoxide metabolite (see Figure 2–1 in Chapter 2, "Pharmacokinetics, Pharmacodynamics, and Pharmacogenomics").

Divalproex

Mild, asymptomatic leukopenia occurs in rare instances with divalproex (0.4% point prevalence in the McLean Hospital pharmacoepidemiological study by Tohen et al. [1995]) and typically reverses upon dosage reductions or drug cessation. Thrombocytopenia has typically been defined on the basis of serum platelet counts <140,000×10^9 per liter. Initial case reports and case series in the late 1970s and early 1980s suggested that thrombocytopenia could be an immune-mediated reaction to divalproex caused by structural similarities between the drug and the cell membrane constituents. Later studies have suggested that the phenomenon reflects a dose-related toxicity rather than peripheral destruction or a dose-independent immunologically based event. Risk may be mediated by duration of exposure and may be higher in elderly patients and in women. Thrombocytopenia caused by divalproex typically remits after dosage reductions, without the need for drug discontinuation. No formal recommendation exists for surveillance monitoring of platelet counts during acute or ongoing therapy with divalproex, but periodic assessment (e.g., every 6–12 months) is advisable, particularly in older adults or patients taking >1,000 mg/day.

Second-Generation Antipsychotics

Clozapine is the most widely recognized SGA that carries a risk for developing agranulocytosis (~1%) (■). The mechanism by which clozapine can suppress leukocyte counts is not well understood but is thought to involve an immunologically mediated cytotoxic effect of clozapine or its metabolites; however, research efforts have not demonstrated immunologically associated features such as eosinophilia. Clozapine-associated myelosuppression is most likely to occur within the first 6 months of treatment, although exceedingly rare single case reports have been published involving the development of clozapine-induced agranulocytosis after 17 months, 2.5 years, or even 11 years, lengthy time frames that represent the exception rather than the rule. Research efforts have not identified predictors of eventual agranulocytosis, although risk may increase somewhat with age and female sex. An earlier literature also suggested that rises in total white blood cell (WBC) counts by ~15% may sometimes precede agranulocytosis from clozapine.

Guidelines for WBC monitoring during clozapine therapy are presented in Table 14–1. In October 2015, the FDA began a centralized Risk Evaluation and Mitigation Strategy (REMS) program to oversee monitoring of hematological parameters and drug dispensing for all U.S. patients taking clozapine.

In July 2009, the FDA imposed a class effect on FGAs and SGAs, warning of an association with leukopenia/neutropenia and possible agranulocytosis. The clinical significance of the warning does not involve a need for widespread or routine monitoring of CBCs among patients taking SGAs, but rather an awareness that this drug class should be considered in the differential diagnosis of individuals who may present with low WBC counts. Antipsychotics should be discontinued in the setting of an ANC of <1,000/mm^3, with subsequent close monitoring of WBC counts until recovery.

The risk for agranulocytosis may increase whenever a new antipsychotic agent is introduced and may be mediated in part by a longer duration of high-dose therapy.

Clinicians sometimes think of using lithium as a strategy to promote leukocytosis and boost WBC counts. At one time, it was thought that leukocytosis during lithium therapy merely reflected increased demargination of WBCs from blood vessel endothelial linings, rather than truly

TABLE 14–1.   **Monitoring of white blood cell counts during clozapine treatment**

Event	Complete blood count (CBC) monitoring
0–6 months	Monitor weekly.
6–12 months	Monitor biweekly.
>12 months	Monitor monthly.
Substantial drop within 3 weeks (WBC≥3,000/mm^3 or ANC≥1,500/mm^3)	Repeat CBC. If WBC=3,000–3,500/mm^3 and ANC<2,000/mm^3, monitor twice weekly.
WBC=3,000–3,500/mm^3 or ANC=1,500–2,000/mm^3	Monitor twice weekly until WBC>3,500/mm^3 and ANC>2,000/mm^3.
WBC=2,000–3,000/mm^3 or ANC=1,000–1,500/mm^3	Monitor CBC daily until WBC > 3,000/mm^3 and ANC>1,000/mm^3; then twice weekly until WBC > 3,500/mm^3 and ANC>2,000/mm^3; then weekly. May then rechallenge and monitor weekly for 1 year.
WBC<2,000/mm^3 and ANC<1,000/mm^3	Discontinue clozapine. Monitor CBC daily until WBC>3,000/mm^3 and ANC>1,500/mm^3; then twice weekly until WBC>3,500/mm^3 and ANC>2,000/mm^3; then weekly.
ANC≤500/mm^3 (agranulocytosis)	Discontinue clozapine. Monitor CBC daily until WBC>3,000/mm^3 and ANC>1,500/mm^3; then twice weekly until WBC>3,500/mm^3 and ANC>2,000/mm^3; then weekly.

Note.   ANC=absolute neutrophil count; WBC=white blood cell (count).

increasing the new production and differentiation of granulocytes from bone marrow. However, more recent efforts suggest that lithium may indeed foster a true myeloproliferative response (rather than demargination) by increasing granulocyte colony–stimulating factor and augmenting its effects (Focosi et al. 2009).

Although product information from clozapine's manufacturer does not prohibit the reintroduction of clozapine after development of neutropenia, rechallenge is controversial and has not been systematically studied. Manu and colleagues (2012) identified 112 reported cases of clozapine rechallenge after neutropenia, occurring from 1 to 156 weeks after initial drug cessation. In about 30% of clozapine-rechallenged cases, the patient again developed neutropenia (about half the time resulting in even more severe agranulocytosis than had occurred previously), occurring at a mean of about 4 weeks after its reintroduction. After severe neutropenia (ANC < 500 / mm³), hematologically successful outcomes after clozapine rechallenge occurred in only 3 of 15 cases.

Granulocyte colony–stimulating factor (GCSF) itself is often used to treat neutropenia from myelodysplastic syndromes or myelosuppression caused by antineoplastic agents, although its use to counteract drug-induced agranulocytosis is less well established except in cases of severe bone marrow hypoplasia. Reports exist using the injectible GCSF compound filgrastim (dosed at > 0.3 mg/ week) to rechallenge patients with clozapine after their having developed agranulocytosis, although the efficacy of this strategy appears variable. Generally, psychotropic-induced agranulocytosis resolves after cessation of a causal agent, and new granulocytes arise within 21 days, obviating the need for further intervention other than supportive measures (as in the setting of fever or infection).

Other Agents

Thrombocytopenia has been described as a rare event with SSRIs, clonazepam, and diazepam. Agranulocytosis has been described as a rare, potentially immune-mediated occurrence during long-term treatment with chlordiazepoxide, diazepam, midazolam, and modafinil. Rare reports exist of pancytopenia, including aplastic anemia and pure red blood cell aplasia, occurring during treatment with lamotrigine. In premarketing studies of mirtazapine, agranulocytosis was observed in 2 of 2,796 patients, with one-third developing severe neutropenia, yielding a crude incidence of 1.1 per 1,000 exposed patients. All observed cases resolved after drug cessation. Mirtazapine should be stopped in patients who develop signs of an infection with an accompanying low WBC count.

Platelet Aggregation Disorders and Bleeding Risk

General Recommendations

Individuals with a history of gastrointestinal bleeding or other risk factors for bleeding (e.g., use of anticoagulants or NSAIDs, liver disease) may have a low but statistically significantly increased risk for bleeding during therapy with serotonergic antidepressants. The presence of clear, identifiable increased risk factors for bleeding may favor the use of nonserotonergic over serotonergic antidepressants when feasible, possible cotherapy with a proton pump inhibitor in individuals at particular risk for gastrointestinal bleeding, and the temporary discontinuation of serotonergic antidepressants before elective surgery on a case-by-case basis.

There is unresolved controversy surrounding the potential for bleeding disorders due to platelet serotonin dysfunction during therapy with serotonergic antidepressants. Some reports suggest a roughly 2-fold increased risk for upper gastrointestinal bleeding with SSRIs, particularly when combined with NSAIDs, anticoagulants including aspirin, or antiplatelet drugs (e.g., Andrade et al. 2010), whereas other studies have failed to replicate such concerns and dispute their validity. Short-term (rather than long-term) SSRI exposure also has been associated with intracranial and intracerebral hemorrhage as an extremely rare event (estimated as one additional case per 10,000 persons treated for a year (Hackam and Mrkobrada 2012). SSRI-induced thrombocytopenia also represents a separate mechanism by which some serotonergic antidepressants, such as citalopram, have reportedly been associated with bleeding disorders (Andersohn et al. 2010).

Clinicians should keep in mind that the differential diagnosis of iatrogenic abnormal bleeding extends beyond pharmacologically induced disruption of platelet aggregation and may include hepatic failure (e.g., diminished production of clotting factors, elevated prothrombin time), disseminated intravascular coagulopathy (which may rarely occur in the setting of serotonin syndrome), and inherited bleeding disorders (e.g., von Willebrand disease), among other factors.

Red Blood Cells

General Recommendations

Decreased red blood cell production is rarely iatrogenic and should prompt a comprehensive review of risk factors for anemia or suppression of other cell lines.

Although a number of psychotropic agents may cause fulminant aplastic anemia, relatively few have been associated solely with the suppression of red blood cell production (reticulocytopenia). Macrocytic anemia has been described in case reports following treatment with divalproex, oral contraceptives, sulfa antibiotics, and reverse transcriptase inhibitors, among other drugs. Drug-induced hemolytic anemias seldom are associated with psychotropic drugs (e.g., levodopa) and more often may result from antibiotics (e.g., cephalosporins or penicillins) or from NSAIDs. The evaluation and differential diagnosis of reticulocytopenia is extensive, and in addition to iron deficiency, may include liver or renal failure, myelodysplastic syndromes, nutritional deficiencies, toxicities (e.g., lead, arsenic), and endocrinopathies (e.g., hypothyroidism, hyperparathyroidism), among other causes. Table 14–2 identifies key considerations in the initial assessment of anemia.

TABLE 14–2.   Considerations in the assessment of anemia

Parameter	Relevance
Is patient's anemia macrocytic or microcytic?	Most common causes of macrocytic anemias are alcoholism, malnutrition, or malabsorption disorders leading to vitamin B_{12} or folic acid deficiency. The most common cause of microcytic anemia is iron deficiency. Drug-induced hemolytic anemias are usually normocytic.
Is the reticulocyte count elevated?	A compensatory increase in reticulocytes would be expected due to blood loss, hypoxia, or hemolytic anemia.
Are there indications of jaundice (e.g., icteric sclerae)?	Jaundice may indicate a hemolytic process.
Are chronic inflammatory (e.g., rheumatoid arthritis) or neoplastic conditions present?	These conditions may indicate anemia of chronic disease.

15

Metabolic Dysregulation and Weight Gain

Dyslipidemias

General Recommendations

Patients who develop dyslipidemias while taking SGAs or some antidepressants may warrant cotherapy with lipid-lowering agents prescribed in conjunction with the primary care physician or cardiologist. Decisions must be made on a case-by-case basis about the relative merits of switching from an existing SGA to an alternative agent with potentially lesser risk for lipid dysregulation versus treating abnormal lipids with statins, depending on assessment of atherosclerotic cardiac disease risk versus the magnitude of benefit with an existing psychotropic agent, and the likelihood that a replacement drug would yield at least comparable efficacy. Melatonin agonists have shown preliminary evidence of lowering total serum cholesterol levels among atypical antipsychotic recipients.

The symbol ■ is used in this chapter to indicate that the FDA has issued a boxed warning for a prescription medication that may cause serious adverse effects.

Abnormal elevations of total serum cholesterol and serum triglycerides have been linked directly with most SGAs and represent a key aspect of metabolic syndrome. The mechanisms by which SGAs may cause dyslipidemias, other than as a secondary consequence of obesity caused by increased caloric intake, remain elusive. In addition, abdominal obesity and hypercholesterolemia have been associated with some SSRIs—notably, sertraline, fluoxetine, and fluvoxamine—but not with citalopram, whereas weight gain with paroxetine appears to be independent of new-onset dyslipidemias (Raeder et al. 2006).

The CATIE study (Lieberman et al. 2005) in chronic schizophrenia found the greatest rises in serum cholesterol with olanzapine and the greatest reductions from baseline with ziprasidone (Table 15–1).

Several studies have reported a lower incidence of hypertriglyceridemia and elevations in serum leptin levels in patients with schizophrenia during treatment with quetiapine, and a minimal change during risperidone therapy, as compared with during therapy with clozapine or olanzapine (Atmaca et al. 2003).

Hypertriglyceridemia is generally thought to pose a less direct atherosclerotic risk than other lipid parameters (e.g., high LDL cholesterol or low HDL cholesterol), and it carries an increased risk mainly for pancreatitis or cholelithiasis. Hypertriglyceridemia also has been identified as a risk factor for the development of hyperglycemia and eventual non-insulin-dependent diabetes mellitus (NIDDM) (Tirosh et al. 2008), although hypertriglyceridemia is thought to be a covariate (rather than a cause) of NIDDM that becomes evident before the emergence of frank diabetes. Nevertheless, moderate or greater hypertriglyceridemia alters lipoprotein metabolism and still represents an independent risk factor for coronary artery disease, especially in women (McBride 2007). By convention, normal triglycerides are generally defined as <150 mg/dL, borderline-high triglycerides as 150–199 mg/dL, high triglycerides as 200–499 mg/dL, and very high triglycerides as ≥ 500 mg/dL.

The components of metabolic syndrome, summarized in Table 15–2, collectively increase the risk for coronary heart disease, regardless of LDL cholesterol levels. *Metabolic syndrome* is defined by the presence of three or more of these risk factors. To further aid medication risk-benefit decisions, clinicians should calculate a given patient's 10-year risk for ASCVD using the so-called Pooled Cohort Equations (see http://www.cvriskcalculator.com/) based on age, gender, race, total cholesterol, HDL cholesterol, diabetes status, smoking status, and blood pressure. Pooled Cohort Equations have come to replace the FRS, which does not account for diabetes or race. The so-called Reynolds risk score is a similar measure that adds C-reactive protein level and parental history of premature MI

TABLE 15–1. Changes in lipid parameters during U.S. Food and Drug Administration registration trials or randomized studies of second-generation antipsychotics

Agent	Changes in total cholesterol	Changes in serum triglycerides
Aripiprazole	Randomized trials in schizophrenia; median change in total cholesterol across five acute placebo-controlled studies ($n=860$) = +1.0 mg/dL (Marder et al. 2003). LDL declined by ≤1 mg/dL over 26 weeks (Pigott et al. 2003). Acute or long-term schizophrenia FDA trials: no differences from placebo.	In 6-week adjunctive trials for major depression: 5% increase from baseline. In 26-week randomized trial in schizophrenia: −37.2 mg/dL (Pigott et al. 2003).
Asenapine	Acute bipolar or schizophrenia trials: mean changes from +1.1 to +0.4 mg/dL; 1-year open extension trial in schizophrenia: −6.0 mg/dL.	Acute bipolar or schizophrenia trials: mean changes from −3.5 to +3.8 mg/dL; 1-year open extension trial in schizophrenia: −9.8 mg/dL.
Brexpiprazole	Major depression adjunctive therapy and schizophrenia acute trials: no differences from placebo; in long-term open-label phases, 9% of major depression and 6% of schizophrenia patients had categorical shifts in total cholesterol from "normal" to "high."	Categorical shifts from "normal" to "high" occurred in 5%–13% of major depression patients across dosages over 6 weeks during acute adjunctive therapy and up to 17% of patients during long-term open-label treatment; and in 8%–10% of schizophrenia patients during 6-week acute trials as well as 13% during long-term open label treatment.

TABLE 15–1. Changes in lipid parameters during U.S. Food and Drug Administration registration trials or randomized studies of second-generation antipsychotics (continued)

Agent	Changes in total cholesterol	Changes in serum triglycerides
Cariprazine	Acute schizophrenia and bipolar mania trials: no significant differences from placebo in categorical shifts from "normal" to "high."	Acute schizophrenia and bipolar mania trials: no significant differences from placebo in categorical shifts from "normal" to "high."
Iloperidone	Acute schizophrenia trials: net 0 mg/dL change (Weiden et al. 2008).	−26.5 mg/dL (Weiden et al. 2008).
Lurasidone	Manufacturer's short-term trials in schizophrenia: across dosages, −8.2 mg/dL. Manufacturer's longer-term studies: at 24 weeks, −4.2 mg/dL; at 36 weeks, −1.9 mg/dL; at 52 weeks: −3.6 mg/dL. Monotherapy in bipolar depression: +1.2 mg/dL (dosing 20–60 mg/day) or −4.6 mg/dL (dosing 80–120 mg/day) over 6 weeks (Loebel et al. 2014a). Adjunctive therapy in bipolar depression: −3.0 mg/dL over 6 weeks (Loebel et al. 2014b).	Manufacturer's collective short-term trials in schizophrenia: across dosages, −9.3 mg/dL. Manufacturer's longer-term studies: at 24 weeks, −13.6 mg/dL; at 36 weeks, −3.5 mg/dL; at 52 weeks, −6.5 mg/dL. Monotherapy in bipolar depression: +5.6 mg/dL (dosing 20–60 mg/day) or +0.4 mg/dL (dosing 80–120 mg/day) over 6 weeks (Loebel et al. 2014a). Adjunctive therapy in bipolar depression: +9.0 mg/dL over 6 weeks (Loebel et al. 2014b).

TABLE 15–1. Changes in lipid parameters during U.S. Food and Drug Administration registration trials or randomized studies of second-generation antipsychotics *(continued)*

Agent	Changes in total cholesterol	Changes in serum triglycerides
Olanzapine	+21.1 mg/dL over 24 weeks (Newcomer et al. 2009). +9.4±2.4 mg/dL in CATIE (Lieberman et al. 2005).	+30.9 mg/dL over 24 weeks (Newcomer et al. 2009). +40.5±8.9 mg/dL in CATIE (Lieberman et al. 2005).
Paliperidone	<0.1 mg/dL across three 6-week trials in schizophrenia (Meltzer et al. 2008).	<0.1 mg/dL across three 6-week trials in schizophrenia (Meltzer et al. 2008).
Pimavanserin	Not reported	Not reported
Quetiapine	+13.1 mg/dL over 24 weeks (Newcomer et al. 2009). +6.6±2.4 mg/dL in CATIE (Lieberman et al. 2005).	+21.2±9.2 mg/dL in CATIE (Lieberman et al. 2005).
Risperidone	−1.3±2.4 mg/dL in CATIE (Lieberman et al. 2005).	−2.4±9.1 mg/dL in CATIE (Lieberman et al. 2005).
Ziprasidone	−8.2±3.2 mg/dL in CATIE (Lieberman et al. 2005); median change of −14.5 mg/dL from baseline in acute industry trials for psychosis.	−16.5±12.2 mg/dL in CATIE (Lieberman et al. 2005); median change of −37.0 mg/dL from baseline in acute industry trials for psychosis.

Note. CATIE=Clinical Antipsychotic Trials of Intervention Effectiveness; FDA=U.S. Food and Drug Administration; LDL=low-density lipoprotein.

to the calculated risk score. Current guidelines from the American College of Cardiology and the American Heart Association (ACC/AHA; Stone et al. 2014) advise physicians to base their decisions about statin initiation (and dosing intensity) according to Pooled Cohort Equation scores when 10-year risk for an MI equals or exceeds 7.5% (and in some cases even ≥5%). Previously, decisions about initiating statins were driven more narrowly by LDL-cholesterol scores per se rather than by global ASCVD risk.

Longitudinal studies indicate that risk factors for the development of diabetes or prediabetes during treatment with an SGA include HDL concentrations <28 mg/dL, age >58 if HDL is ≥28 mg/dL, serum glucose levels ≥92 mg/dL, posttreatment rises in triglyceride values ≥145 mg/dL (for diabetes) or ≥59 mg/dL (for prediabetes), and rapid weight gain (within 2 weeks) of ≥6.1 kg in conjunction with a triglyceride increase of ≥145 mg/dL (Reaven et al. 2009). On the basis of the nontrivial risks for coronary heart disease caused by iatrogenic dyslipidemias, many psychiatrists often favor replacing an SGA that is suspected of causing dyslipidemia or metabolic dysregulation with a different SGA of presumed lower risk, or possibly even an FGA, regardless of possible differences in psychotropic efficacy. However, the risk-benefit analysis of this proposition is not always straightforward. A significant dyslipidemia certainly presents a compelling rationale for considering a switch to alternative agents. The main uncertainties in doing so involve whether the substituted new agent indeed possesses more benign metabolic effects for a given patient, and has at least comparable efficacy to sustain the benefit of a previous agent. Unless there are no viable alternatives to a known effective SGA with substantial cardiovascular adverse effects, patients with significant cardiovascular risk factors generally should receive psychotropic agents with minimal metabolic or cardiovascular adverse effects (e.g., aripiprazole, ziprasidone, asenapine, iloperidone, lurasidone, or FGAs with minimal glycemic or lipid-altering effects).

On the other hand, circumstances may arise in which the benefit of a particular agent is so dramatic and unique (e.g., in the case of patients with schizophrenia in whom clozapine exerts unequivocally greater efficacy than other antipsychotics) that active treatment of an iatrogenic dyslipidemia may be advisable. In the case of clozapine, metabolic dysregulation has been linked with serum norclozapine but not serum clozapine levels—a finding that led to a preliminary randomized study of adjunctive fluvoxamine (50 mg/day) or placebo added to clozapine (≤250 mg/day with fluvoxamine or ≤600 mg/day with placebo), yielding greater reductions in weight, serum glucose, and triglycerides (but not cholesterol) with fluvoxamine cotherapy (Lu et al. 2004). Such a

TABLE 15–2.   Risk determinants for metabolic syndrome[a]

Risk factor	Defining level
Central obesity[b]	Waist circumference
Men	≥90 cm in South Asians, Chinese, or Japanese; ≥94 cm in Europids
Women	≥80 cm
plus any two of the following factors:	
Triglycerides	≥150 mg/dL
HDL cholesterol	
Men	<40 mg/dL
Women	<50 mg/dL
Blood pressure	≥130/≥85 mm Hg
Fasting glucose	≥100 mg/dL

Note.   HDL=high-density lipoprotein.
[a]Based on the International Diabetes Foundation Consensus Worldwide Definition of the Metabolic Syndrome. Brussels, Belgium, IDF Communications, 2006, pp. 1–24.
[b]Can be assumed if BMI >30 kg/m².

strategy demands careful monitoring of other adverse effects (e.g., lowered seizure threshold, anticholinergic effects), signs of toxicity, and clozapine levels, due to the potential for marked increases in serum clozapine levels.

To date, surprisingly little study has been done on efforts to treat hypercholesterolemia or hypertriglyceridemia using lipid-lowering drugs in patients who have developed dyslipidemias secondary to SGA therapy. Landry et al. (2008) retrospectively examined outcomes in 18 clozapine-treated schizophrenia patients with hyperlipidemia who were followed for a mean of 4.4 years while taking lipid-lowering medications (either pravastatin, atorvastatin, fenofibrate, gemfibrozil, or lovastatin). Mean triglyceride and total cholesterol levels declined significantly from baseline. Similarly, a 28-day open trial of omega-3 fatty acids (~10 g/day of fish oil, containing 1.8 g/day of eicosapentaenoic acid and 1.2 g/day of docosahexaenoic acid) among 28 clozapine recipients was associated with a significant (22%) reduction in LDL and a 22% reduction in triglycerides (Cantiano et al. 2006). These dosages are higher than the more customary 2–4 g/day of omega-3 fatty acids sometimes recommended by primary care physicians for hyperlipidemia. Notably, however, the clinical end-point data do not robustly demonstrate the efficacy of omega-3 fatty acids to reduce the risk for coronary heart disease, and they are not considered first-line therapies for diagnosed hyperlipidemia.

The first level of intervention for weight gain and dyslipidemias continues to be lifestyle modification (i.e., aerobic exercise lasting about 4 hours/week, dietary changes that include the minimization of simple sugars such as fructose, and elimination of smoking). The 2013 ACC/AHA guideline (Stone et al. 2014) advises that statin therapy may benefit patients with the following characteristics:

- Clinical presence of atherosclerotic cardiovascular disease (ASCVD)
- Low-density lipoprotein cholesterol (LDL-C)>190 mg/dL
- Diabetic patients ages 40–75 with LDL-C of 70–189 mg/dL and without signs of clinical ASCVD
- Nondiabetic patients ages 40–75 with an estimated 10-year risk (e.g., Pooled Cohort Equations score)>7.5%

Statins vary in the extent to which they reduce LDL, and the magnitude of desired LDL reduction may depend on the presence and extent of other cardiac risk factors. Dosages may vary depending on the presence of additional factors (e.g., comorbid hypothyroidism), and all statins may require monitoring of liver enzymes and the clinical emergence of myalgias (which could reflect rhabdomyolysis).

Psychiatrists need to be aware of the risks and benefits of psychotropic drugs that may cause dyslipidemias, weight gain, or glycemic dysregulation, and they should collaborate proactively with primary care physicians when the observed psychiatric benefits are substantial and not easily re-created by an alternative medication. To that end, psychiatrists should be conversant with the use of available lipid-lowering agents, their specific indications (e.g., including dosing variations and the extent to which statins can reduce triglycerides as well as LDL), and relative safety profiles (Table 15–3). It is important to note that the 2014 ACC/AHA guideline favors statins (and their optimized dosages when necessary) as first-line lipid-lowering strategies rather than other cholesterol-lowering agents such as fibrates (e.g., gemfibrozil, clofibrate) or niacin, since controlled data are lacking for the use of nonstatins in lowering ASCVD mortality.

Additionally, preliminary controlled trial data suggest a possible lipid-lowering benefit from daily melatonin 3 mg/day or the melatonin agonist ramelteon 8 mg/day (Wang et al. 2016). Use of adjunctive lis-

TABLE 15–3. Lipid-lowering medications

Agent	Indication or usual clinical profile	Dosing range, mg/day	Common adverse effects	Laboratory monitoring
Statins (HMG-CoA reductase inhibitors)	First-line therapies, usually recommended for LDL ≥190 mg/dL or LDL≥160 mg/dL and positive family history of premature coronary artery disease or ≥2 coronary risk factors present in adolescents.	—	Myalgias; rare risk for rhabdomyolysis or diabetes mellitus	Serum ALT monitoring is recommended at baseline and periodically thereafter.
Atorvastatin	—	10–80	—	—
Fluvastatin	—	20–80	—	—
Lovastatin	—	20–80	—	—
Pravastatin	—	20–40	—	—
Rosuvastatin	The most potent statin; FDA approved for men > age 50 or women > age 60 with normal LDL but elevated CRP and one other risk factor for coronary artery disease (e.g., smoking, low HDL, family history).	5–40	—	—

TABLE 15–3.   Lipid-lowering medications *(continued)*

Agent	Indication or usual clinical profile	Dosing range, mg/day	Common adverse effects	Laboratory monitoring
Statins (HMG-CoA reductase inhibitors) *(continued)*				
Simvastatin	Lowers LDL by >30%; appropriate in diabetes or known heart disease as well as primary or secondary prevention indications.	20–80	—	—
Omega-3 fatty acids	Reduce triglycerides (FDA approved for triglycerides >500 mg/dL) and may increase HDL; have not been shown to reduce LDL or to lower risk for myocardial infarction or cardiovascular mortality.	≥1,000	Fishy aftertaste, GI upset, eructation, potential risk for increased bleeding time	None
Lovaza[a]	Hypertriglyceridemia.	—	—	None

TABLE 15–3. Lipid-lowering medications *(continued)*

Agent	Indication or usual clinical profile	Dosing range, mg/day	Common adverse effects	Laboratory monitoring
Combination regimens				
Atorvastatin/ amlodipine	Combination treatment for hypercholesterolemia and hypertension.	2.5/10–10/80	Constipation, diarrhea, nausea, headaches, dizziness, flushing, fatigue, weakness	As per statins
Ezetimibe/ simvastatin	Decreases total cholesterol, LDL cholesterol, apolipo-protein B, triglycerides, and non-HDL cholesterol; increases HDL.	10/10–10/80	Headache, arthralgias, GI upset	As per statins

Note. ALT=alanine aminotransferase; CRP=C-reactive protein; ER=extended release; FDA=U.S. Food and Drug Administration; GI=gastrointestinal; HDL=high-density lipoprotein; HMG-CoA=3-hydroxy-3-methylglutaryl coenzyme A; LDL=low-density lipoprotein; VLDL=very-low-density lipoprotein.
[a]A 1-g capsule contains 47% eicosapentaenoic acid and 38% docosahexaenoic acid.

dexamfetamine for bipolar depression also has been associated with reductions in total cholesterol, fasting LDL, and triglycerides (McElroy et al. 2015). Use of these agents, when psychiatrically appropriate, may thus have an added benefit of at least partly countering hypercholesterolemia, although neither would be a strategy aimed to reduce ASCVD and its associated risk for mortality.

Glycemic Dysregulation and Diabetes Mellitus

General Recommendations

Patients taking SGAs should have fasting blood glucose assessments before or upon the initiation of therapy, after 12 weeks of treatment, and annually thereafter while continuing an SGA. Measurement of hemoglobin A_{1c} also may be informative regarding patterns of hyperglycemia and assessment of diabetes or risk for the development of diabetes. The introduction of oral hypoglycemic agents such as metformin may be useful to counter weight gain and possible insulin resistance caused by psychotropic agents. Progression of insulin resistance or glycemic dysregulation may warrant discontinuation of a presumptive causal agent, particularly in the setting of other risk factors for coronary artery disease—unless a particular psychiatric agent appears to exert a unique benefit that outweighs metabolic risk, in which case active management of glycemic dysregulation to permit continued pharmacotherapy may be warranted.

Impaired glucose homeostasis is a known risk with SGAs and a number of other psychotropic compounds. Pharmaceutical manufacturers are quick to point out that individuals with serious mental illnesses such as bipolar disorder and schizophrenia have an inherently increased risk for the eventual development of diabetes and cardiovascular disease, independent of pharmacotherapies. Such observations, however, provide clinicians with little perspective on the independent contributions of specific psychotropic agents to a given patient's cumulative metabolic risk.

Above and beyond the increased vulnerability to diabetes caused by bipolar disorder or schizophrenia, SGAs can to varying degrees disrupt glucose metabolism by causing insulin resistance. For example, short-term (8-day) exposure of olanzapine in healthy men has been shown to impair insulin-mediated glucose metabolism, as well as to impede insulin-induced declines of free fatty acids and triglycerides (Vidarsdottir et al. 2010) — a finding at variance with earlier industry-sponsored reports that claimed to find no adverse effects on glucose disposal rate or insulin sensitivity among healthy volunteers after 3 weeks of exposure to olanzapine or risperidone (Sowell et al. 2003). Preclinical studies also indicate that the acute infusion of olanzapine in animals leads to rapid increases in blood sugar and marked reductions of plasma insulin and C-peptide in response to glucose challenge (Chintoh et al. 2008). In patients with schizophrenia treated over 24 months with an SGA, significant reductions from baseline in insulin sensitivity have been shown with olanzapine (~19%) or risperidone (~16%) but not with quetiapine (Newcomer et al. 2009). At least in schizophrenia, antipsychotic polypharmacy does not appear to increase the risk for metabolic syndrome over and above the risk incurred by use of a single SGA.

The reporting of changes in fasting blood glucose levels from short-term randomized trials is far less informative than long-term data, given that impaired glucose tolerance is a phenomenon that arises over the course of months to years, rather than weeks to months. In addition, pharmaceutical manufacturers of SGAs sometimes imply that their own reported fasting glucose rates may be overstated because some study participants may not reliably be tested under fasting conditions. By contrast, obviously, clinicians and patients are more concerned with manufacturers' underestimation rather than overestimation of metabolic parameters.

The American Diabetes Association (2010) identifies diabetes mellitus on a continuum based on degrees of hyperglycemia and impaired glucose tolerance, as summarized in Table 15–4.

Current recommendations from the American Diabetes Association and the American Psychiatric Association for patients taking an SGA include monitoring of fasting glucose and blood pressure at baseline, at 12 weeks, and annually thereafter. Metabolic monitoring for SGA recipients also includes weight or BMI measurement at baseline and at 4, 8, and 12 weeks, followed by quarterly assessments, waist circumference measurement at baseline and annually thereafter, and fasting lipid profiles at baseline, 12 weeks, and every 5 years thereafter (American Diabetes Association et al. 2004).

Insulin resistance refers to the body's inability to transport and use glucose from the vascular to the intracellular compartment. One theory to account for hyperglycemia associated with SGAs involves their apparent capacity to increase insulin resistance. An elevated ratio of serum triglycerides to HDL cholesterol (specifically, >3.8) is predictive of coronary disease and is sometimes taken as a rough proxy for insulin resistance (although the relationship appears less robust among blacks than whites). Insulin resistance and pancreatic beta-cell function also can be

TABLE 15–4. Operational definitions of diabetes mellitus

Category	Operational definition
Increased risk for diabetes	Fasting blood glucose of 100–125 mg/dL *or* 2-hour blood glucose of 140–199 mg/dL during a 75-g oral glucose tolerance test *or* Hemoglobin A_{1C} of 5.7%–6.4%
Diabetes mellitus	Hemoglobin $A_{1C} \geq 6.5\%$ *or* Fasting (≥ 8 hours) blood glucose ≥ 126 mg/dL *or* 2-hour blood glucose ≥ 200 mg/dL during 75-g oral glucose tolerance test *or* Random blood glucose > 200 mg/dL

Source.   American Diabetes Association 2010.

quantified using the homeostatic model assessment of insulin resistance (HOMA-IR) defined by the following equation:

$$\text{HOMA-IR} = \frac{\text{fasting glucose (nmol/L)} \times \text{fasting insulin (}\mu\text{U/L)}}{22.5}$$

HOMA-IR values ≥ 2.6 are sometimes viewed as a threshold cutoff to define insulin resistance (Ascaso et al. 2003).

Table 15–5 reports incidence rates for changes in blood glucose levels identified in randomized clinical trials of SGAs.

Since 2003, manufacturers' package inserts for all SGAs have carried a class warning from the FDA regarding their potential to increase blood sugar. Hyperglycemia may arise after short-term exposure to SGAs and may occur independently of weight gain (which separately can contribute to peripheral insulin resistance). Both clozapine and olanzapine inhibit glucose-induced insulin release from pancreatic beta cells (Chintoh et al. 2009), posing an independent cause of iatrogenic hyperglycemia.

In addition to the risk factors for metabolic syndrome previously identified above in Table 15–5, a personal or family history of non-insulin-

TABLE 15–5. Changes in blood sugar reported in FDA registration and other representative randomized trials of second-generation antipsychotics

Agent	Observations
Aripiprazole	In a 26-week randomized trial in schizophrenia, +0.13 mg/dL from baseline (Pigott et al. 2003); mean of 4.1 mg/dL less than seen with olanzapine across three schizophrenia trials (N=1,487) (Rummel-Kluge et al. 2010).
Asenapine	In 3-week registration trials for bipolar mania and 6-week registration trials for schizophrenia, mean change from baseline=–0.6 mg/dL and +3.2 mg/dL, respectively. In 52-week open extension data in schizophrenia, mean change from baseline=+2.4 mg/dL.
Brexpiprazole	In 6-week schizophrenia or major depression adjunctive trials, no significant differences from placebo in categorical changes from "normal" (<100 mg/dL) to "high" (≥126 mg/dL) fasting glucose; in long-term open trials, 9% of major depression patients and 10% of schizophrenia patients had categorical shifts from "normal" or "borderline" to "high."
Cariprazine	Across pooled 3-week registration trials in bipolar I mania (N=1,065), changes from baseline in fasting glucose levels were only nominally higher with cariprazine (3–6 mg/day=6.6 mg/dL; 9–12 mg/day=7.2 mg/dL) than placebo (1.7 mg/dL) (Earley et al. 2017b). In 48-week open-label extension data in schizophrenia, categorical shifts from normal (<100 mg/dL) to high (≥126 mg/dL) fasting glucose levels were comparable across cariprazine doses (2.6%–4.5%) to those seen with placebo (3.8%) (Nasrallah et al. 2017).
Iloperidone	Mean serum glucose: +7.2 mg/dL to +16.2 mg/dL (dose dependent and greater than seen with placebo) (Weiden et al. 2008).

TABLE 15–5. **Changes in blood sugar reported in FDA registration and other representative randomized trials of second-generation antipsychotics *(continued)***

Agent	Observations
Lurasidone	Fasting glucose levels across dosages from manufacturer's pooled short-term trials in schizophrenia = +1.3 mg/dL. From open-label extension data: at 24 weeks: +1.6 mg/dL; at 36 weeks: +0.3 mg/dL; at 52 weeks: +1.2 mg/dL. In bipolar depression monotherapy or adjunctive therapy trials: −0.8 mg/dL to +0.9 mg/dL (Loebel et al. 2014a, 2014b).
Olanzapine	In CATIE, mean change in fasting glucose = +15.0 mg/dL (Lieberman et al. 2005).
Paliperidone	Mean change from baseline in serum glucose level = +0.1 mg/dL across three pooled 6-week randomized trials in schizophrenia (Meltzer et al. 2008).
Pimavanserin	Not reported.
Quetiapine	Incidence of fasting glucose ≥126 mg/dL = 2%–12% across indications in FDA randomized trials. In CATIE, mean change in fasting glucose = +6.8 mg/dL (Lieberman et al. 2005); mean of 9.3 mg/dL less than olanzapine across four schizophrenia trials (N=986) (Rummel-Kluge et al. 2010).
Risperidone	In CATIE, mean change in fasting glucose = +6.7 mg/dL (Lieberman et al. 2005); mean of 5.9 mg/dL less than olanzapine across nine schizophrenia trials (N=986) (Rummel-Kluge et al. 2010).
Ziprasidone	In CATIE, mean change in fasting glucose = +2.3 mg/dL (Lieberman et al. 2005); mean of 8.35 mg/dL less than olanzapine across four schizophrenia trials (N=1,420) (Rummel-Kluge et al. 2010).

Note. CATIE=Clinical Antipsychotic Trials of Intervention Effectiveness; FDA=U.S. Food and Drug Administration.

dependent diabetes (e.g., gestational diabetes) increases the risk specifically for hyperglycemia or the eventual development of diabetes. Racial/ethnic differences also may contribute to differential effects on metabolic dysregulation. For example, the risk for metabolic syndrome during treatment with aripiprazole appears higher in black or Hispanic subjects than in white subjects, whereas no such racial/ethnic differences have been observed in the case of olanzapine (Meyer et al. 2009) even though weight gain may be significantly greater during olanzapine treatment among black versus white patients with primary psychotic disorders (Stauffer et al. 2010).

Although no absolute contraindication exists for the use of SGAs among individuals with known type 2 diabetes, minimal literature is available on the safety and efficacy of using such agents in this population. The CATIE study (Lieberman et al. 2005) included about 10% of subjects with known type 2 diabetes at baseline, but all were treated with oral hypoglycemics or additional antidiabetic regimens, which would have confounded post hoc analyses regarding differential effects of antipsychotics on blood glucose levels. No prospective randomized studies of SGAs have been undertaken specifically among individuals with preexisting type 2 diabetes; consequently, decisions about the relative risks versus benefits of SGAs for diabetic patients must be individualized on the basis of the magnitude and extent of metabolic dysregulation and cardiovascular risk versus the severity of psychopathology and availability of other effective, metabolically neutral pharmacotherapies.

Certain antidepressants, including SSRIs, venlafaxine, and TCAs, have also been implicated in the development of impaired glucose homeostasis and diabetes, particularly during long-term treatment in patients under age 44. In patients with diabetic neuropathic pain, for example, duloxetine significantly increased fasting glucose (by 12.5 mg/dL over 52 weeks) and hemoglobin A_{1C} (by 0.5%) versus placebo. A nested case-control study of 165,958 patients with major depression in the United Kingdom found that over a period of at least 2 years' exposure, recipients of an SSRI or TCA had an approximate twofold increased risk for new-onset diabetes mellitus compared with matched comparison subjects who did not take an antidepressant (Andersohn et al. 2009); among studied agents, the highest rates were seen with amitriptyline (risk ratio=9.05) or venlafaxine (risk ratio=3.01), and the lowest rates were seen with fluvoxamine (risk ratio=1.75). The risk for developing type 2 diabetes with an SSRI was lower in patients whose exposure was shorter and in whom dosages were lower. In this study, glycemic dysregulation was thought to arise secondarily to weight gain rather than other mechanisms (e.g., time spent depressed).

The oral hypoglycemic agent metformin is perhaps the most extensively studied of adjunctive pharmacotherapies used for patients who gain significant weight or develop increased metabolic risk due to psychotropic drugs, most notably SGAs. Metformin belongs to a drug class known as biguanides; two other biguanides, buformin (never approved by the FDA) and phenformin, have been withdrawn from most worldwide markets due to high risks for lactic acidosis. By comparison, the risk for either significant hypoglycemia or lactic acidosis among type 2 diabetics taking metformin appears extremely low (i.e., 6 cases in total identified among 50,048 subjects in one nested case-control study, yielding a crude incident rate of 3.3 cases per 100,000 person-years); in fact, recognized cases of lactic acidosis during metformin therapy for diabetes typically appear linked to the presence of other risk factors for lactic acidosis, such as congestive heart failure, acute renal failure, or sepsis (Bodmer et al. 2008). Metformin does not directly stimulate insulin secretion, and this likely accounts for its low risk for causing hypoglycemia.

A meta-analysis by Ehret et al. (2010) showed that although metformin added to SGAs did not significantly lower the risk for the eventual development of type 2 diabetes, it was associated with significant reductions in weight, body mass index, and waist circumference. Metformin's presumptive mechanism for weight loss appears related to helping overcome insulin resistance caused by antipsychotics and decreasing hepatic glucose production. Studies have not, as yet, examined whether metformin could help counteract weight gain caused by psychotropic drugs other than SGAs, although to the extent that its mechanism of action appears linked with counteracting drug-induced insulin resistance, it might not be expected to cause weight loss unless the proximal cause of weight gain involved increased insulin resistance.

A number of other agents have been developed in recent years that function as oral hypoglycemics or insulin-sensitizing drugs relevant to patients with, or at risk for, diabetes. These drugs vary in the extent to which they have been found to promote weight loss, and most have not been formally studied to counteract iatrogenic metabolic dysregulation specifically caused by psychotropic medications. Such agents include three main classes:

- *Thiazolidinediones* (also known as *glitazones* or *peroxisome proliferator-activated receptor gamma [PPARγ] agonists*), including pioglitazone and rosiglitazone, decrease insulin resistance and reduce leptin levels (potentially *increasing* appetite, posing greater likelihood of weight gain than loss); they may shift fat distribution from visceral to subcutaneous adipose tissue, thereby improving insulin sensitivity.

- *Selective dipeptidyl peptidase–4 inhibitors* (*DPP-4 inhibitors*, also known as *gliptins*), such as alogliptin, linagliptin, saxagliptin, and sitagliptin, increase levels of incretins (metabolic hormones that augment insulin release to enhance lowering of postprandial blood sugar). DPP-4 inhibitors as a class may cause severe joint pain. There is unresolved controversy about whether they may also increase the risk for pancreatitis and pancreatic cancer, based mainly on data in rodents.
- *Glycogen-like peptide–1 (GLP-1) agonists*, such as luraglutide and dulaglutide, which mimic the action of incretins to lower blood sugar, slow gastric emptying and increase insulin release from pancreatic beta cells. Some SGAs appear to increase glucagon levels and suppress GLP-1 activity in preclinical studies.

A summary of findings regarding oral hypoglycemics and their potential value for managing obesity and metabolic dysregulation is provided in Table 15–6.

Weight Gain

General Recommendations

Interventions focused on diet and exercise appear to have the greatest overall efficacy in helping to counteract psychotropic-induced weight gain, particularly in patients with poor nutritional habits and sedentary lifestyles. Pharmacological strategies that have demonstrated clinically meaningful weight loss include metformin (for atypical antipsychotics), topiramate, zonisamide, amantadine, lamotrigine, and either switches to or augmentation with aripiprazole or ziprasidone. Psychostimulants or phentermine may be useful when appropriate. Adjunctive orlistat has shown modest benefit in men with psychotropic-induced weight gain. Liraglutide may promote weight loss particularly among patients with at-risk status for diabetes.

Iatrogenic obesity and overweight are among the most common and difficult-to-treat problems that confront prescribers of almost all classes of psychotropic medications and represent a leading cause of medication cessation. Differences may exist across types of medicines regarding probable mechanisms of weight gain, time course to weight gain, and risk factors, although particular risk factors for weight gain with a specific psychotropic agent have not been well described in the literature. Many agents that cause significant weight gain (e.g., lithium, divalproex) do so only after extended periods of treatment, and this limits

TABLE 15–6.   Oral hypoglycemics and other insulin-sensitizing agents relevant to managing metabolic dysregulation

Drug class	Dosing range/route	Relevant findings
Oral hypoglycemics/biguanides		
Metformin	500–2,550 mg po qDay	A meta-analysis of 12 studies involving 743 antipsychotic-treated schizophrenia or schizoaffective disorder patients revealed a mean weight change of −3.27 kg (95% CI=−4.66 to −1.89 kg), significantly reduced BMI, and improved insulin resistance (de Silva et al. 2016). May also decrease blood lipids.
Thiazolidinediones		
Pioglitazone	15–30 mg po qDay	Improves fasting glucose levels, insulin resistance, and HDL levels in antipsychotic-treated schizophrenia patients with dyslipidemias or glycemic dysregulation, but weight loss has not been demonstrated (Smith et al. 2013).
Rosiglitazone	4–8 mg po qDay	Preliminary trials suggest improved glucose utilization and trends toward improved insulin sensitivity in clozapine-treated schizophrenia patients (Henderson et al. 2009b) and improved glycemic control but no weight reduction in olanzapine-treated schizophrenia patients (Baptista et al. 2009).

TABLE 15–6. Oral hypoglycemics and other insulin-sensitizing agents relevant to managing metabolic dysregulation (*continued*)

Drug class	Dosing range/route	Relevant findings
DPP-4 inhibitors		
Alogliptin	25 mg po qDay	No data in psychotropic-induced weight gain or metabolic dysregulation. In NIDDM patients, improves glycemic control, but there is no evidence of weight loss. May increase the risk of heart failure.
Linagliptin	5 mg po qDay	No data in psychotropic-induced weight gain or metabolic dysregulation. In NIDDM patients, improves glycemic control, but there is no evidence of weight loss.
Saxagliptin	2.5–5 mg po qDay	No data in psychotropic-induced weight gain or metabolic dysregulation. In NIDDM patients, improves glycemic control, but there is no evidence of weight loss. May increase the risk of heart failure.
Sitagliptin	100 mg po qDay	No data in psychotropic-induced weight gain or metabolic dysregulation. In NIDDM patients, improves glycemic control, but there is no evidence of weight loss. Rare cases of renal failure and pancreatitis in humans have been reported.
GLP-1 agonists		
Albiglutide	30–50 mg SC once weekly	Modest weight loss in overweight adults with diabetes.

TABLE 15–6. Oral hypoglycemics and other insulin-sensitizing agents relevant to managing metabolic dysregulation (continued)

Drug class	Dosing range/route	Relevant findings
GLP-1 agonists (*continued*)		
Liraglutide	Begun at 0.6 mg/day SC, increased by 0.6 mg/day each week to target dose of 1.8 mg/day SC	In prediabetic and overweight/obese clozapine- or olanzapine-treated schizophrenia spectrum patients, significantly better glucose tolerance, greater weight loss (−5.3 kg), and reductions in waist circumference (−4.1 cm), visceral fat (−250.19 grams), and LDL cholesterol levels (−15.4 mg/dL) after 16 weeks (Larsen et al. 2017); may also reduce insulin resistance and weight gain in olanzapine-treated obese rats.
Lixisenatide	10 µg/day SC × 14 days, then 20 µg/day SC	In otherwise healthy adults with NIDDM, may improve glycemic control as well as promote weight loss (−2.96 to +0.3 kg in acute trials; Trujillo and Goldman 2017). No data as yet for managing psychotropic-induced weight gain or metabolic dysregulation.
Dulaglutide	0.75 mg–1.5 mg SC once weekly	Weak but significant correlation between improvements in HbA$_{1C}$ and weight loss over 26 weeks in otherwise healthy adults with NIDDM (weight loss range=−0.87 kg to −3.18 kg; Umpierrez et al. 2016). No data as of yet for managing psychotropic-induced weight gain or metabolic dysregulation.
Exenatide	2 mg SC once weekly	No difference from placebo in weight loss over 3 months in obese antipsychotic-treated schizophrenia patients (Ishøy et al. 2017).

Note. BMI=body mass index; DPP-4=dipeptidyl peptidase-4; GLP-1=glycogen-like peptide-1; HbA$_{1C}$=hemoglobin A$_{1C}$; NIDDM= non-insulin-dependent diabetes mellitus; po=by mouth; SC=subcutaneously.

the extent to which short-term randomized controlled trials of FDA registration studies are able to detect long-term risk. Risks also may differ with a given compound across varying disease states (e.g., schizophrenia vs. bipolar disorder; major depression vs. anxiety disorders), within a given disease state (e.g., atypical depression vs. agitated or melancholic depression), in the presence or absence of common comorbidities (e.g., alcohol abuse), or when used as a monotherapy versus in conjunction with other agents.

As a rule of thumb, ideal body weight for men is 47.7 kg for the first 5 feet and an additional 2.7 kg for each inch above 5 feet; in women, ideal body weight is 45 kg at 5 feet with 2.3 kg added per inch above 5 feet. Medically, clinicians should assure the absence of other causes of weight gain before assuming it is the result of psychotropic medications. Careful assessment includes the following considerations:

- Differentiating weight gain caused by adipose tissue versus fluid retention (rapid and substantial weight gain should prompt examination for edema)
- Assuring the absence of hypothyroidism
- Assessing dietary habits, including alcohol
- Differentiating hyperphagia due to depression or anxiety from appetite stimulation caused by medications
- Identifying all medications, both psychiatric and nonpsychiatric, that may predispose to weight gain (Table 15–7)
- Identifying any nonprescribed nutritional supplements, such as high-dose vitamins, minerals, and antioxidants, that potentially could interfere with treatment

Industry-sponsored clinical trials typically define substantial weight gain by convention as increases of ≥7% from baseline weight, but this metric can be clinically uninformative if it is not normalized by baseline weight or BMI (i.e., less weight gain is needed to fulfill this criterion in subjects with low initial weight). In adults, but not children, absolute weight gain offers a more robust and clinically useful statistic. In addition, although weight gain has been reported in some industry clinical trials as being more likely among subjects with low rather than high pretreatment BMI, this distinction has not been borne out in naturalistic studies.

Second-Generation Antipsychotics

Representative rates of weight gain with SGAs as reported in clinical trials, stratified by psychiatric disorders, are summarized in Table 15–8.

TABLE 15–7. Weight changes associated with common medications

Minimal or no weight gain	Moderate or variable weight gain	Substantial weight gain
ACE inhibitors	Aripiprazole	Clozapine
·Asenapine	Brexpiprazole	Mirtazapine
Atomoxetine	Divalproex	Olanzapine
Beta-blockers	Duloxetine	Quetiapine
Bupropion	Gabapentin	Risperidone
Buspirone	Lithium	
Carbamazepine	MAOIs	
Desvenlafaxine	Pregabalin	
Fluoxetine	SSRIs other than	
H$_2$ blockers	fluoxetine or	
Iloperidone	vilazodone	
Lamotrigine	Tricyclic antidepressants	
Levomilnacipran	Venlafaxine	
Lurasidone		
Naltrexone		
Psychostimulants		
Topiramate		
Transdermal selegiline		
Vilazodone		
Vortioxetine		
Ziprasidone		

Note. ACE=angiotensin-converting enzyme; MAOI=monoamine oxidase inhibitor; SSRI=selective serotonin reuptake inhibitors.

Appetite Stimulation

In the case of SGAs, it is thought that weight gain, to varying degrees, may occur from appetite stimulation caused by blockade of histamine H$_1$ receptors and antagonism of serotonin type 2C (5-HT$_{2C}$) receptors, which together disrupt hypothalamic satiety control. SGAs may induce lipogenic genes (Kristiana et al. 2010) and activate protein kinase C-beta, which in turn may foster the differentiation and proliferation of preadipocytes (Pavan et al. 2010). Other proposed mechanisms of weight gain

TABLE 15–8. Representative rates of weight gain with SGAs as reported in FDA registration trials and other randomized studies[a]

Drug	Disorder	NNH[b]	Short-term		Long-term	
			Mean weight changes	Incidence of clinically significant weight ↑[c]	Mean weight changes	Incidence of clinically significant weight ↑[b]
Aripiprazole	Schizophrenia	21	+0.7 kg across 4- to 6-week trials	8%	+0.3 kg over 28 weeks (oral) −0.2 kg over 52 weeks (long-acting injectible) (Kane et al. 2012)	16% (oral) (Kane et al. 2009) 6.4% (long-acting injectible) (Kane et al. 2012)
	Bipolar disorder	ND	+0.1 kg across 3-week trials	2%	+0.4 kg across three randomized trials	20% (McIntyre 2010)
	Major depression	22	+1.7 kg across two randomized 6-week trials (Fava et al. 2009)	5.2%	—	—

TABLE 15–8. Representative rates of weight gain with SGAs as reported in FDA registration trials and other randomized studies[a] *(continued)*

Drug	Disorder	NNH[b]	Short-term		Long-term	
			Mean weight changes	Incidence of clinically significant weight ↑[c]	Mean weight changes	Incidence of clinically significant weight ↑[b]
Asenapine	Schizophrenia	35	+1.1 kg	4.9%	+0.7 kg over 26 weeks of randomized monotherapy (Kane et al. 2010)	8.0% (Kane et al. 2011)
	Bipolar disorder	19	+1.3 kg	5.8%	—	—
Brexpiprazole	Major depressive disorder	52	+1.3 kg to +1.6 kg across doses in acute adjunctive trials	2%–5%	+2.9 kg at 26 weeks; +3.1 kg at 52 weeks	30%
	Schizophrenia	17	+1.0 to +1.2 kg across doses in acute trials	10%–11%	+1.3 kg at 26 weeks; +2.0 kg at 52 weeks	20%
	Bipolar mania	ND	+0.5 to +0.6 kg across doses in 3-week trials	3%	+0.9 kg over 16-week open-label trial (Ketter et al. 2018)	9.3% after 16 weeks (Ketter et al. 2018)

TABLE 15–8. Representative rates of weight gain with SGAs as reported in FDA registration trials and other randomized studies[a] *(continued)*

Drug	Disorder	NNH[b]	Short-term		Long-term	
			Mean weight changes	Incidence of clinically significant weight ↑[c]	Mean weight changes	Incidence of clinically significant weight ↑[b]
Cariprazine	Bipolar depression	ND	+0.6 to +1.1 kg across doses (no clear dose relationship) in 8-week randomized trial (Durgam et al. 2016)	2%–7% across doses (no clear dose relationship)	No data	No data
	Schizophrenia	34	+0.8 to +1.0 kg across doses in 6-week trials	8%–17%	+1.2 kg at 12 weeks; +1.7 kg at 24 weeks; +2.5 kg at 48 weeks	—
	Schizophrenia	ND	+1.1 kg (dose-related across four acute trials (Earley et al. 2017a)	9.2%	+1.58 kg over 48 weeks (Nasrallah et al. 2017)	27% (Nasrallah et al. 2017)

TABLE 15–8. Representative rates of weight gain with SGAs as reported in FDA registration trials and other randomized studies[a] (continued)

Drug	Disorder	NNH[b]	Short-term		Long-term	
			Mean weight changes	Incidence of clinically significant weight ↑[c]	Mean weight changes	Incidence of clinically significant weight ↑[b]
Clozapine	Schizophrenia	NR	+4.5 kg (meta-analysis of acute trials; Allison et al. 1999)	—	+7.7 kg; 75% gained ≥4.5 kg over 6 months (Lamberti et al. 1992); +11.7 kg over 8 years (Bai et al. 2006)	—
Iloperidone	Schizophrenia	10	+1.5 kg to +2.1 kg (Weiden et al. 2008)	12%–18%	—	—
Lurasidone	Schizophrenia	67	+0.5 kg to +0.9 kg (Meltzer et al. 2011)	5.6%	–0.4 kg to –0.7 kg (24- to 52-week open-label extension data)	—

TABLE 15–8. Representative rates of weight gain with SGAs as reported in FDA registration trials and other randomized studies[a] *(continued)*

| Drug | Disorder | NNH[b] | Short-term | | Long-term | |
			Mean weight changes	Incidence of clinically significant weight ↑[c]	Mean weight changes	Incidence of clinically significant weight ↑[b]
Lurasidone *(continued)*	Bipolar depression	58	Monotherapy: +0.6 kg (20–60 mg/day) or 0.0 kg (80–20 mg/day) (Loebel et al. 2014a) Adjunctive therapy: +0.2 kg (Loebel et al. 2014b)	2.4% (monotherapy) 3.1% (adjunctive therapy)	–0.2 kg (24-week open-label extension data)	—

TABLE 15–8. Representative rates of weight gain with SGAs as reported in FDA registration trials and other randomized studies[a] *(continued)*

Drug	Disorder	NNH[b]	Short-term		Long-term	
			Mean weight changes	Incidence of clinically significant weight ↑[c]	Mean weight changes	Incidence of clinically significant weight ↑[b]
Olanzapine	All indications	3–6	Across 13 acute placebo-controlled FDA registration trials, mean change of +2.6 kg; +4.2 kg in meta-analysis of acute trials (Allison et al. 1999)	22%	+4.3 to +13.2 kg over 6 months to 2.5 years (Kinon et al. 2001; Lieberman et al. 2005; Newcomer et al. 2009; Vanina et al. 2002); +5.6 kg over 48 weeks in FDA registration trials	30% (Lieberman et al. 2005) to 75% (Perez-Iglesias et al. 2008)

TABLE 15–8. Representative rates of weight gain with SGAs as reported in FDA registration trials and other randomized studies[a] *(continued)*

Drug	Disorder	NNH[b]	Short-term		Long-term	
			Mean weight changes	Incidence of clinically significant weight ↑[c]	Mean weight changes	Incidence of clinically significant weight ↑[b]
Paliperidone	Schizophrenia	35	+0.6 to +1.1 kg across three 6-week acute trials	6%–9%	+1.4 kg across 24 weeks; +2.6 kg at 52 weeks in open-label extension trials	32% (52-week open-label extension data)
Quetiapine	Schizophrenia	6	+2.0 kg	23%	+0.5 kg to +3.7 kg (up to 18 months) (Lieberman et al. 2005; Newcomer et al. 2009)	16% (Lieberman et al. 2005)
	Bipolar disorder	8–20	+1.7 kg (mania) +1.0 kg to +1.6 kg (depression; Calabrese et al. 2005)	21% 3.5%–9%	In maintenance trials, +3.1 kg as monotherapy in first 36 weeks, then +0.5 kg as adjunct to lithium or divalproex in weeks 37–104 (Suppes et al. 2009)	11.5% as adjunct to lithium or divalproex over 104 weeks (Suppes et al. 2009)

TABLE 15–8. Representative rates of weight gain with SGAs as reported in FDA registration trials and other randomized studies[a] *(continued)*

Drug	Disorder	NNH[b]	Short-term		Long-term	
			Mean weight changes	Incidence of clinically significant weight ↑[c]	Mean weight changes	Incidence of clinically significant weight ↑[b]
Risperidone	All indications	18	+2.1 kg (meta-analysis of acute trials; Allison et al. 1999)	18% (acute schizophrenia trials); 2.5% (bipolar mania trials)	+0.4 kg to +9.5 kg (up to 18 months) (Lieberman et al. 2005; Newcomer et al. 2009; Perez-Iglesias et al. 2008; Vanina et al. 2002)	14% (Lieberman et al. 2005) to 71% (Perez-Iglesias et al. 2008)
Ziprasidone	All indications	16–58	Stratifies by BMI: baseline BMI <23:1.4-kg gain; BMI >27: 1.3-kg loss	10%	−0.7±0.5 kg (CATIE; Lieberman et al. 2005)	7% (Lieberman et al. 2005)

Note. −=no data; BMI=body mass index; CATIE=Clinical Antipsychotic Trials of Intervention Effectiveness; FDA=U.S. Food and Drug Administration; ND=no different from (or less than reported with) placebo; NR=not reported.
[a]Data based on FDA registration trial data as reported in manufacturers' package insert information, unless otherwise noted.
[b]NNH for significant weight gain as reported by Citrome (2009a, 2010, 2011a, 2014, 2015).
[c]"Clinically significant weight gain" defined as ≥7% increase of initial weight.

include decreased thermogenesis and decreased energy expenditure. Weight gain associated with some SGAs also has been associated with changes in levels of the appetite-stimulating peptide hormone ghrelin and the appetite-suppressing hormones leptin and adiponectin. However, the relationships between changes in these hormones and appetite increases induced by SGAs are not straightforward. Several studies have identified increases in serum leptin after administration of some SGAs—notably, clozapine (Atmaca et al. 2003) and olanzapine (Atmaca et al. 2003; Hosojima et al. 2006), with a lesser effect from risperidone (Atmaca et al. 2003). Serum ghrelin levels have been shown to decrease during treatment with olanzapine in some studies (Hosojima et al. 2006; B. J. Kim et al. 2008), whereas adiponectin levels appear unaffected during the first few weeks after initiation of an SGA (Hosojima et al. 2006). Still other investigators have found elevated ghrelin levels with relatively unchanged leptin levels in connection with weight gain related to clozapine, olanzapine, or risperidone (Esen-Danaci et al. 2008). In all likelihood, leptin levels rise as a result of (rather than cause) the increased fat stores induced by some SGAs, and persistent hunger fails to override the leptin signal that would otherwise promote satiety.

Predictors of Weight Gain

The literature is surprisingly sparse in identifying robust predictors of weight gain caused by SGAs, with few exceptions. Substantial weight gain appears more likely to occur during treatment with olanzapine in patients who are younger, are nonwhite, have a low BMI, have a non-rapid-cycling course of bipolar illness, and have psychotic features (Lipkovich et al. 2006). Weight gain seems to correlate with clinical response (which may be an artifact of the amount and duration of exposure to therapy), as well as rises in blood pressure, total serum cholesterol, and nonfasting blood glucose levels (Hennen et al. 2004). In short-term (~6-week) trials of olanzapine or risperidone in patients with schizophrenia, predictors of weight gain included younger age, male gender, nonwhite race, and favorable clinical response (Basson et al. 2001). Longer-term randomized trials (≥39 weeks) of olanzapine in schizophrenia identified low baseline BMI as a robust predictor of weight gain (Kinon et al. 2001). Other reported predictors of weight gain with olanzapine, risperidone, or clozapine include female gender, parents' BMI, younger age, and nonsmoking status (Gebhardt et al. 2009). In bipolar disorder, lower cognitive function (notably, attention, verbal memory, working memory, and global cognition) appear to be associated with weight gain during pharmacotherapy, independent of other clinical predictors (Bond et al. 2017).

Time Course and Magnitude of Weight Gain

The time course and magnitude of weight gain with SGAs can vary. In the case of olanzapine in the treatment of schizophrenia, weight gain appears to persist for up to 39 weeks before eventually plateauing (see Kinon et al. 2001). During a 1-year follow-up of 351 psychiatric patients taking a variety of antipsychotics, antidepressants, and mood stabilizers associated with weight gain, an increase from baseline weight of >5% after one month was highly predictive of more serious subsequent weight gain (≥15% after 3 months) (Vandenberghe et al. 2015). While most SGAs carry some liability for weight gain, they may vary considerably in magnitude and extent. In the CATIE chronic schizophrenia trial (Lieberman et al. 2005), for example, premature study termination due to weight gain or metabolic effects was significantly more likely among subjects taking olanzapine (9%) than all other agents (1%–4%).

Zydis Formulations

Anecdotal observations and reports from small case series have suggested that the Zydis orally dissolving formulation of olanzapine may cause less weight gain than the conventional formulation (for review, see Karagianis et al. 2008). At least one rather speculative mechanism has been proposed to account theoretically for this possibility, involving the faster absorption of orally dissolving olanzapine when administered sublingually (Markowitz et al. 2006), which in turn may lead to decreased ghrelin signaling, possibly because of the lesser quantity of olanzapine coming into proximity with ghrelin-containing cells in the fundus of the stomach (Chawla and Luxton-Andrew 2008).

A preliminary 6-week randomized comparison of orally dissolving olanzapine versus standard olanzapine in 38 first-onset psychosis patients found significantly less weight gain occurring in those taking the orally dissolving formulation (Arranz et al. 2007), although a larger and more definitive industry-sponsored 16-week multisite randomized trial, involving 149 bipolar or primary psychotic disorder patients who had gained at least 5 kg with standard olanzapine tablets, found no significant differences between conventional olanzapine and the Zydis formulation in any parameters related to weight gain (Karagianis et al. 2009).

Long-Acting Injectable SGA Formulations

Metabolic changes, including potential weight gain, during treatment with long-acting injectable (LAI) formulations of SGAs, are generally comparable to those observed during short- and long-term use of oral

SGA formulations. Changes in weight as reported from clinical trials with SGA LAIs are presented in Table 15–9.

Lithium, Anticonvulsants, and Antidepressants

Tables 15–10 and 15–11 summarize information from controlled trials, including FDA registration trials, regarding the incidence and correlates of weight gain during treatment with lithium or anticonvulsants and with antidepressants, respectively.

Mechanisms for iatrogenic weight gain with lithium or anticonvulsants are less well understood than appears to be the case with SGAs or antidepressants. Notably, however, divalproex may increase body mass via raising serum leptin levels (Verrotti et al. 1999) as well as by reducing thermogenesis and increasing long-chain fatty acids through competitive binding to serum albumin (Vanina et al. 2002). Lithium-induced weight gain (unrelated to peripheral edema or hypothyroidism) has been suggested to result from thirst-related increased consumption of high-sugar beverages and increased body stores of carbohydrates and lipids (Vanina et al. 2002). Lithium also may decrease plasma adiponectin levels, in turn contributing to weight gain. Compared with olanzapine, weight gain with lithium or divalproex may follow a more gradual trajectory and result in less total weight gain than seen with certain SGAs.

Studies that report weight gain with anticonvulsants other than divalproex (e.g., gabapentin; DeToledo et al. 1997) typically have focused on high doses in epilepsy populations rather than in psychiatric patients. Extended-release carbamazepine and lamotrigine each appear to be weight-neutral during long-term treatment for bipolar disorder (Ketter et al. 2004; Sachs et al. 2006a). In fact, lamotrigine has been associated with weight loss in obese nonpsychiatric patients as well as obese patients with bipolar disorder (see Table 15–2).

Data from FDA registration studies have important limitations regarding inferences for patients treated in routine clinical practice: 1) trials are generally brief, providing no information on weight gain with long-term use; 2) most trials involve monotherapy, whereas many patients with mood or anxiety disorders take combinations of drugs with additive or synergistic risks for weight gain; and 3) subjects enrolled in FDA registration trials often are already overweight and lack risk factors for weight gain that pertain to the general population. These include the absence of unstable medical problems (e.g., diabetes, nonalcoholic steatohepatitis or nonalcoholic fatty liver disease; see the section "Hepatic Impairment and Transaminitis" in Chapter 12, "Gastrointestinal System"); an absence of concurrent psychiatric disorders (e.g., eating disorders) or

TABLE 15–9. Weight changes with long-acting injectable second-generation antipsychotic formulations

Agent	Study	Total weight change	Proportion with > 7% weight gain
Aripiprazole extended-release injectable suspension	Schizophrenia (12-week placebo-controlled trial) (Kane et al. 2014)	+3.5 kg	21.5%
	Schizophrenia (52-week placebo-controlled trial) (Kane et al. 2012)	+0.1 kg during acute stabilization; −0.2 kg at end of maintenance phase	5.4% during acute stabilization; 6.4% at end of maintenance phase
	Bipolar disorder (52-week placebo-controlled trial) (Calabrese et al. 2017)	+1.3 kg	18%
Paliperidone palmitate	Schizophrenia (Four 9–13-week placebo-controlled trials (manufacturer's product information)	+0.4 to +1.4 kg across dosages and trials	6.0%–13.1% across dosages and trials
	Schizophrenia (24-week placebo-controlled trial) (Hough et al. 2010)	+1.9 kg	23%
	Schizophrenia (53-week open label trial) (manufacturer's product information)	+2.4 kg at week 29; +4.3 kg at week 53	Not reported

TABLE 15–9. Weight changes with long-acting injectable second-generation antipsychotic formulations *(continued)*

Agent	Study	Total weight change	Proportion with >7% weight gain
Paliperidone palmitate *(continued)*	Schizoaffective disorder (25-week open label trial) (manufacturer's product information)	+2.2 kg	18.4%
Risperidone long-acting injectable	Schizophrenia (12-week placebo-controlled trial) (manufacturer's product information)	+0.5 kg to +1.2 kg	8%–10%
	Schizophrenia (50-week open label trial) (manufacturer's product information)	+2.1 kg (week 24); +2.8 kg (week 50)	Not reported
	Bipolar I disorder (12-week open label, then 18-week placebo-controlled trial) (Vieta et al. 2012)	24% reported "weight increase"	14%
Olanzapine long-acting injectable	Schizophrenia (8-week placebo-controlled trial) (Lauriello et al. 2008)	+3.2 to +4.8 kg across doses	23.6%–35.4% across doses
	Schizophrenia (24-week placebo-controlled trial) (Kane et al. 2010)	+0.67 to +1.70 kg across doses	8%–24% across doses
	Schizophrenia (6-year open label) (Anand et al. 2015)	+2.19 kg	40.8%

TABLE 15–10. Representative rates of weight change with lithium or anticonvulsants reported in FDA registration trials and other randomized studies

Agent	Weight change and time course	Notable risk factors
Lithium	Up to 66% of patients gained an average of 10 kg over 2–10 years (Vanina et al. 2002); 13% of bipolar I patients had weight gain with monotherapy over 1 year (Bowden et al. 2000). In a 1-year comparison of lithium with lamotrigine or placebo for bipolar relapse prevention, mean weight changes with lithium monotherapy were +6.1 kg among initially obese subjects and +1.1 kg in initially nonobese subjects (Bowden et al. 2006a).	Obesity at baseline; mechanism of weight gain may be related to lithium-induced decreases in serum leptin levels (Atmaca et al. 2002) or direct serotonergic effects; no clear dose relationship.
Carbamazepine	Weight gain is not identified as an adverse effect in FDA registration trials, although isolated case reports of weight gain have been described in the epilepsy literature.	None known.
Divalproex	21% of bipolar I patients had weight gain during divalproex maintenance treatment over 1 year (Bowden et al. 2000).	Serum valproate levels >125 ng/mL (Bowden et al. 2000).
Gabapentin	2% of patients had weight gain in trials for postherpetic neuralgia; 3% of patients had weight gain in add-on therapy trials for epilepsy.	None known.

TABLE 15–10. Representative rates of weight change with lithium or anticonvulsants reported in FDA registration trials and other randomized studies *(continued)*

Agent	Weight change and time course	Notable risk factors
Lamotrigine	In trials for bipolar disorder, weight gain was reported in 1%–5%. Mean weight change at 52 weeks was –4.2 kg among initially obese patients and –0.5 kg among nonobese patients (Bowden et al. 2006a).	None known.
Oxcarbazepine	1%–2% incidence of any weight gain during trials of adjunctive therapy for epilepsy. Postmarketing case reports also identify weight loss.	None known.

Note. FDA=U.S. Food and Drug Administration.

TABLE 15–11. Representative rates of weight changes across antidepressants reported in clinical trials

Agent	Weight changes in FDA registration trials	Additional studies and observations
Bupropion	Major depression Bupropion IR: 9% gained weight over 3–6 weeks; 28% had weight loss of >2.3 kg. Bupropion SR: 2%–3% gained >2.3 kg in 4–6 weeks (300 or 400 mg/day); 14% (300 mg/day) to 19% (400 mg/day) had weight loss >2.3 kg. Seasonal affective disorder: Bupropion XL: 11% gained >2.3 kg; 23% lost >2.3 kg.	Mean weight loss identified in meta-analysis was 2.8 kg (95% CI, 1.1–4.5 kg) over 6–12 months (Li et al. 2005).
Citalopram	*Major depression:* Mean weight change was −0.5 kg over 4–6 weeks.	Meta-analysis suggests greater weight loss than gain (Li et al. 2005).
Desvenlafaxine	*Major depression:* 1%–2% of subjects reported weight loss across dosages (50–400 mg/day). Mean weight change ranged from −0.4 to −1.1 kg in acute trials at dosages up to 400 mg/day. Mean weights did not differ significantly from those with placebo by the end of a 6-month placebo-controlled extension phase for acute responders.	None.

TABLE 15–11. Representative rates of weight changes across antidepressants reported in clinical trials *(continued)*

Agent	Weight changes in FDA registration trials	Additional studies and observations
Duloxetine	*Major depression:* Weight loss in 2% (cf. <1% with placebo). *Major depression and GAD:* Mean weight change over 10 weeks of −0.5 kg (cf. +0.2 kg with placebo). *All other indications:* Mean weight change over 26 weeks was −0.6 kg (cf. +0.2 kg with placebo).	*Major depression:* A 7-week open trial (N=128) yielded a mean weight loss of −1.2 kg, which then normalized by 20 weeks and subsequently increased to a gain of +2.4 kg at 1 year and +3.1 kg after 2 years (Wohlreich et al. 2007). *Major depression:* Mean +2.4-kg weight gain over 1 year (N=1,279) (Raskin et al. 2003).
Escitalopram	*Major depression:* No difference from placebo in weight change.	In three 8-month placebo-controlled trials for GAD, mean weight gain was +1.4 kg (Davidson et al. 2005).
Fluoxetine	*Major depression:* Decreased appetite in 11% and weight loss in 1.4%. *OCD:* Decreased appetite in 17%, weight loss in 2%. *Bulimia nervosa:* Decreased appetite in 8% with mean weight loss of −0.45 kg, with dosages of 60 mg/day over 15 weeks.	*Major depression:* −0.4 kg weight loss in first 4 weeks; no significant weight differences from placebo over 50 weeks of continuation/ maintenance therapy for depression (Michelson et al. 1999); meta-analysis of studies using fluoxetine to treat obesity shows weight changes from −14.5 to +0.4 kg after 12 or more months (Li et al. 2005). *(Note:* Studies of fluoxetine targeting weight loss have typically involved higher dosages [~60 mg/day] than generally used for major depression [Li et al. 2005].)

TABLE 15–11. Representative rates of weight changes across antidepressants reported in clinical trials *(continued)*

Agent	Weight changes in FDA registration trials	Additional studies and observations
Fluvoxamine	*OCD:* Decreased appetite in >5%; specific weight changes not reported in manufacturer's package insert, other than no differences from placebo were observed.	None.
Levomilnacipran	*Major depression:* –0.5 to –0.8 kg across doses in 8-week acute depression trials (Asnis et al. 2013).	Mean weight change in 48-week open-label extension study for MDD: –0.6 kg; 10% gained >7% of initial body weight while 17% lost >7% of initial body weight (Citrome 2013a).
MAOIs other than transdermal selegiline: isocarboxazid, phenelzine, tranylcypromine	Incidence rates for weight change are not reported in manufacturers' product information materials.	Weight gain during treatment for depression reportedly more common with phenelzine than tranylcypromine (Cantú and Korek 1988).
Mirtazapine	*Major depression:* Increased appetite in 17% of subjects in acute trials (cf. 2% with placebo); 7.5% of mirtazapine recipients gained ≥7% of their baseline weight (cf. 0% with placebo), as did 49% of subjects in pediatric trials (cf. 5.7% with placebo).	None.
Nefazodone	*Major depression:* Weight gain in >1% of subjects. No significant differences from placebo in incidence of substantial weight gain (i.e., ≥7% of initial body weight). Weight loss occurred in <1% of subjects.	None.

TABLE 15–11. Representative rates of weight changes across antidepressants reported in clinical trials *(continued)*

Agent	Weight changes in FDA registration trials	Additional studies and observations
Paroxetine	*Across indications:* Increased appetite in 2%–4%; decreased appetite in 6%–9%. Average weight change in short-term trials was approximately –2.2 kg. Weight gain occurred in >1% across indications.	None.
Sertraline	Incidence rates for weight changes not reported in manufacturer's product information materials (although weight increase reported as occurring in >1% of subjects across all FDA registration trials).	*OCD:* Mean +1.6-kg weight gain (+2.5% of baseline weight) over 2.5 years (Maina et al. 2004).
TCAs	Acute trials of tertiary-amine TCAs (e.g., imipramine or amitriptyline) have been associated with mean weight gains of 2.0–7.0 kg; secondary-amine TCAs (e.g., desipramine, nortriptyline) have shown minimal weight gain in trials, presumably because of lower H_1 histamine or anticholinergic effects (Vanina et al. 2002).	None.
Transdermal selegiline	*Major depression:* Over 6–8 weeks, 2.1% of subjects gained ≥5% of their initial body weight, and 5.0% lost ≥5% of their baseline weight. Mean weight change was –0.5 kg (cf. +0.1 kg with placebo).	None.

TABLE 15–11. Representative rates of weight changes across antidepressants reported in clinical trials *(continued)*

Agent	Weight changes in FDA registration trials	Additional studies and observations
Venlafaxine	*Major depression:* 7% of patients lost ≥5% of their initial body weight. *GAD, social anxiety disorder, or panic disorder:* 3%–4% of subjects lost ≥7% of their initial body weight. *Across indications:* Weight gain occurred in ≥1% of subjects.	None.
Vilazodone	*Major depression:* In 8-week placebo-controlled trials, no observed differences from placebo (+0.2 kg with either drug or placebo; gains of ≥7% from baseline weight occurred in 0.9% of vilazodone recipients and 1.2% of placebo recipients).	None.
Vortioxetine	*Major depression:* In published 8-week placebo-controlled trials, mean weight changes were –0.10 to +0.19 kg across dosages (no different from placebo; +0.46 kg).	In a 52-week open-label extension trial for completers of a randomized acute trial in major depression, mean weight change at study end was +0.67 kg (Alam et al. 2014).

Note. CI=confidence interval; FDA=U.S. Food and Drug Administration; GAD=generalized anxiety disorder; IR=immediate release; MAOI=monoamine oxidase inhibitor; OCD=obsessive-compulsive disorder; SR=sustained release; TCA=tricyclic antidepressant; XL=extended release.

substance use disorders (notably, alcoholism) that may influence body weight and nutritional intake; and minimal if any contribution from cotherapies that may pose additive weight gain, such as anticholinergic drugs or sedative-hypnotics. A further consideration regarding iatrogenic weight gain in both research trials and routine treatment for mood disorders involves the distinction between the restoration of lost appetite attributable to the treatment of depression versus the stimulation of appetite and weight gain above and beyond changes caused by treating depression.

The prevalence and magnitude of weight gain associated with antidepressants is less extensive than with SGAs, even though almost all classes of antidepressants — with the notable exception of bupropion — have been associated with some weight gain. FDA registration trials for most antidepressants involve relatively short durations of treatment (typically 4–8 weeks) for acute major depressive episodes, but changes in weight may be more likely to occur during long-term rather than short-term therapy. Among SSRIs, fluoxetine may have a lower incidence of weight gain than other agents, based mainly on early studies involving its use for the treatment of obesity. A few randomized trials comparing SSRIs over approximately 6–9 months found more weight gain with paroxetine than with sertraline, and often the least amount with fluoxetine. Significant weight gain also was more extensive during short- and long-term treatment with SSRIs or TCAs than with nefazodone (Sussman et al. 2001).

Lifestyle Modification

Lifestyle modification remains the first line, and arguably safest and best studied, level of intervention to counteract psychotropic-induced weight gain, although in real life it is often very hard to achieve. The evidence base in support of this statement includes the following:

- STRIDE, a 12-month group- and individually based dietary and lifestyle modification program for overweight or obese adults taking antipsychotic medications, reported a mean weight loss of 4.4 kg at 6 months and 2.6 kg at 12 months alongside an approximate 6-point reduction in fasting glucose levels as compared with control subjects receiving usual care (Green et al. 2015).
- A 12-week randomized study of overweight or obese outpatients with psychotic disorders receiving a variety of SGAs, comparing usual care with individual twice-weekly exercise training plus nutritional counseling, found significant weight loss and decreased cholesterol: HDL ratio (Blouin et al. 2009).

- A 24-week intensive program of diet, exercise, and nutritional counseling in 22 obese or overweight patients with chronic psychotic disorders yielded an average 6-kg weight loss (5.7% of baseline weight) and 11% reduction in blood pressure; 77% of subjects completed the program (Centorrino et al. 2006).
- A 12-week program of exercise (20 minutes three times per week) plus nutritional and behavioral counseling (e.g., learning to read food labels, meal planning, portion control, healthy snacking) in 31 overweight or obese schizophrenia or schizoaffective disorder patients taking SGAs led to a 2.7-kg weight loss; 87% of participants completed the program (Vreeland et al. 2003). Notably, a 40-week extension of this program (completed by 65% of subjects) further demonstrated significant reductions from baseline in hemoglobin A_{1C}, blood pressure, and hip and waist circumference, but not lipid parameters, and most of the observed weight loss occurred in the first 3 months with a subsequent plateau despite continued SGA therapy (Menza et al. 2004).
- A 12-week study in 48 obese or overweight schizophrenia or schizoaffective subjects who had been taking olanzapine for at least 12 weeks and gained >7% of their pretreatment weight compared usual care versus a program of diet management (i.e., keeping a food diary, diet planning with a nutritionist, learning about food exchange tables, reading food labels, healthy snacking, and low-calorie food preparation) combined with exercise management (i.e., keeping an exercise diary and pursuing a tailored exercise plan with an exercise manager). Subjects randomly assigned to the weight management program lost a mean of 4 kg, with significant differences visible at week 8. No significant reductions in lipid parameters were observed. The protocol was completed by 75% of enrollees (Kwon et al. 2006).
- An 18-month open, prospective comparison of usual treatment versus a supervised, facility-based exercise program with dietary counseling in 110 schizophrenia, schizoaffective disorder, or bipolar disorder patients with antipsychotic-induced weight gain revealed a 3.5% reduction in body weight; subjects in the weight management arm had significantly greater reductions in total cholesterol, LDL, triglycerides, and fasting glucose, as well as significantly greater increases in HDL when compared with subjects receiving usual care (Poulin et al. 2007).
- In a 10-week open weight-control program involving 33 Taiwanese schizophrenia patients with obesity resulting from SGAs, observed weight loss was 2.1 kg after 10 weeks, 3.7 kg at 6 months, and 2.7 kg at 12-month follow-up, with significant declines in triglycerides but not other lipid or glycemic parameters (Chen et al. 2009).

Among the comprehensive issues relevant to weight management and metabolic risk, nutritional factors should be considered alongside pharmacological and lifestyle factors. Foods with a higher content of protein, fiber, and water have been associated with greater satiety. Efforts toward improving nutritional intake can often be aided by consultation with a registered dietitian, who can make specific recommendations tailored to an individual patient. Monitoring caloric intake and increasing physical activity can help to maintain a stable weight. Diet recommendations often include eating small, frequent meals throughout the day to minimize rebound hunger from prolonged daytime periods of not eating, as well as incorporating lean sources of protein with every meal and snack for satiety and more stable blood glucose levels following intake (spikes in blood sugar after high-carbohydrate meals lead to quick drops, and the patient will feel hungry soon after).

In addition to monitoring food intake, increasing physical activity should be strongly emphasized. Strategies include finding activities that patients enjoy (e.g., walking, dancing, tennis, gardening) so as to minimize the likelihood that exercise could feel like a chore. Before patients begin a new exercise regimen, the clinician must ensure the absence of any physical health constraints, such as unstable cardiopulmonary diseases. For weight loss, at least 60 minutes/day is recommended, whereas 45–60 minutes most days of the week is usually recommended to maintain a stable weight.

Pharmacological Management of Psychotropic-Induced Weight Gain

The management of weight gain caused by serotonergic antidepressants has received comparatively less attention than the weight gain caused by SGAs, for which more pervasive metabolic disturbances appear to be more extensive. Adjunctive topiramate represents one of the best studied remedies for weight gain associated with SSRI treatment, as well as with a range of other psychotropic agents. These studies, summarized in Table 15–12, are all limited by their small sample sizes, use of concomitant therapies, lack of treatment randomization, and heterogeneity of diagnostic groups and clinical states. Potential benefits also may be countered by other adverse effects caused by topiramate, such as cognitive impairment (see Table 17–1 in Chapter 17, "Neurological System") or paresthesias (see the section "Paresthesias and Neuropathies" in Chapter 17). Nevertheless, the studies provide convergent data supporting weight loss with adjunctive topiramate for psychotropically induced weight gain.

TABLE 15–12.   Open-label studies of adjunctive topiramate and weight loss in patients with mood and anxiety disorders

Study population	N	Duration	Dosing	Mean weight loss
Weight gain induced by SSRIs for anxiety disorders (Van Ameringen et al. 2002)	15	10 weeks, open label	Mean dose=135±44 mg/day	4.2±6.0 kg.
Bipolar or unipolar depressed patients (Kirov and Tredget 2005)	12	6–12 months	Begun at 25 mg/day and increased by 25–50 mg every 1–2 weeks to a maximum of 600 mg/day; mean dose=296 mg/day	At 3 months, 5.0±3.3 kg; at 6 months, 7.8±6.9 kg; patients completing 12 months lost a mean of 9.6±6.7 kg.
Bipolar I or schizoaffective manic patients (Chengappa et al. 1999)	20	5 weeks	Begun at 25 mg/day, increased by 25–50 mg every 3–5 days; mean dose at week 5=211 mg/day	–4.3 kg (range: –1.4 to –10.5 kg by 5 weeks).
Bipolar I, II, not otherwise specified, or schizoaffective bipolar disorder patients (Vieta et al. 2002)	31	≤6 months	Mean dose=202±65 mg/day	–2.3±1.3 kg.

TABLE 15–12. Open-label studies of adjunctive topiramate and weight loss in patients with mood and anxiety disorders *(continued)*

Study population	N	Duration	Dosing	Mean weight loss
Bipolar I, II, or schizoaffective bipolar disorder patients (Vieta et al. 2004)	26	12 months	Topiramate (25- to 50-mg/day weekly increases) plus olanza-pine concurrently begun; mean modal topiramate dose = 271.1±117.6 mg/day	−0.5±1.1 kg.
Refractory bipolar disorder patients (Guille and Sachs 2002)	14	1–64 weeks (mean = 22.4 weeks)	Mean dose=100±72 mg/day	4 subjects with a baseline BMI>28 had a mean weight loss of 13.5±7.4 kg.

TABLE 15–12.   Open-label studies of adjunctive topiramate and weight loss in patients with mood and anxiety disorders *(continued)*

Study population	N	Duration	Dosing	Mean weight loss
Diversity of mood, anxiety, psychotic, and personality disorders (Cates et al. 2008)	41	1–39 months (mean = 16.2 months)	Begun at 50 mg/day; median maximum dosage of 100 mg/day	Any weight loss occurred in 59% (mean weight loss = 2.2 kg); modest reductions from baseline weight or BMI (<2%); more substantial weight loss occurred among those who had any weight loss (7.2 kg); any weight loss was more likely among heavier subjects (i.e., baseline weight >91 kg at topiramate initiation); 76% completed at least 6 months, 59% completed at least 1 year; 27% completed 2 years. Adverse effects, reported in 17% of subjects, included cognitive dulling, appetite increase, behavioral activation, and gastrointestinal disturbances.

Note.   BMI = body mass index; SSRI = selective serotonin reuptake inhibitor.

Psychostimulants, which are sometimes used to promote weight loss, have not been extensively studied specifically for counteracting psychotropic-induced weight gain. In patients with primary psychotic disorders, stimulants pose obvious concerns for the potential psychotomimetic effects. In children and adolescents receiving SGAs for aggression and disruptive behavioral disorders, no differences were found over 12 weeks in body weight or metabolic parameters among those who did ($N=71$) or did not ($N=82$) also receive stimulants under naturalistic conditions (Penzer et al. 2009). Notably, unlike amphetamine or methylphenidate, the novel stimulants modafinil or armodafinil do not appear to be associated with clinically meaningful weight loss.

A number of pharmacotherapies have been described to help counter obesity in otherwise healthy adults for whom weight gain was not the result of psychotropic medications. Such medications, which by extrapolation may warrant consideration as possible strategies for psychotropic weight gain, include the following:

- **Bupropion SR:** A 24-week randomized comparison of placebo versus bupropion SR (300–400 mg/day) in obese, otherwise healthy adults found significantly greater reductions from baseline weight among those receiving bupropion SR 300 mg/day (7.2% loss from baseline) or 400 mg/day (10.1% loss from baseline) than among those receiving placebo (Anderson et al. 2002). In addition, a 26-week randomized placebo-controlled trial in 193 subsyndromally depressed subjects yielded a significantly greater mean weight loss in those taking bupropion SR (4.4 kg, or 4.6% of baseline weight) than placebo (1.7 kg, or 1.8% of baseline weight), with a significant correlation observed between improvement in depressive symptoms and weight loss (Jain et al. 2002). Among a small group ($N=8$) of diagnostically diverse outpatients with olanzapine-associated weight gain, an open trial of bupropion 150–300 mg/day resulted in a mean weight loss of 3.4 kg over 24 weeks (Gadde et al. 2006).
- **Bupropion SR plus naltrexone:** This combination was examined on the basis of the ability of bupropion to activate hypothalamic pro-opiomelanocortin neurons and the theoretical ability of naltrexone to block opioid-mediated pro-opiomelanocortin autoinhibition. The combination of bupropion SR (360 mg/day) plus naltrexone (16 or 32 mg/day) was associated with substantial reductions from baseline weight over 56 weeks (half of subjects lost 5% of their baseline weight with the 16 mg/day naltrexone dose; a mean 6% loss from baseline weight occurred with the 32 mg/day naltrexone dose) in a 34-site study

of 1,742 overweight or obese adults in the United States (Greenway et al. 2010).

- **Zonisamide plus bupropion:** A 12-week open-label randomized study was conducted in 18 psychiatrically healthy obese women comparing the anticonvulsant zonisamide (begun at 100 mg/day and increased to 400 mg/day over 4 weeks) alone or with bupropion (the latter begun at 100 mg/day and then increased to 200 mg/day after 2 weeks). Combination therapy yielded significantly more weight loss (mean=7.2 kg) than zonisamide alone (mean=2.9 kg) (Gadde et al. 2007).

- **Phentermine:** This amphetamine-like stimulant is an appetite suppressant used for the short-term management of obesity. In a pooled analysis of nine randomized trials occurring from 2 to 24 weeks, with dosages of 15–30 mg/day, subjects lost a mean of 3.6 kg (95% CI, 0.6–6.0 kg) (Li et al. 2005). Side effects of phentermine appear modest and bear mainly on its sympathomimetic effects (e.g., tachycardia, hypertension).

- **Phentermine plus topiramate:** In a 56-week trial with 2,487 obese or overweight adults, the combination of phentermine (7.5 or 15 mg/day) plus topiramate (46 or 92 mg/day) produced significantly greater mean weight loss (–8.1 kg [95% CI, –8.5 to –7.1 kg] and –10.2 kg [95% CI, –10.4 to –9.3 kg] at each respective dose pairing) as compared with placebo (mean weight loss=–1.4 kg [95% CI, –1.8 to –0.7 kg]), with 62% and 70% losing at least 5% of their initial weight with each respective dose pairing of active drug arms; adverse effects that were more common with active drug than placebo included dry mouth, paresthesias, constipation, insomnia, dizziness, and dysgeusia (Gadde et al. 2011).

Clozapine-induced weight gain may at least partly derive from the more potent 5-HT_{2C} antagonism caused by its metabolite norclozapine. Lu et al. (2004) capitalized on the pharmacokinetic effect of coadministering fluvoxamine (50 mg/day) with clozapine (250 mg/day), which raises clozapine levels by ~2.3-fold while decreasing norclozapine levels, to demonstrate significantly less weight gain over 12 weeks than with clozapine alone. Careful monitoring of serum clozapine levels during deliberate coadministration of fluvoxamine is important to minimize the risk of toxicity and seizures.

Finally, it is important to keep in mind that some psychiatric disorders, such as bipolar disorder, may involve an intrinsic risk for developing obesity or substantial weight gain, posing a confounding factor when attempting to apportion the etiology of weight gain to a treatment versus a disease state itself.

Among studies of pharmacotherapies used to counteract psychotropic-induced weight gain, a meta-analysis of 32 studies involving 1,482 subjects and 15 medications or medication combinations to remedy antipsychotic-associated weight gain, used over diverse time periods, found the most extensive mean weight loss as compared with placebo with metformin (2.9 kg), followed by D-fenfluramine (2.6 kg), sibutramine (2.6 kg), topiramate (2.5 kg), and the noradrenergic reuptake inhibitor reboxetine (1.9 kg) (Maayan et al. 2010). (D-Fenfluramine was withdrawn from the U.S. market by the FDA in 1997 due to reports of cardiac valve disease and pulmonary hypertension, and sibutramine was withdrawn from the U.S. market in 2010 because of excessive cardiovascular events [e.g., nonfatal heart attacks and strokes]; however, these agents are included here because of their historical role and known efficacy for weight loss.)

Table 15–13 summarizes major findings with randomized pharmacological intervention studies to counteract psychotropic-induced weight gain in patients with primary mood or psychotic disorders. Alternatively, psychiatrically stable patients who have gained weight from an SGA with high risk for weight gain (e.g., olanzapine) have been shown to lose significantly more weight and lower their total cholesterol levels by switching within class to another agent that may be less prone to cause weight gain (e.g., aripiprazole or ziprasidone); however, stable psychiatric symptoms have been shown to worsen after switching from olanzapine to aripiprazole (Newcomer et al. 2008), and clinicians cannot assume comparable efficacy among SGAs for patients with primary psychotic disorders. Significant weight loss also has been demonstrated after switching stable schizophrenic outpatients from olanzapine to ziprasidone (median ziprasidone dose=90 mg/day; mean weight loss=1.8 kg) or from risperidone to ziprasidone (median ziprasidone dose=92 mg/day; mean weight loss=0.9 kg) (Weiden et al. 2003a). Stable but symptomatic schizophrenia patients who were switched from either olanzapine or risperidone to ziprasidone demonstrated weight loss but neither improvement nor decline in global symptoms (Weiden et al. 2003b).

Finally, it is worth noting that the selective 5-HT$_{2A}$ inverse agonist pimavanserin, FDA-approved to treat psychosis in Parkinson's disease, has been associated with weight loss; FDA registration trials reported significant reductions in BMI (42%) more often than increases (2%), although clinically significant weight gain was more likely in subjects with a low baseline BMI. Data with pimavanserin outside of its use for psychosis in Parkinson's disease are not extensive; however, in one 6-week trial of risperidone for non-first-episode schizophrenia patients, coadministration with pimavanserin was associated with significantly

TABLE 15–13. Pharmacological strategies with at least one randomized trial to manage psychotropic-induced weight gain

Agent	Rationale	Study designs and findings
Amantadine	Possible dopaminergic and noradrenergic anorexic effect; or via effects of adrenal and gonadal steroids through reduction of prolactin.	Randomized comparison of adjunctive amantadine (up to 300 mg/day) ($N=60$) or placebo ($N=65$) over 16 weeks in schizophrenia, schizoaffective, schizophreniform, or bipolar disorder patients who gained ≥5% of their initial body weight with olanzapine. Significantly greater weight loss with amantadine (mean=−0.2±4.6 kg) than placebo (+1.3±4.3 kg) (Deberdt et al. 2005). Randomized comparison of adjunctive amantadine ($N=12$) or placebo ($N=9$) for 12 weeks in schizophrenia, schizoaffective, or bipolar disorder patients who had gained ≥2.3 kg from olanzapine; amantadine recipients lost a mean of 0.4±3.5 kg, whereas placebo recipients gained a mean of 4.0±5.9 kg (Graham et al. 2005).
Aripiprazole	Considered among the more weight-neutral SGAs, potentially via its modest H_1 antihistamine blockade and serotonin type 2C (5-HT_{2C}) agonism; may promote weight loss despite concomitant treatment with other weight-promoting agents.	10-week placebo-controlled double-blind crossover study of adjunctive aripiprazole (15 mg/day) in overweight schizophrenia patients ($N=15$) stable on olanzapine for at least 1 month; aripiprazole was associated with significantly more weight loss (mean=−1.3±2.1 kg) than placebo (mean gain=+1.0±1.5 kg), as well as greater reduction in triglycerides (−52 mg/dL vs. −48 mg/dL, respectively) and very-low-density lipoprotein reductions (Henderson et al. 2009a).

TABLE 15–13. Pharmacological strategies with at least one randomized trial to manage psychotropic-induced weight gain *(continued)*

Agent	Rationale	Study designs and findings
Lamotrigine	Apparent weight neutrality or weight loss observed in clinical trials for bipolar disorder.	18-month maintenance comparison of lamotrigine (*N*=217), lithium (*N*=166), or placebo (*N*=190); mean weight changes were −1.2 kg (lamotrigine), +2.2 kg (lithium), and +0.2 kg (placebo) (Sachs et al. 2006a). Among obese subjects in this group (*N*=155), mean weight changes at 52 weeks were −4.2 kg (lamotrigine), +6.1 kg (lithium), and −0.6 kg (placebo) (Bowden et al. 2006a).
	Weight loss observed in obese nonpsychiatric patients.	26-week study involving 40 obese psychiatrically healthy adults; significantly greater weight loss with lamotrigine (200 mg/day) than placebo (−2.9±4.7 kg vs. −0.5±3.2 kg, respectively) and mean changes in BMI from baseline to endpoint (−1.5±2.8 and −0.1±1.1 for lamotrigine and placebo, respectively) (Merideth 2006).
α-Lipoic acid (ALA)	Antioxidant associated with weight loss in rodent studies.	12-week placebo-controlled randomized trial involving 22 stable schizophrenia patients; ALA dosing 600–1,800 mg/day. Significantly greater weight loss with ALA (−1.3±1.6 kg) than placebo (+0.7±1.9 kg) (Kim et al. 2016).

TABLE 15–13.   **Pharmacological strategies with at least one randomized trial to manage psychotropic-induced weight gain** *(continued)*

Agent	Rationale	Study designs and findings
Metformin[a]	Oral hypoglycemic agent; decreases insulin sensitivity and prolongs the duration of postprandial falls in plasma levels of ghrelin, the gastrointestinal hormone that promotes satiety (English et al. 2007); inhibits expression of neuropeptide Y and may increase expression of hypothalamic leptin receptors (Aubert et al. 2011).	12-week comparison of placebo, metformin (250 mg tid with meals), metformin plus lifestyle intervention, or lifestyle intervention alone in 128 adults with schizophrenia in China whose weight increased >10% from antipsychotics. Mean reductions in BMI were greatest among subjects randomly assigned to metformin plus lifestyle intervention (1.8), followed by metformin alone (1.2), and lifestyle alone (0.5) (Wu et al. 2008). 16-week comparison of placebo or metformin (initially 500 mg with dinner for 1 week, then 500 mg with breakfast and dinner for 1 week, then 850 mg with breakfast and dinner) in 39 children and adolescents who had >10% weight increase from olanzapine, risperidone, or quetiapine. Placebo recipients gained an additional mean of +4.0±6.2 kg, whereas metformin recipients lost a mean of −0.1±2.9 kg (Klein et al. 2006). 14-week double-blind placebo-controlled trial in 40 schizophrenia patients taking olanzapine; glucose levels declined significantly with metformin but no significant changes observed in weight gain or insulin resistance (Baptista et al. 2006).

TABLE 15–13. Pharmacological strategies with at least one randomized trial to manage psychotropic-induced weight gain *(continued)*

Agent	Rationale	Study designs and findings
Naltrexone	Antipsychotics may disrupt endorphin-mediated food reward.	8-week randomized comparison of naltrexone 25 mg/day (N=11) or placebo (N=12) in overweight women with schizophrenia or schizoaffective disorder. Significantly greater weight loss with naltrexone (mean=−3.4 kg) than placebo (mean=+1.4 kg) (Tek et al. 2014).
Nizatidine	H_2 receptor antagonism may exert a direct appetite-suppressant effect or an indirect weight loss effect by reducing gastric acid secretion.	16-week comparison of nizatidine 150 mg or 300 mg bid versus placebo in 175 schizophrenia patients beginning treatment with olanzapine; significantly less weight gain with high-dose nizatidine than placebo at weeks 3 and 4, but not at week 16 (Cavazzoni et al. 2003). 8-week randomized comparison of adjunctive nizatidine or placebo in 35 schizophrenia patients who gained > 2.3 kg from SGAs; significant weight loss and reduction in serum leptin levels (Atmaca et al. 2004). 2.5-month open-label adjunctive nizatidine (N=47) 150 mg bid followed by 8-week randomized adjunctive nizatidine or placebo (N=28) for quetiapine-associated weight gain in schizophrenia patients; no significant reductions in weight or serum leptin levels (Atmaca et al. 2004).

TABLE 15–13.　Pharmacological strategies with at least one randomized trial to manage psychotropic-induced weight gain (*continued*)

Agent	Rationale	Study designs and findings
Orlistat	Interferes with absorption of intestinal fat.	16-week randomized, placebo-controlled study of orlistat dosed at 360 mg/day in 63 obese or overweight schizophrenia patients taking clozapine or olanzapine. Men (but not women) had significantly greater weight change with orlistat (loss of −2.36 kg) than with placebo (gain of +0.62 kg) (Joffe et al. 2008). A 16-week open-label extension phase trial in 44 of these subjects yielded significant further weight loss (−1.29±3.04 kg), with men but not women showing the most robust declines (Tchoukhine et al. 2011).
Topiramate	Direct appetite suppressant effect by unknown mechanism; may reduce fat deposition by stimulating energy expenditure.	24-week randomized comparison of flexibly dosed topiramate (mean dose=209±145 mg/day) or sibutramine (mean dose=12±7 mg/day) in 46 overweight bipolar disorder outpatients; statistically similar magnitude of weight loss with topiramate (−2.8±3.5 kg) or sibutramine (−4.1±5.7 kg) but high dropout rates in both groups (McElroy et al. 2007). 12-week double-blind comparison of olanzapine plus topiramate (100 mg/day) or placebo in first-episode schizophrenia: mean weight loss of −1.3±2.3 kg with topiramate (significantly greater than placebo) alongside significantly greater reductions in serum leptin and other metabolic parameters (Narula et al. 2010).

TABLE 15–13. Pharmacological strategies with at least one randomized trial to manage psychotropic-induced weight gain (*continued*)

Agent	Rationale	Study designs and findings
Zonisamide	Possible dopaminergic and serotonergic effects may affect satiety.	In randomized study, 60 obese, psychiatrically healthy adults had significantly more weight loss (mean=−5.9 kg at 16 weeks and −9.2 kg at 32 weeks) with zonisamide (initially 100 mg/day increased to a maximum of 600 mg/day) than with placebo (Gadde et al. 2003). In a 16-week randomized comparison of zonisamide (mean dose=380 mg/day) versus placebo in obese bipolar patients taking olanzapine, significantly less weight gain occurred with zonisamide (mean=0.9 kg) than with placebo (5.0 kg) (McElroy et al. 2012). In a 10-week double-blind randomized comparison of zonisamide 150 mg/day (*n*=21) or placebo (*n*=20), there was significantly greater weight loss with zonisamide (mean=−1.1±1.4 kg) than with placebo (mean=+1.9±2.2 kg) (Ghanizadeh et al. 2013). Open trial of adjunctive zonisamide (final mean dose of 375±206 mg/day; range: 75–800 mg/day) in 25 obese recovered bipolar I or II patients over a mean of 14 weeks; mean weight loss of 1.2±1.9 BMI points; notably, 44% of subjects prematurely discontinued participation due to worsening mood symptoms (Wang et al. 2008).

Note. bid=twice daily; BMI=body mass index; SGA=second-generation antipsychotic; tid=three times daily.
[a]In the United States, only 500-mg nonscored tablets of metformin are manufactured, and these cannot easily be split.

less weight gain and lower rises in fasting glucose than was seen in patients taking risperidone plus placebo (Meltzer et al. 2012).

Weight Loss Supplements

There are a number of over-the-counter supplements that people sometimes use in attempts to hasten weight loss. Although evidence to support the efficacy of such approaches is often inconsistent, clinicians should be aware of safety considerations relevant to commonly used supplements, as summarized in Table 15–14.

Weight Loss

General Recommendations

Stimulants and some antidepressants (certain SSRIs or SNRIs, bupropion, nefazodone) may be associated with weight loss. If significant or undesirable weight loss occurs, drug discontinuation and substitution may be advisable (e.g., switching methylphenidate or amphetamine to atomoxetine, guanfacine, or modafinil/armodafinil).

Psychotropic-induced weight loss is a generally less common phenomenon than weight gain but nevertheless may pose an obstacle to treatment with a number of causal agents. The most well known among medications that can exert a proanorectic effect are psychostimulants (i.e., methylphenidate and amphetamine). No clear differences exist among specific preparations of these compounds (e.g., methylphenidate preparations Ritalin LA vs. Concerta vs. Focalin) or between methylphenidate versus amphetamine. In the treatment of attention-deficit disorder, nonstimulant treatment options such as atomoxetine or guanfacine may be viable alternatives with relatively lesser risk of weight loss. Among antidepressants, some SSRIs (notably, fluoxetine or bupropion) are thought to promote weight loss in some patients, and controlled trials with SNRIs such as duloxetine, venlafaxine, or desvenlafaxine also tend to show somewhat less weight gain than occurs with other antidepressant classes.

The evaluation of weight loss or appetite reduction should include careful assessment of possible noniatrogenic causes, both medical and psychiatric, including the presence of 1) depression, 2) anorexia nervosa or other eating disorders, 3) hypothyroidism, or 4) malignancy.

TABLE 15–14. Nutritional supplements commonly used to promote weight loss

Supplement	Rationale	Evidence	Possible adverse effects
Caffeine	Modest appetite suppression and stimulation of thermogenesis.	Most trials involve combinations of caffeine with thermogenic drugs such as ephedra or ephedrine.	Hypertension; reduces glucose tolerance.
L-Carnitine	Carnitine deficiency impairs fatty acid β-oxidation.	No differences from placebo in controlled trials.	None known.
Chromium picolinate	Trace element that can decrease insulin sensitivity and reduce carbohydrate craving in patients with atypical depression.	12-week randomized trial in overweight healthy adults found no differences in BMI or central adiposity (measured by computed tomography) between chromium picolinate (1,000 µg/day) and placebo (Yazaki et al. 2010).	Reports of acute renal failure, concerns about potential for causing chromosomal damage (clastogenicity).
Cissus quadrangularis (CQ) or CQ plus *Irvingia gabonensis* (CQ-IG)	Unknown.	10 weeks of CQ (150 mg bid) or CQ-IG (250 mg bid) in 72 obese or overweight adults led to an 8.8% reduction from baseline weight with CQ and an 11.9% reduction with CQ-IG (both superior to placebo) (Oben et al. 2008).	Headache, insomnia, GI upset.

TABLE 15–14. Nutritional supplements commonly used to promote weight loss (*continued*)

Supplement	Rationale	Evidence	Possible adverse effects
Citrus aurantium and synephrine alkaloids	Direct appetite suppression.	Case reports but only one (negative) placebo-controlled trial (Bent et al. 2004).	Headache, tachycardia, and hypertension (although touted as a safer alternative to ephedra); cerebrovascular and cardiovascular events reported; tyramine content poses hazard when taken with MAOIs.
Ephedra (*ma huang*)	Increased metabolic rate.	Modest short-term weight loss (about 0.9 kg/month) for up to 6 months, based on meta-analysis of 284 reports (Shekelle et al. 2003).	Hypertension, excessive cardiovascular stress leading to strokes or arrhythmias; consumer alert issued by the FDA in 2008.
Garcinia atroviridis	Thought to block lipogenesis and promote lipid oxidation.	Favorable animal studies (for review, see Hasani-Ranjbar et al. 2009).	None known.
Garcinia cambogia–derived (–)hydroxy-citric acid (HCA)	Competitive inhibitor of ATP citrate lyase, which in turn facilitates fatty acid synthesis.	Meta-analysis of 12 placebo-controlled trials revealed a small, significantly greater short-term weight loss with HCA than placebo (mean difference= 0.88 kg) (Onakpoya et al. 2011).	GI upset.

TABLE 15–14. Nutritional supplements commonly used to promote weight loss (*continued*)

Supplement	Rationale	Evidence	Possible adverse effects
Green tea catechins with caffeine	270–1,200 mg/day empirically observed to reduce appetite; may promote thermogenesis and fat oxidation.	Meta-analysis of 15 studies indicates statistically but not clinically significant reductions in BMI (~0.55) or weight (~1.4 kg) (Phung et al. 2010).	Tachycardia, insomnia, dizziness, nausea.
Hydroxycut	Nutraceutical mixture containing *Garcinia cambogia*, *Gymnema sylvestre*, chromium polynicotinate, caffeine, and green tea.	No peer-reviewed published efficacy data.	Liver failure, rhabdomyolysis, death; recalled by the manufacturer after the FDA issued a warning in May 2009; reformulated and placed back on market.
Sambucus nigra (elderberry)	Antioxidant; possible weight loss mechanism unknown.	Favorable animal studies (for review, see Hasani-Ranjbar et al. 2009).	None known.

Note. ATP=adenosine triphosphate; bid=twice daily; BMI=body mass index; FDA=U.S. Food and Drug Administration; GI=gastrointestinal; MAOI=monoamine oxidase inhibitor.

16

Musculoskeletal System

Joint Pain

General Recommendations

Joint pains are rarely iatrogenic. Clinicians should determine whether such complaints may reflect other medical causes. Persistent idiosyncratic joint pains may warrant discontinuation of suspected causal agents to help clarify etiologies.

Joint pain or stiffness has been identified as a rare, idiosyncratic adverse effect that can occur in connection with virtually every existing psychotropic drug at any time in the course of treatment. However, it is difficult to articulate a pharmacodynamic mechanism by which any antidepressant, antipsychotic, anxiolytic, or anticonvulsant would plausibly cause musculoskeletal pain. Clinicians should assure that the emergence of joint pain is not the mere result of trauma or an intensification of existing arthritis; determine by physical examination the presence of an effusion, inflammation, or tenderness on movement; and obtain a history of rheumatoid or connective tissue diseases, including autoimmune diseases (e.g., systemic lupus erythematosus), gout, thyroid disease and other endocrinopathies, Lyme disease and other infectious processes, fibromyalgia, malignancies, and inflammatory conditions such as sarcoidosis.

No evidence has been reported in the literature attaching medical significance or consequences to idiosyncratic iatrogenic joint pain. However, if symptoms do not resolve spontaneously or with conservative interventions, such as acetaminophen or NSAIDs, cessation of the suspected offending agent may be warranted to assuage patient concerns. Persistent joint discomfort after drug cessation would further indicate the role for independent medical evaluation and diagnostic assessment.

Leg Cramps

General Recommendations

Leg cramps rarely result from psychotropic medications and more often result from endocrine or electrolyte abnormalities or from nutritional or mineral deficiencies. Possible underlying medical etiologies should be investigated (e.g., dehydration, hypothyroidism, hypocalcemia, hypomagnesemia) and corrected as appropriate.

Lower-extremity muscle cramps may result from a wide range of causes, including dehydration, hypomagnesemia, hypocalcemia, hypokalemia, hypothyroidism, or abrupt discontinuation of an SSRI or SNRI. Primarily nonpsychotropic medications often used in psychiatry that are known to cause muscle cramps include albuterol, amlodipine, clonidine, clorazepate, donepezil, galantamine, ibuprofen and other NSAIDs, nimodipine, nifedipine, and selegiline.

Quinine was long considered a viable treatment for leg cramps until the FDA banned all prescription formulations of it in 2007—other than the antimalarial agent Qualaquin—because of the drug's dubious efficacy and serious risks for causing extensive hematological, cardiac, neurological, and renal toxicities. Tonic water, which contains minute quantities of quinine (e.g., ~20 mg in 6 fluid ounces of tonic water, in contrast to 324 mg of active ingredient in quinine sulfate capsules), has been described as a popular remedy for leg cramps but has received little formal study of its safety and efficacy for that purpose.

Alternative evidence-based treatments for noniatrogenic leg cramps (i.e., those resulting from vascular, neurological, or arthritic underlying causes) include verapamil ($\leq$120 mg qid), gabapentin ($\leq$400 mg tid), carisoprodol, and orphenadrine (Guay 2008), in addition to carbamazepine (200 mg tid), vitamin E 400–800 IU/day, vitamin B complex capsules (fursultiamine 50 mg/day, hydroxocobalamin 250 µg/day, pyridoxal phosphate 30 mg/day, and riboflavin 5 mg/day), and calcium 0.5–1.0 g qid.

Although some clinicians advocate supplemental magnesium for leg cramps, randomized trials in the absence of known deficiencies have found no differences from placebo.

Myalgias

General Recommendations

Myalgias may be common, nonspecific, and often benign phenomena associated with numerous psychotropic drugs. Clinicians should determine whether myalgias entail muscle rigidity (suggestive of NMS), signs of metabolic acidosis (e.g., lactic acidosis secondary to oral hypoglycemics), cramping (suggestive of dehydration or electrolyte [e.g., calcium and magnesium] deficiencies), or myopathy attributable to other medicines (e.g., statins, steroids).

Muscle spasms or myalgias are often listed by drug manufacturers as rare side effects (typically with an incidence of <5%) of numerous psychotropic agents (e.g., acamprosate, atomoxetine, certain antidepressants [e.g., bupropion, citalopram, duloxetine, escitalopram, paroxetine, sertraline, venlafaxine], many anticonvulsants [e.g., carbamazepine, divalproex, lamotrigine, tiagabine, topiramate], some benzodiazepines [e.g., alprazolam, clonazepam], some antipsychotics [e.g., aripiprazole, clozapine, olanzapine, paliperidone, pimozide, risperidone, ziprasidone], clonidine, modafinil, nimodipine, some dopamine agonists [e.g., pramipexole, ropinirole], triptans [e.g., sumatriptan, zolmitriptan], phosphodiesterase inhibitors [e.g., sildenafil, tadalafil, vardenafil], and some benzodiazepine agonists [e.g., zaleplon, zolpidem]). In patients taking paliperidone for schizoaffective disorder, those taking 9–12 mg/day experienced more myalgias than did those taking 3–6 mg/day (manufacturer's product information).

Several important points require consideration in the evaluation of patient complaints about muscle aches or discomfort. Because antidepressant discontinuation syndromes may involve myalgias and other flulike symptoms, consideration should be given to erratic treatment adherence among patients being prescribed short-acting SSRIs or SNRIs. Among patients taking antipsychotic drugs, probably the most critical concern is the potential for NMS to manifest as muscle pain or stiffness (see "Neuroleptic Malignant Syndrome" in Chapter 20, "Systemic Reactions"). A diagnosis of fibromyalgia may warrant consideration in patients whose examinations reveal multiple "trigger" points of musculoskeletal tenderness. Myalgias or even rhabdomyolysis can be caused by a number of nonpsychotropic medications, including statins, metformin (due to lactic acidosis, usually at high doses), and corticosteroids such as prednisone.

Myalgia is a general term that refers to muscle pain; *myopathy* refers to any form of muscle disease, while *myositis* is a distinct, relatively rare inflammatory disorder of muscle fibers thought to be autoimmune in origin.

Randomized trials report incident rates of statin-associated myalgias in <5% of recipients, although observational studies identify rates of up to 20% during routine practice. Atorvastatin and simvastatin have been associated with higher myotoxicity rates than have other statins. Patient-specific risk factors for statin-related myotoxicity (SRM) have been identified (Oskarsson 2011):

- Family history of myopathy
- Advanced age (>80 years old)
- Low body weight
- Female sex
- Hypertension
- Diabetes mellitus
- Renal or liver disease
- Small body frame
- Preexisting muscle disease

A classification system for SRM, as described by Babu and Li (2015), is summarized in Table 16–1. Its evaluation and treatment, typically done by a primary care physician, involve discontinuation of the statin, hydration, and measurement of serum CK along with renal functioning.

Rhabdomyolysis (which by definition involves a serum CK level of >1,000 IU/L) is rare but possible from SRM. Rhabdomyolysis also can occur from excessive alcohol use, as well as use of methamphetamine, cocaine, 3,4-methylenedioxymethamphetamine (MDMA, or Ecstasy), and cannabis.

Evaluation of myalgias should address possible noniatrogenic causes and other associated symptoms, as well as the time course of their onset relative to changes in a psychotropic drug regimen. Treatment, if any, should target identifiable underlying medical etiologies.

TABLE 16–1. Classification of statin-related myotoxicity (SRM)

Classification	Description and terminology	Creatine kinase level	Incidence
SRM 0	Asymptomatic	<4× ULN	1.5%–26%
SRM 1	Myalgia, tolerable	Normal	190/100,000 patient years
SRM 2	Myalgia, intolerable	<4× ULN	0.2–2/1,000
SRM 3	Myopathy	>4× but <10× ULN	5/100,000 patient years
SRM 4	Severe myopathy	>10× but <50× ULN	0.11%
SRM 5	Rhabdomyolysis	>50× ULN or >10× ULN with signs of impaired kidney function	0.1–8.4/1,000 patient years
SRM 6	Autoimmune-mediated necrotizing myositis (presence of HMGCR antibodies)	Variable; may correlate with HMGCR levels (Werner et al. 2012)	~2 million/year

Note. HMGCR = 3-hydroxy-3-methylglutaryl-coenzyme A reductase; ULN = upper limit of normal.
Source. Adapted from Babu and Li 2015.

17

Neurological System

Cognitive Complaints

General Recommendations

Clinicians should carefully evaluate patients to determine whether subjective cognitive complaints reflect true cognitive deficits, psychiatric symptoms, or other deficits (e.g., learning disabilities). Clinicians should recognize common cognitive adverse effects of specific psychotropic agents and reduce dosages or eliminate likely offending agents when possible. Clinicians also should address other exogenous factors that may contribute to cognitive problems (e.g., alcohol or substance abuse, sleep disorders). Psychostimulants (amphetamine, methylphenidate, and modafinil or armodafinil) may aid attentional processing and verbal fluency in patients who are suitable candidates. Dopamine agonists (e.g., pramipexole) also may help attention in some patient groups.

Numerous factors in addition to psychotropic medications can contribute to subjective cognitive complaints and include affective or psychotic symptoms, anxiety disorders or symptoms, substance abuse,

---

The symbol ■ is used in this chapter to indicate that the FDA has issued a boxed warning for a prescription medication that may cause serious adverse effects.

attention-deficit disorder, and a variety of comorbid medical conditions. Furthermore, at least in some conditions (e.g., bipolar disorder), subjective cognitive complaints often correlate poorly with objective deficits in cognitive performance, making it essential for clinicians to discern the nature of cognitive complaints beyond patients' superficial reports of their presence.

Any psychoactive drug may impair judgment, thinking, or motor skills, although demonstrated adverse cognitive effects related to psychiatric medications are relatively circumscribed. Cognitive dulling that is plausibly attributable to sedating psychotropics (e.g., anticholinergic drugs, benzodiazepines, FGAs, SGAs, and certain anticonvulsants [in particular, topiramate]) poses difficult obstacles that are not easily overcome short of dosage reductions, or when necessary, eliminating a causal agent. In the case of topiramate, adverse cognitive effects may be dose-related and typically include psychomotor slowing, word-finding problems, impaired working memory, poor attention and concentration, and decreased verbal and nonverbal fluency (reviewed in Goldberg 2008). In some instances, agents with a high potential for cognitive dulling or disorganization can be replaced with other, more cognitively neutral medications (e.g., replacing the anticholinergic drug benztropine with the dopamine agonist amantadine as an alternative method to counteract extrapyramidal side effects of antipsychotic drugs).

Few if any rigorous data implicate antidepressants as having adverse cognitive effects, with the exception of anticholinergic effects related to TCAs (especially tertiary-amine TCAs such as amitriptyline or imipramine) or paroxetine. In fact, given their potential neuroprotective effects as demonstrated from preclinical studies (e.g., increasing brain-derived neurotrophic factor), nonanticholinergic antidepressants conceivably may have some potential benefit for enhancing neuronal viability and function. Most notably, the novel serotonergic antidepressant vortioxetine has been shown to improve aspects of cognitive functioning in major depression patients independent of its antidepressant effects (McIntyre et al. 2014), potentially mediated in part through its antagonism of the 5-HT_7 receptor. Among SGAs, 5-HT_7 antagonism may also contribute to the observed improvement in global cognition, visual memory, and visuospatial working memory seen in euthymic bipolar patients who were randomly assigned to receive adjunctive lurasidone (added to existing pharmacotherapy, vs. receiving only treatment as usual) (Yatham et al. 2017).

A summary of known adverse cognitive effects associated with psychotropic medications is provided in Table 17–1.

TABLE 17–1. Adverse cognitive effects of common psychotropic agents

Agent	Cognitive effects
Atomoxetine	None known.
Buspirone	None known.
Anticonvulsants and lithium	
Carbamazepine	In epilepsy studies, reports of subtle adverse effects on learning, delayed visuospatial processing, and impaired visual memory (reviewed in Goldberg 2008).
Divalproex	Subtle dose-related attentional and memory deficits, impaired verbal memory, and delayed decision time (reviewed in Goldberg 2008).
Gabapentin	Minimal adverse cognitive effects.
Lamotrigine	"Concentration disturbance" noted as an adverse event in 2% of epilepsy patients during premarketing studies; clinical trials in bipolar disorder suggest *improvement* (rather than worsening) of working and verbal memory, verbal fluency, and immediate recall (reviewed in Goldberg 2008); lamotrigine toxicity may manifest with diffuse cognitive impairment (Bouman et al. 1997).
Lithium	Diminished creativity, associative fluency, and verbal memory; no significant effects on visual memory, attention, executive function, processing speed, and psychomotor performance (Wingo et al. 2009).
Oxcarbazepine	No adverse effects on memory seen acutely in healthy volunteers (taking 300–600 mg/day); possible enhanced attention and motor speed, which may decline with dosages ≥1,200 mg/day (reviewed in Goldberg 2008).
Topiramate	Possible marked impairment (not clearly dose related) of global cognitive functioning, including attention, concentration, verbal and nonverbal fluency, processing speed, language skills, working memory, and perception; in epilepsy patients, cognitive deficits were shown to attenuate with time in some studies but not others (reviewed in Goldberg 2008).

TABLE 17–1. Adverse cognitive effects of common psychotropic agents *(continued)*

Agent	Cognitive effects
Antidepressants	
Bupropion	None known.
MAOIs	None known.
Mirtazapine	None known.
Nefazodone	Dose-dependent increased reaction time (van Laar et al. 1995).
SNRIs	None known.
SSRIs	None known.
Trazodone	None known.
TCAs	Possible impaired attention, psychomotor speed and coordination, and memory.
Vilazodone	None known.
Vortioxetine	No known adverse effects; may improve processing speed and recall.
Benzodiazepines	Possible impaired attention, arousal, and verbal or nonverbal memory, as well as motor speed and reaction time; anterograde amnesia may be common (reviewed by Buffett-Jerrott and Stewart 2002).
SGAs	Possible impaired attention, spatial working memory and visuospatial function, processing speed, verbal memory, verbal fluency, set shifting, and other executive functions — all independent of sedative effects or severity of psychopathology in bipolar or schizophrenia patients (reviewed by Goldberg 2008).

Note. MAOI=monoamine oxidase inhibitor; SGA=second generation antipsychotic; SNRI=serotonin-norepinephrine reuptake inhibitor; SSRI=selective serotonin reuptake inhibitor; TCA=tricyclic antidepressant.

Few strategies have been formally studied to address remedies for adverse cognitive effects caused by psychotropic agents. Interest and curiosity surround the potential for cognitive enhancement associated with procholinergic agents (e.g., donepezil or galantamine) or glutamate antagonists (e.g., memantine), although the efficacy of these agents has not been examined for purposes of counteracting cognitive deficits caused by psychotropic agents. In our clinical experience, it is unlikely for pro-cholinergic drugs or glutamate antagonists to ameliorate the cognitive dulling caused by benzodiazepines, anticholinergic drugs, or sedating antipsychotics.

In 2012, a large, 15-year prospective naturalistic study of elderly French patients found an approximate 50% increased risk for developing dementia among those who had taken a benzodiazepine several years before being assessed (Biliotti de Gage et al. 2012). Similarly, a second larger, age- and sex-matched case-control study by the same investigators using Canadian insurance claims data found a 1.3-fold increased risk for Alzheimer's dementia among patients taking benzodiazepines (particularly longer-acting agents, such as diazepam or flurazepam) for 3–6 months, and a 1.8-fold increased risk after >6 months' exposure (Biliotti de Gage et al. 2012). While these findings are provocative, the nonrandomized study designs from which they were derived make it impossible to attribute a causal relationship between benzodiazepine use and development of dementia. It is equally plausible that adults who are at greater risk for dementia may be more likely to be prescribed benzodiazepines prior to manifesting clear signs of dementia (such as undiagnosed mood or anxiety disorders, which in themselves may predispose to eventual dementia).

By contrast, a later, 8.3-year follow-up study of 3,433 older adults found only a modest increased risk for developing dementia among ever- versus never-users of benzodiazepines, but no significantly in-creased risk among those with greatest cumulative exposure (Gray et al. 2016). Findings from this latter study also indicated that chronic use of anticholinergic drugs (including tricyclic antidepressants) separately increased the risk for developing dementia by 19%–54% (increasing with duration exposure) (Gray et al. 2015). On the other hand, a separate report from the Baltimore Epidemiologic Catchment Area (ECA) study found no evidence of gross cognitive decline, using the MMSE, among adults (mean age=54 years) who took TCAs over an 11.5-year follow-up period (Podewils and Lyketsos 2002).

Our interpretation of these studies is that benzodiazepines and anticholinergic drugs may indeed pose cognitive hazards, particularly among older adults, but it is difficult to attribute to either drug class an indisputable independent risk alongside the many other known contributing risks for dementia, such as smoking status, untreated hypertension, concomitant medications, substance misuse, and preexisting psychiatric disorders. Cautious observation, rather than dogmatic avoidance, would seem prudent in risk-benefit decision making regarding the long-term use of either drug class.

With respect to other psychotropic drugs linked with adverse cognitive effects, all SGAs carry an FDA warning label identifying the potential for cognitive and motor impairment; however, the absence of head-to-head comparison studies focusing on changes in cognitive function makes it difficult to judge whether some SGAs may be more cognitively sparing than others.

The novel stimulant modafinil, as well as its enantiomer armodafinil, has been the subject of interest as a strategy to counteract sedation and possible adverse cognitive effects, although few formal studies have addressed that specific purpose. The dopamine D_2/D_3 agonist pramipexole has been suggested to improve attentional processing in euthymic bipolar disorder patients and could potentially be of value for iatrogenic cognitive dysfunction (Burdick et al. 2011).

The oral hypoglycemic agent liraglutide (1.8 mg/day administered subcutaneously) was found in one preliminary open-label trial to improve multiple dimensions of (presumably noniatrogenic) cognitive dysfunction in mood disorder patients (Mansur et al. 2017).

The root and leaf extract of the herb *Withania somnifera* (also known as ashwagandha, or Indian ginseng), dosed at 500 mg/day, has been reported to improve working memory, reaction time, and social cognition better than placebo in patients with bipolar disorder (Chengappa et al. 2013) and may offer broader utility for safely addressing cognitive complaints in other patient groups.

Delirium and Encephalopathy

General Recommendations

Acute mental status changes that involve disorientation, a waxing-and-waning level of arousal, and other focal neurological signs rarely result from psychotropic drugs apart from specific toxicity states (e.g., anticholinergic delirium, serotonin syndrome). Underlying etiologies (including systemic infections or neurological processes and toxic-metabolic states) should be thoroughly evaluated in the assessment of delirium or related acute changes in mental status.

Relatively rare reports exist of individual psychotropic agents or combinations of agents that may cause delirium or encephalopathy. Among the best known of these is the possible adverse interaction between lithium and FGAs, based on a handful of anecdotal case observations beginning in the mid-1970s. Some authors of retrospective case reviews subsequently suggested that dose-dependent neurotoxicity (notably, delirium with extrapyramidal signs, and more rarely, cerebellar signs) could result from lithium, antipsychotics, or their combination. Modern interpretations of this anecdotal literature have been tempered by vast experience for several decades with the safe and effective use of combination therapy involving lithium with FGAs and SGAs. The possibility of idiosyncratic neurotoxic interactions between these drugs is considered remote.

Clinicians should be aware, however, of more common causes of delirium or acute encephalopathic states; these include drug toxicities, acute cerebral events, hypoxia, infection, and neoplasm. Anticholinergic delirium typically manifests with associated signs of antimuscarinic (M_1) anticholinergic toxicity, commonly described as follows:

- "Mad as a hatter" (i.e., altered mental states),
- "Dry as a bone" (i.e., dry skin and mucous membranes),
- "Red as a beet" (i.e., flushing),
- "Blind as a bat" (i.e., mydriasis with loss of accommodation),
- "Full as a flask" (i.e., urinary retention), and
- "Hot as a hare" (i.e., fever).

Anticholinergic delirium must be recognized in patients receiving drugs such as diphenhydramine, TCAs, antispasmodics (e.g., dicyclomine), low-potency FGAs, histamine H_2 blockers, and some calcium channel blockers (e.g., nifedipine). Certain systemic neurological drug reactions—notably, serotonin syndrome—also may manifest with delirium.

Rare reports (approximately 2%) exist of profound somnolence following intramuscular administration of the long-acting injectable formulation of olanzapine (termed "post-injection delirium/sedation syndrome [PDSS]"), characterized by sedation or somnolence, confusion, dysarthria, dizziness, and disorientation. The phenomenon typically occurs within 1 hour of injection and characteristically resolves spontaneously within 72 hours.

Fatigue and Sedation

General Recommendations

Sedation from psychotropic drugs, particularly those that are antihistaminergic, may or may not tolerize with time or dosage reductions. Effective management involves identifying and eliminating or managing additional potential causes of sedation (e.g., sleep apnea, alcohol abuse, concomitant pharmacotherapies, comorbid medical conditions). Adjunctive stimulants, including modafinil, armodafinil, amphetamine, or methylphenidate, may help to alleviate persistent or significant sedation in patients for whom stimulants may be safe and appropriate short-term adjunctive treatments.

Fatigue encompasses a wide range of phenomena that may include the soporific effects of a drug (e.g., drowsiness, somnolence, sedation), loss of energy, and physical weakness independent of level of arousal. In premarketing FDA registration trials, MedDRA terms such as *sedation* or *somnolence* are differentiated by a matter of relative degree. Most randomized trials do not report information on the longitudinal trajectory of sedation (i.e., whether it is an early or late phenomenon, whether it plateaus over time), variations in severity, or timing during the day (e.g., sedation arising shortly after administration vs. excessive daytime sleepiness following nighttime administration).

A summary of reported incidence rates of sedation or somnolence across major psychotropic drug classes in FDA registration trials is presented in Table 17–2. For comparative purposes, Table 17–2 also includes information regarding drug-associated insomnia, a topic further discussed in the section "Insomnia" in Chapter 19, "Sleep Disturbances."

Histamine H_1 antagonism is considered to be one of the most common causes of sedation or somnolence caused by psychotropic agents. Some authors have proposed that tolerance may develop to the sedating effects of H_1 blockade over time during continued treatment with psychotropic drugs that have antihistaminergic properties; however, in our experience this often does not routinely occur.

Adjunctive psychostimulants likely represent the most obvious pharmacological strategy to counteract sedation from other psychiatric medicines. Many clinicians consider the wakefulness-promoting agent modafinil (or armodafinil) to be among the safest and best tolerated therapeutic options for treating somnolence or cognitive dulling. However, randomized trials have generally failed to demonstrate an advantage for adjunctive modafinil over placebo in diminishing either fatigue or cognitive functioning in patients with schizophrenia. In studies of patients with major depression, open-label trials have suggested some value for adjunctive modafinil in reducing associated symptoms of fatigue and sleepiness, although subsequent randomized placebo-controlled trials have failed to replicate earlier open-label findings. Some studies also suggest an advantage for adjunctive modafinil over placebo during the

TABLE 17–2. Reported incidence rates of somnolence, sedation, and insomnia across U.S. Food and Drug Administration registration trials

Agent	Somnolence or sedation	Insomnia
Anticonvulsants		
Carbamazepine	32% (Equetro in bipolar mania; 12% in open-label extension)	≤5% (Equetro in bipolar mania)
Divalproex	17% (migraine), 19% (bipolar mania), 27% (epilepsy)	≤5% (all indications)
Gabapentin	21% (postherpetic neuralgia)	>1% (but ≤placebo)
Lamotrigine	9% (bipolar maintenance), 14% (epilepsy)	6% (epilepsy), 10% (bipolar maintenance)
Oxcarbazepine	20%–36% (epilepsy; apparent dose relationship)	2%–4% (epilepsy; no apparent dose relationship)
Topiramate	15% (epilepsy; no apparent dose relationship)	4% (epilepsy; no apparent dose relationship)
Antidepressants		
Bupropion	2%–3% (MDD, 300–400 mg/day)	11%–16% (MDD, 300–400 mg/day); 20% (seasonal affective disorder, 150–300 mg/day)
Citalopram	18%	15%
Desvenlafaxine	4%–12% (MDD, 50–400 mg/day)	9%–15% (MDD, 50–400 mg/day)
Escitalopram	6% (MDD), 13% (GAD)	9% (MDD), 12% (GAD)
Fluoxetine	13%–17% across disorders	16%–33% across disorders
Fluvoxamine	32%–35% across disorders	26%–27% across disorders

TABLE 17–2. **Reported incidence rates of somnolence, sedation, and insomnia across U.S. Food and Drug Administration registration trials** *(continued)*

Agent	Somnolence or sedation	Insomnia
Antidepressants *(continued)*		
Levomilnacipran	<2% (MDD)	<2% (MDD)
Mirtazapine	54%	0%
Paroxetine	19%–24% across disorders	18%–24% across disorders
Sertraline	13%–15% across disorders	12%–28% across disorders
Venlafaxine	12%–20%	15%–24% across disorders
Vilazodone	3%	6%
Vortioxetine	<2% (MDD)	<2% (MDD)
Sedative-hypnotics[a]		
Eszopiclone	8%–10%	Not identified
Ramelteon	3%	Not identified
Suvorexant	8%	Not identified
Tasimelteon	Not reported	Not identified
Zaleplon	6%	Not identified
Zolpidem	5%–8%	Not identified
SGAs		
Aripiprazole	11% (across acute adult indications)	18% (across acute adult indications)
Asenapine	13% (schizophrenia), 24% (bipolar disorder) in acute trials	6% (bipolar mania), 16% (schizophrenia)
Brexpiprazole	2%–3% (schizophrenia), 4%–6% (MDD)	<2% (all indications)
Cariprazine	7%–8% (bipolar mania), 5%–10% (schizophrenia)	8%–9% (bipolar mania), 11%–13% (schizophrenia)
Clozapine	39%	2%
Iloperidone	9%–15% (schizophrenia, across doses)	Not reported

TABLE 17–2. Reported incidence rates of somnolence, sedation, and insomnia across U.S. Food and Drug Administration registration trials *(continued)*

Agent	Somnolence or sedation	Insomnia
SGAs *(continued)*		
Lurasidone	22% (combined data for 20–120 mg/day over 6 weeks), 13%–15% (adolescent schizophrenia)	8% (combined data for 20–120 mg/day over 6 weeks)
Olanzapine	29% (across acute trial indications)	12% (across acute trial indications)
Paliperidone	6%–11% (acute schizophrenia, across doses); 9%–26% (adolescent schizophrenia); 12% (schizoaffective disorder, across doses)	<2% (across indications)
Quetiapine	Quetiapine XR: 25% (acute schizophrenia), 50% (bipolar mania), 52% (bipolar depression)	Quetiapine XR: ≥1% (acute mania or schizophrenia), 9% (long-term placebo-controlled schizophrenia trials)
Risperidone	2%–7% (acute schizophrenia, across doses); 5% (1–6 mg/day, as monotherapy for bipolar mania)	25%–32% (acute schizophrenia. across doses); 4% (adjuvant therapy in acute bipolar mania)
Ziprasidone	14% (schizophrenia acute trials), 31% (bipolar acute mania trials)	Not reported

Note. GAD=generalized anxiety disorder; MDD=major depressive disorder; SGA=second-generation antipsychotic; XR=extended release.
[a]Refers specifically to excessive daytime sedation.

first few weeks of antidepressant treatment, but these effects may attenuate over time.

In our experience, initial sedation that persists from antihistaminergic medications can be effectively managed with adjunctive modafinil dosed at 100–300 mg/day (in one or two divided doses) or armodafinil dosed at 150–250 mg/day (in one or two divided doses). Traditional psychostimulants such as methylphenidate or amphetamine are also sometimes considered as viable adjunctive treatments to counteract iatrogenic sedation from other medications, although concerns about abuse potential as well as tolerance and dose-related sympathomimetic or psychotomimetic effects from traditional stimulants sometimes limit enthusiasm for their use for such purposes. One must also recognize that because (ar)modafinil potently inhibits CYP2C19, it may increase blood levels of other psychotropic drugs that are substrates for this enzyme, such as clozapine, citalopram, escitalopram, levomilnacipran, amitriptyline, and nortriptyline (see Chapter 2, Table 2–7).

Headache

General Recommendations

Headaches are common, nonspecific side effects that often occur initially and transiently with many psychotropic agents and are best treated, if necessary, with over-the-counter analgesics as needed. Persistent headaches merit careful evaluation for other (i.e., noniatrogenic) etiologies. Psychotropic agents that are suspected of causing persistent headaches (notably, lamotrigine or some SSRIs) may warrant discontinuation for the purposes of diagnostic clarification as well as relief of the presumed side effect.

Headache is among the most commonly reported adverse effects in both active drug and placebo arms in randomized trials of psychotropic compounds. The often nonspecific nature of headache can pose some difficulties in determining its iatrogenic from noniatrogenic etiologies, particularly in the absence of other neurological or systemic symptoms. Incidence rates of headache from controlled trials of common psychotropic drugs are reported in Table 17–3.

Importantly, because headache is among the most frequently occurring of all adverse effects from placebo (see the section "The Nocebo Phenomenon and Proneness to Adverse Effects" in Chapter 1, "The Psychiatrist as Physician"), the incidence rates with active drug reported from controlled trials in Table 17–3 likely highly overestimate true drug ef-

TABLE 17–3. Associations between psychotropic agents and treatment-emergent headaches

Agent	Comments
Atomoxetine	Incidence of 19% in acute (≤18-week) child and adolescent ADHD studies (cf. 15% with placebo).
Buspirone	Incidence of 6% in FDA registration trials.
Anticonvulsants	
Carbamazepine	Incidence of 22% in manufacturer's 6-month open-label trial of Equetro in bipolar disorder.
Divalproex	Incidence of 31% in FDA registration trials as adjunctive therapy for complex partial seizures (cf. 21% incidence with placebo); reported incidence >5% but no different from placebo in trials for acute mania.
Gabapentin	Incidence of 3.3% in postherpetic neuralgia (monotherapy); >1% (but no different from placebo) as add-on therapy in epilepsy.
Lamotrigine	Incidence of ~30% of migraine-like headaches in clinical trials for bipolar disorder; however, case reports also support efficacy of lamotrigine to prevent migraine with aura.
Oxcarbazepine	Incidence of 26%–32% (no clear dose relationship) in add-on therapy studies for epilepsy.
Topiramate	Not reported.
Antidepressants	
Bupropion	Incidence of 25% (bupropion SR 400 mg/day)–26% (bupropion SR 300 mg/day) (cf. 23% incidence with placebo) and 34% (bupropion XL across doses; cf. 26% with placebo).
Citalopram	Incidence of >2% but less than seen with placebo in FDA registration trials for major depression.
Desvenlafaxine	Incidence of 20%–22% (doses of 50–100 mg/day) in FDA registration trials for major depression (no different from placebo).

TABLE 17–3.   **Associations between psychotropic agents and treatment-emergent headaches** *(continued)*

Agent	Comments
Antidepressants *(continued)*	
Duloxetine	Incidence of 14% across indications in FDA registration trials (no different from placebo).
Escitalopram	Incidence of 24% in FDA registration trials for GAD; in FDA registration trials for MDD, incidence of ≥2% but comparable or higher with placebo than escitalopram; specific incidence rate in MDD trials not reported.
Fluoxetine	Approximate incidence of 20% in FDA registration trials for all indications.
Fluvoxamine	Incidence of 22% in FDA registration trials for combined adult OCD and major depression.
Levomilnacipran	Not reported (aside from a general risk for transient headaches with abrupt cessation).
Mirtazapine	Incidence of ≥1% in FDA registration trials.
Paroxetine	Approximate incidence of 18% in FDA registration trials for GAD or major depression.
Sertraline	Approximate incidence of 25% in FDA registration trials for all indications.
Venlafaxine	Incidence of 38% in social anxiety disorder (but no different from placebo across other indications).
Vilazodone	Migraine reported in ≥1% in FDA registration trials for major depression.
Vortioxetine	Not reported (aside from a general risk for transient headaches with abrupt cessation).

Note. ADHD=attention-deficit/hyperactivity disorder; FDA=U.S. Food and Drug Administration; GAD=generalized anxiety disorder; MDD=major depressive disorder; OCD=obsessive-compulsive disorder; SR=sustained release; XL=extended release.

fects. For example, in the case of escitalopram for GAD, the active drug incidence rate of 24% is counterbalanced by a nocebo incidence rate for headache of 17%.

In patients taking lithium, chronic headaches have been associated, rarely, with pseudotumor cerebri, a syndrome that also involves bilateral papilledema and increased intracranial pressure on lumbar puncture but no localized neurological signs or structural abnormalities visible on neuroimaging.

Movement Disorders

Akathisia and Extrapyramidal Adverse Effects

General Recommendations

Centrally acting β-blockers (e.g., propranolol) or benzodiazepines remain the most evidence-based adjunctive strategies to counteract antipsychotic-induced akathisia. Preliminary studies also support the adjunctive use of gabapentin, trazodone, and mirtazapine, as well as amantadine, although benefits with amantadine may be transient. The use of anticholinergic drugs such as benztropine is less well-established for akathisia than for pseudoparkinsonism.

Extrapyramidal adverse effects broadly encompass abnormal motor movements that originate outside of the motor cortex, including akathisia and parkinsonian symptoms, as well as bradykinesia, akinesia, tremor, choreiform movements, and dystonias. *Akathisia* — either the objective manifestation or the subjective experience of physical restlessness — is a common, usually dose-related problem related to treatment with most dopamine antagonists. It has in some instances been linked with violence and suicidal thinking or behavior. *Tardive akathisia* describes chronic akathisia, lasting for at least 1 month and often persisting for months or even years after antipsychotic discontinuation. A handful of case reports also suggest that true akathisia may also be inducible by lithium, mirtazapine (with chronic use), and some SSRIs, possibly in dose-related fashion (presumably via striatal dopamine antagonism resulting from the inhibitory effects of serotonin). Pseusoparkinsonism describes EPS resembling Parkinson's disease, usually caused by antipsychotic-induced disruption of dopaminergic tracts in the nigrostriatal pathway (which, when intact, normally modulate motor coordination through the extrapyramidal system). Rare case reports of de novo parkinsonian symptoms have also been described among epilepsy patients taking either divalproex or lamotrigine, while other reports suggest efficacy for lamotrigine to treat parkinsonian symptoms in bipolar disorder patients. Sertraline is thought to be the most potent dopamine reuptake inhibitor among the SSRIs, and as such, its potential for causing adventitious movements may be minimal.

Incidence rates of akathisia and other forms of EPS from antipsychotics have been reportedly lower with agents that dissociate rapidly and are thus considered "loose" binders of the dopamine D_2 receptor (Kapur and Seeman 2001), such as quetiapine and clozapine, and higher among agents with "tight" D_2 receptor binding affinities, such as risperidone and aripiprazole (Table 17–4). Patient-specific risk factors for akathisia vary across studies and in some, but not all, may include older age, female sex, negative symptoms, cognitive deficits, and affective symptoms. Akathisia also may be more likely to occur in patients taking two or more antipsychotics simultaneously (Berna et al. 2015), or during combination therapy with mood-stabilizing drugs or antidepressants in bipolar disorder or major depression, respectively, than might otherwise occur as monotherapy. EPS from high-potency antipsychotics might be less likely to occur when significant initial improvement is evident within the first 2 weeks of treatment (Rasmussen et al. 2017).

Physiological mechanisms to explain the pathogenesis of akathisia are complex and not fully understood, but prevailing theories include hypodopaminergic activity in the ventral striatum, with compensatory upregulation of noradrenergic terminals from the locus coeruleus to the shell of the nucleus accumbens and prefrontal cortex. In other words, striatal dopamine blockade may lead to diminished noradrenergic tone, likely accounting for the potential benefits of noradrenergic agents.

Centrally acting lipophilic β-blockers such as propranolol have become traditional cornerstones of treatment for akathisia, alongside benzodiazepines. Propranolol nonselectively antagonizes both β_1 and β_2 CNS receptors and is usually dosed from 30 to 90 mg/day in two or three divided doses. Betaxolol, another centrally acting antagonist that is selective for β_1 receptors, dosed from 10 to 20 mg/day, has shown efficacy comparable to that of propranolol (20–40 mg/day), suggesting possible specificity of β_1 receptors in the mechanism of akathisia (Dumon et al. 1992; Dupuis et al. 1987). By contrast, non–centrally acting hydrophilic β-blockers that do not cross the blood-brain barrier (e.g., atenolol, metoprolol, nadolol, sotalol) show little efficacy in akathisia (Dumon et al. 1992; Dupuis et al. 1987). One must obviously avoid β-blockers (particuarly β_2 blockers) in patients with asthma, bradycardia, or sick sinus syndrome, although β_1-blockers (which are cardioselective) pose no bronchopulmonary hazard.

TABLE 17–4. Reported rates of akathisia and number needed to harm among second-generation antipsychotics in U.S. Food and Drug Administration registration trials[a]

Agent	NNH[b]	Incidence
Aripiprazole	12 (BM) 25 (SZ) 5 (MDD)	10%–13% in acute monotherapy trials across indications; 19%–25% when added to lithium or divalproex (bipolar disorder) or antidepressants (major depression)
Asenapine	34 (SZ) 50 (BM)	4%–11% across indications
Brexpiprazole	15 (MDD) 112 (SZ)	4%–7% in pooled schizophrenia trials, dosed 1–4 mg/day; 4%–14% in pooled MDD adjunctive trials, dosed 1–3 mg/day
Cariprazine	7 (BM) 15 (SZ)	9%–14% in acute trials for schizophrenia (dosed 1.5–6 mg/day); 20% or 21% in acute trials for bipolar mania (dosed at 3–6 mg/day or 9–12 mg/day, respectively)
Clozapine	NR	3%
Iloperidone	~100–~250 (SZ)	1.7%–2.3%; parkinsonism in 0.2%–0.3%
Lurasidone	10 (SZ) 12–18 (BD)	6%–22% in acute trials for schizophrenia
Olanzapine	25 (SZ) 167 (MDD)	3% in acute trials across indications
Paliperidone	39 (SZ)	6%–9% in acute schizophrenia trials
Quetiapine	91 (MDD) 143 (BM) 188 (SZ)	1%–4% across indications
Risperidone	15 (SZ) 17 (BM)	5%–9% (across indications); parkinsonism in 12%–20% across indications
Ziprasidone	20 (BM) 100 (SZ)	8%–10% (across indications); other extrapyramidal symptoms in 14%–31% across indications

Note. BD=bipolar depression; BM=bipolar mania; MDD=major depressive disorder; NNH=number needed to harm; NR=not reported; SZ = schizophrenia.
[a]Based on manufacturers' product information.
[b]NNH as calculated by Citrome (2009b, 2014, 2015).

Increased noradrenergic tone also can arise from $\alpha_1\beta$ agonism, which likely accounts for the extremely low incident rate of akathisia (but also high rate of orthostatic hypotension) with iloperidone.

Among dopamine agonists, amantadine, dosed from 100 to 200 mg bid, has been shown to rapidly improve akathisia, but its effects may dissipate within several weeks of initiation. Its value may be more robust in pseudoparkinsonism than in akathisia, and as an alternative to benztropine, diphenhydramine, or trihexyphenidyl, it spares the cognitive and adverse effects of anticholinergic drugs. Preliminary controlled data also support use of rotigotine (mean dose=~3 mg/day; range=2–8 mg/day) for akathisia and extrapyramidal signs.

Case reports have suggested potential value with adjunctive gabapentin up to 1,200 mg/day for antipsychotic-induced akathisia, as well as instances of akathisia induced by abrupt cessation of gabapentin.

Benzodiazepines are also commonly used to manage acute akathisia. A 2002 Cochrane Database analysis based on two small randomized trials (N=27) found clonazepam superior to placebo for reducing symptoms of akathisia within 7–14 days of initiation (Resende Lima et al. 1999).

Akathisia associated with SSRIs as well as some antipsychotics has been hypothesized to result from undesired 5-HT_{2A} agonism, prompting interest in the use of 5-HT_{2A} antagonists such as trazodone (50–100 mg/day) or mirtazapine (15 mg/day); however, case reports also link mirtazapine with causing akathisia.

Some investigators have reported low serum iron levels in association with chronic akathisia, with case reports of improvement following intravenous iron therapy.

Use of the antiserotonergic drug cyproheptadine (16 mg/day) also has demonstrated efficacy comparable to that of propranolol (up to 80 mg/day) for treating akathisia in preliminary randomized trials.

Preliminary randomized controlled data show high tolerability and greater improvement in antipsychotic-associated parkinsonism with adjunctive modafinil (50–200 mg/day) than placebo (Lohr et al. 2013).

Vitamin B_6 dosed at 600 mg twice daily also has been reported in small, preliminary randomized trials to ameliorate subjective, but not objective, restlessness and distress associated with akathisia (Lerner et al. 2004).

Finally, anticholinergic drugs such as benztropine are sometimes used in the treatment of akathisia, although their value for this intended purpose appears less well established than in the amelioration of antipsychotic-induced pseudoparkinsonism. Indeed, a 2006 Cochrane Database review found no relevant randomized controlled trials from which to draw broad recommendations or that support or refute the efficacy of anticholinergic drugs to treat akathisia (Rathbone and Soares-Weiser 2006).

Dystonic Reactions

General Recommendations

Acute dystonic reactions should be treated promptly with an oral or intramuscularly dosed anticholinergic drug such as diphenhydramine 50–100 mg or benztropine 1–2 mg. Dystonias typically occur due to excessive dosing of high-potency antipsychotics but may also reflect motor sensitivity to usual dosages in some patients.

Dystonia refers to "sustained or intermittent muscle contractions causing abnormal, often repetitive movements, postures or both" that are "typically patterned, twisting, and (possibly) tremulous… often initiated or worsened by voluntary action" (Albanese et al. 2013, p. 866). Involuntary spasmodic "pulling" of large muscle groups also is often a descriptive term. Acute dystonic reactions to antipsychotic drugs most often occur within the first week of starting (or raising the dose of) a dopamine-blocking drug. In some studies, younger age and male sex have been reported as possible risk factors. Dystonic reactions can, rarely, be life-threatening (e.g., due to airway obstruction from laryngospasm) and require urgent attention.

Administration of anticholinergic medications is the usual treatment of choice. For acute dystonic reactions, this may involve benztropine 1–2 mg or diphenhydramine 1–2 mg/kg (up to 100 mg); in children, dosing is typically 0.02 mg/kg. Alternatively, biperiden 1–5 mg IM typically renders relief within 20 minutes of administration. Intramuscular or slow intravenous administration of anticholinergic drugs renders relief faster than oral administration. Dosing may be repeated after 10–30 minutes if no signs of response are evident. Parenteral (IV but not IM) diazepam 5–10 mg is sometimes used if the interventions described above fail to relieve symptoms promptly. Continued oral dosing of an anticholinergic drug (e.g., benztropine 1–2 mg twice daily) for several days is then usually recommended to prevent recurrence.

Types of acute focal dystonic reactions to antipsychotic drugs include the following:

- *Spasticity*: dystonic reaction in which truncal and sometimes limb muscles develop prolonged increased tone (becoming tight or stiff) that may be painful

- *Torticollis and retrocollis:* movements involving turning the head to one side or backward, respectively
- *Laryngospasm:* sudden contraction and spasm of the vocal cords.
- *Opisthotonos:* often painful hyperextension of the neck, and possibly the back, causing a marked overarching posture
- *Oculogyric crises:* dystonic reactions involving a sustained and involuntary upward deviation of the eyes due to spasm of the extraocular muscles. It may be caused by FGAs or SGAs or by abrupt cessation of antipsychotic agents, and more rarely of other psychotropic agents, including lithium, carbamazepine, oxcarbazepine, amantadine, SSRIs, and benzodiazepines, among other medications. Antipsychotic-induced oculogyric crises have been reported to occur, often in association with autonomic features (e.g., flushing, sweating) and transient exacerbations of psychotic symptoms (e.g., hallucinations, delusions, catatonia). Oculogyric crises are typically self-limited, but their resolution may be hastened by anticholinergic medications such as benztropine or diphenhydramine. Case reports also suggest that oculogyric crises caused by FGAs or some SGAs may not necessarily resolve solely by discontinuation of the antipsychotic but may improve after the initiation of quetiapine. It is unknown whether recurrent or chronic antipsychotic-induced oculogyric crises increase the probability of developing long-term movement disorders such as tardive dyskinesia. Relatively long-acting benzodiazepines, such as clonazepam, may also provide benefit for alleviating antipsychotic-induced oculogyric crises, with clonazepam being among the best studied in case reports (Horiguchi and Inami 1989; Viana Bde et al. 2009).

Motor Tics

General Recommendations

Identification and elimination of the causal agent are advisable if the symptom produces distress. Alpha agonists such as guanfacine or clonidine or low-dose antipsychotics are generally considered the treatment of choice to counteract tics.

Tics are repetitive, intermittent hyperkinetic movements that characteristically can be voluntarily suppressed and are usually associated with an urge to perform the movement. They rarely may be caused by certain psychotropic medications. Obviously, the clinician's first task is to affirm whether the development of a new, sudden repetitive movement or vocalization likely represents a tic (as opposed to a compulsive behavior or motor neuron disease) and whether other more primary etiologies (e.g., Tourette's syndrome, usually in individuals under age 18; head trauma; stroke; infection) are plausible explanations. Tics commonly include coughing, throat clearing, grunting, sniffing, blinking, and head jerking, and they may include more complex behaviors such as shouting or touching objects or people. Rare neurological conditions such as gelastic seizures (sudden paroxysms of laughter) or chorea may also pose unusual symptoms that require differentiation from tics and determination of a primary neurological etiology versus a secondary iatrogenic phenomenon.

Psychotropic drugs that have been reported to cause (or exacerbate) tics most recognizably include stimulants (i.e., amphetamine and methylphenidate) but may also more rarely include bupropion, sertraline, fluoxetine, imipramine, and certain anticonvulsants (notably, carbamazepine and lamotrigine). Although the manufacturer's product information for atomoxetine states that the drug does not worsen tics in patients with ADHD and comorbid Tourette's syndrome, such cases have been reported. In the great majority of case reports involving the emergence or exacerbation of tics with each of the aforementioned medications, subjects were usually those with preexisting tic disorders. Increased dopaminergic tone is thought to contribute to pharmacologically induced or exacerbated tics; mechanisms by which some anticonvulsants may cause tics are less well understood but are thought to involve antiglutamatergic effects that may affect motor control. In general, the recommendation is to discontinue a medication if it is believed to cause or exacerbate a tic.

Alpha agonists such as clonidine (0.1–0.3 mg/day) or guanfacine (0.5–3.0 mg/day) have demonstrated efficacy in tic disorders in children and adolescents, although extended-release guanfacine may show only a modest effect. Outcomes with alpha agonists for tic treatment in adults are less well established. Data also exist to support the utility of both FGAs (e.g., haloperidol, fluphenazine) and SGAs (e.g., aripiprazole) for treatment of tics, again with a stronger evidence base in youth than in adults.

Pharmacotherapies intended to counteract or treat iatrogenic motor tics are generally not undertaken, although medications used to suppress tics include α_2-adrenergic agonists such as clonidine or guanfacine, benzodiazepines such as diazepam, antipsychotic agents (haloperidol and pimozide being among the best studied), and possibly donepezil (2.5–10 mg/day). In children with ADHD and chronic tics, desipramine suppresses tics while reducing ADHD symptoms better than placebo (Spencer et al. 2002), suggesting a broader role for TCAs in managing tics. Of note, discontinuation of any of these agents (or poor adherence) could lead to the reemergence of tics that are no longer being suppressed.

Restless Legs Syndrome

General Recommendations

Adjunctive benzodiazepines or dopamine agonists (e.g., prami-pexole, ropinirole) may help to curtail restless legs caused by psychotropic agents. Restless legs caused by FGAs or SGAs may be a manifestation of dose-related akathisia, which may improve with dosage reductions or, if necessary, a change to an alternative within-in-class agent that may be associated with a lower incidence of akathisia.

Restless legs syndrome (RLS) is sometimes regarded as a form of dyskinesia that reportedly may be provoked by a number of medications in addition to dopamine antagonists, including mirtazapine (particularly when coadministered with tramadol or dopamine antagonists; S. W. Kim et al. 2008), escitalopram, and citalopram. Some authors have suggested that RLS induced by SSRIs may reflect the consequences of SSRI-induced downregulation of dopamine tone in the basal ganglia, for which replacement with bupropion (as a dopaminergic alternative antidepressant) may be useful. Some SGAs have been reported to cause RLS or periodic limb movements during sleep that occur independently of other motor abnormalities and potentially in a dose-related fashion. RLS has been linked with olanzapine and risperidone. Treatment with benzodiazepines or dopamine agonists (e.g., pramipexole or ropinirole) may not be efficacious to counteract RLS induced by SGAs, although changing to an alternative SGA with loose D_2 receptor binding affinity, such as quetiapine, may be ameliorative. Anticholinergic drugs are not known to ameliorate RLS despite the likely pathogenic role of the basal ganglia and related extrapyramidal structures. Gabapentin enacarbil, a pro-drug with nearly twofold greater bioavailability than gabapentin, is an established treatment for primary RLS but has not been studied as a remedy to counteract RLS secondary to psychotopic medications.

Tardive Dyskinesia

General Recommendations

Tardive dyskinesia (TD) is a potentially severe and sometimes irreversible movement disorder caused by long-term use of antipsychotic drugs. The emergence of early signs of TD (e.g., involuntary oral-buccal movements) should prompt the limited use—if not complete cessation—of antipsychotics if clinically feasible, balanced against the risk for worsening underlying psychosis or other psychopathology. A lower incidence of TD may occur with clozapine, quetiapine, or olanzapine than with other antipsychotics. Valbenazine and deutetrabenazine are both human vesicular monoamine transporter type 2 inhibitors that are FDA approved for the treatment of TD. Data from preliminary randomized controlled trials also suggest safety and potential benefit with vitamin B_6, *Ginkgo biloba*, levetiracetam, melatonin, and amantadine.

Tardive dyskinesia is a hyperkinetic, often complex and irregular involuntary movement disorder involving symptoms developing after >3 months' cumulative exposure to antipsychotics or >1 month if older than 60 years (American Psychiatric Association 2013). In a majority of cases, TD involves oral-buccal regions (characterized by tongue thrusts and lip smacking or pursing) and also may encompass abnormal involuntary movements of the head and neck, trunk, and upper and lower extremities. TD movements may be described as

- Choreiform (i.e., abrupt, irregular, nonrepetitive, and nonrhythmic) in all regions, including the tongue when protruded. Fingers may move nonrhythmically as if in a "piano player" fashion.
- Athetotic, involving slow, continuous, sinewy or serpentine-like writhing.
- Tics.
- Myoclonic jerks.
- Focal dystonias, including blepharospasm (i.e., frequent blinking or sustained eyelid closure) and torticollis of the head, neck, and shoulders; botulinum toxin injections may be indicated for blepharospasm if its severity essentially renders a patient functionally blind.

Tardive dystonia is considered a subtype of TD; it manifests with prolonged, nonrhythmic contractions of specific muscle groups that involve increased tone and spasmodic contortions. (In contrast, dyskinesias involve more rhythmic movements of large muscle groups, without increased motor tone.)

The incidence of TD has been estimated at 3%–5% per year during treatment with FGAs; the risk during treatment with SGAs is thought to be somewhat lower but still observable (with a weighted annual mean incidence of 0% in children, 0.8% in adults, 6.8% in adults plus older adults combined, and 5.4% in adults over age 54, according to some estimates; Correll et al. 2004). Although TD risk is widely thought to be lower with newer-generation antipsychotics, meta-analyses suggest that point prevalence rates are substantial with both FGAs (~30%) and SGAs (~21%), independent of age (Carbon et al. 2017). Clinicians must also keep in mind that lifetime risk is cumulative and may be higher in patients taking SGAs as a result of past exposure to FGAs.

Established risk factors for TD include the following:

- Duration of antipsychotic exposure
- Advanced age
- High dosages
- Female sex
- Diagnosis of an affective disorder

African, African American, or Afro-Caribbean race has been linked with a higher risk for developing TD during antipsychotic use; however, these reported associations may be artifacts of higher antipsychotic dosages and durations. Diabetes mellitus and cigarette smoking also have been reported in some, but not all, studies as TD risk factors among antipsychotic recipients. Some studies also suggest that akathisia or EPS in themselves may be a risk factor for developing TD. HIV+ patients have anecdotally been reported to be at higher risk for developing TD from antipsychotics, presumably due to basal ganglia viral penetration involvement.

TD is often irreversible. It can sometimes be masked at least temporarily by increased doses of an antipsychotic. Proposed mechanisms behind TD include dopamine supersensitivity as well as neurotoxic effects related to oxidative stress. A key pharmacological management approach is to reduce the availability of presynaptic central dopamine. One such strategy involves tetrabenazine, which reversibly inhibits vesicular monoamine oxidase 2 (VMAT2), the intracellular apparatus for transporting cytosolic dopamine quanta to axonal terminals for presynaptic release. Less available dopamine in the synaptic cleft is thought to diminish postsynaptic supersensitivity to striatal dopamine release, thereby reducing symptoms of TD. Reserpine, known for its antihypertensive and potential depressogenic effects, is another VMAT2 inhibitor that has been shown to improve TD symptoms in small preliminary trials. Unlike tetrabenazine, reserpine acts irreversibly and binds to both VMAT1 and VMAT2, and also causes peripheral as well as central monoamine depletion as well as orthostatic hypotension. In principle, VMAT2 inhibitors could also treat psychosis — as is, in fact, the case with reserpine — but dosages needed to potentially exert antipsychotic effects would likely pose problems with psychotropic tolerability.

Tetrabenazine was FDA approved in 2008 to treat Huntington's chorea and is occasionally used off-label to treat TD. However, its short half-life requires multiple daily doses, and it carries nontrivial risks for causing or exacerbating depression and suicidal thinking or behavior (■) in Huntington's disease, although this labeled warning has not been extended to patients with TD. Tetrabenazine also has been shown to prolong the QTc by about 8 msec on ECG.

In April 2017, the FDA approved the reversible VMAT2 inhibitor valbenazine for the treatment of TD. Tetrabenazine is metabolized by carbonyl reductase to four distinct stereoisomers of dihydrotetrabenazine, of which only one (R,R,R-dihydrotetrabenazine, or [+]-α-dihydrotetrabenazine) has very high binding affinity for VMAT2. Valbenazine is the valine-esterified analogue of tetrabenazine; peripheral hydrolysis of the valine moiety yields R,R,R-dihydrotetrabenazine, the aforementioned highly active [+]-α-dihydrotetrabenazine isomer (see Figure 17–1). Valbenazine itself has only modest VMAT2 binding affinity (Ki=~150 nM), but its [+]-α-dihydrotetrabenazine metabolite has high VMAT2 selectivity and binding affinity (Ki=~4 nM) (Grigoriadis et al. 2017). As compared with tetrabenazine, valbenazine's longer half-life (15–22 hours) permits once-daily dosing, and the molecule carries a much lower risk for inducing depression or suicidality, or cardiovascular effects, presumably because of its extremely weak binding affinity for D_1, D_2, 5-HT_{1A}, $α_1$ or $α_2$ adrenergic receptors, or for the serotonin, dopamine, or norepinephrine transporters. Valbenazine can prolong the QTc interval if coadministered with a strong CYP2D6 or 3A4 inhibitor, or in poor metabolizers of CYP2D6.

Valbenazine, dosed at 40 mg/day for 1 week, then 80 mg/day, yielded a response rate (defined as >50% reduction in global symptom severity) after 6 weeks of 23.8% (40 mg/day) and 40.0% (80 mg/day), both significantly better than the reduction seen with placebo (8.7%). Its most common adverse effect is sedation (about 10%; NNH=15). Although valbenazine demonstrates a moderate effect size to reduce TD symptoms (NNT=~4), those symptoms often promptly recur if and when valbenazine is stopped.

A second reversible VMAT2 inhibitor, deutetrabenazine (a deuterated form of tetrabenazine; see Figure 17–2), received FDA approval in August 2017 for the treatment of TD. Deuterium, a stable isotope of hydrogen, extends the half lives of tetrabenazine's active metabolites, and deutetrabenazine appears to have fewer adverse effects than tetrabenazine (including less risk for depression, akathisia, sedation, insomnia, and parkinsonism).

Two 12-week placebo-controlled randomized trials have demonstrated the safety and efficacy of deutetrabenazine for TD when dosed at 24 or 36 mg/day (Anderson et al. 2017; Fernandez et al. 2017). Deutetraben-

valine

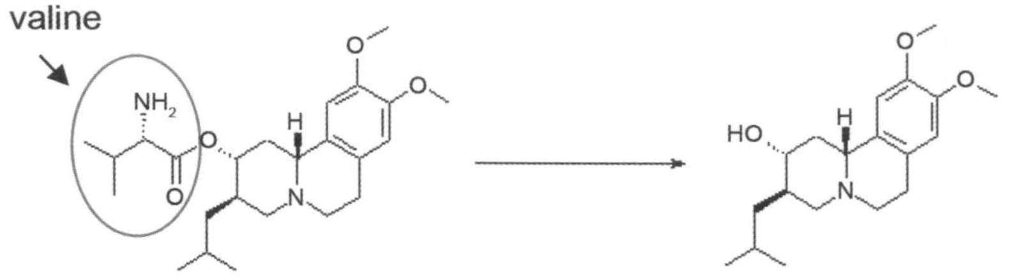

FIGURE 17–1. Metabolism of valbenazine to [+]-α-dihydrotetrabenazine.

azine carries a boxed warning (■) because of its risk for inducing suicidal thoughts or behaviors, based on clinical trials in patients with Huntington's disease, and presumably by virtue of its potential for depletion of catecholamines and indoleamines, analogous to tetrabenazine. In FDA registration trials of deutetrabenazine for TD, the most commonly observed adverse effects were nasopharyngitis (NNH=50) and insomnia (NNH=34), yielding a likelihood of being helped or harmed of 27 (Citrome 2017). Predicted Fridericia-corrected QTc interval prolongation with deutetrabenazine in registration trials for TD (across dosages of 18 mg bid and 24 mg bid) revealed a QTc of 4.69 msec (90% CI=2.03–7.85 msec).

QTc prolongation is listed in the manufacturer's product labeling for deutetrabenazine even though this phenomenon was not observed in its FDA registration trials for TD (likely reflecting the potential for QTc prolongation associated with tetrabenazine). Per the manufacturer, use of deutetrabenazine in patients who are poor metabolizers of CYP2D6, or when coadministered with strong CYP2D6 inhibitors, could cause clinically relevant QTc prolongation.

Among other, non-FDA-approved treatment options for TD, adjunctive vitamin E (dosed from 800 to 1,600 IU/day) was historically regarded as among the few viable strategies for either its treatment or its prevention. However, contemporary reports demonstrate less robust acute efficacy than was once believed and only modest value from taking 800 IU twice daily for delaying the onset of TD during antipsychotic therapy. The U.S. recommended daily allowance of vitamin E is 22 IU/day. A 2001 Cochrane Database review of 10 randomized studies found no evidence for reduction of TD symptoms with vitamin E but less progression of TD symptoms with vitamin E use as compared with placebo (Soares-Weiser et al. 2011). (Of note, only 3 of the 10 studies included in that review involved treatment durations of 5 months or longer.)

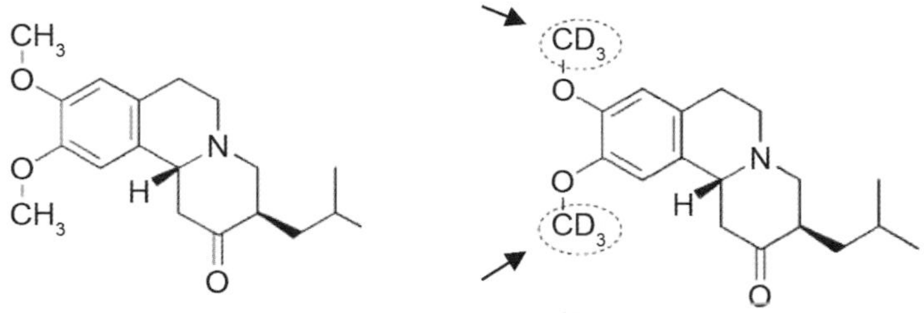

FIGURE 17–2. Tetrabenazine and deutetrabenazine.

High-dose vitamin E in the form of alpha-tocopherol has separately been implicated as a risk factor for prostate cancer, leading some authors to advocate the use of mixed (alpha and gamma) tocopherol formulations of vitamin E along with other antioxidants (e.g., vitamin C) to protect against its possible pro-oxidative effects. Among other antioxidants, vitamin B_6 (dosed at 1,200 mg/day) was found to be superior to placebo in reducing parkinsonian and dyskinetic movements as well as EPS during a 26-week randomized double-blind study involving 50 patients with schizophrenia or schizoaffective disorder and TD (Lerner et al. 2007). Extract of gingko biloba (a putative free-radical scavenger) was studied at a dosage of 240 mg/day ($n=78$) versus placebo ($n=79$) over 12 weeks in Chinese inpatients with schizophrenia and yielded a significantly greater reduction in Abnormal Involuntary Movement Scale (AIMS) scores, with response (defined as $\geq 30\%$ reduction from baseline AIMS) seen in 51% of the patients who were taking active drug versus 5% of the patients who were taking placebo (Zhang et al. 2011). Similarly, the antioxidant piracetam (orally dosed at 4,800 mg/day) was superior to placebo during a 9-week randomized crossover study in 40 patients with schizophrenia or schizoaffective disorder and TD (Libov et al. 2007). Relatedly, a randomized controlled study using the ethylated congener of piracetam, levetiracetam (dosed from 500 to 3,000 mg/day; mean final dosage=2,156 mg/day), was found to be superior to placebo over 12 weeks in reducing moderately severe TD symptoms in 50 patients with schizophrenia, with a mean reduction in AIMS scores of 43.5% (as compared with 18.7% for patients given placebo) (Woods et al. 2008). Consistent with these observations, an open case series of adjunctive levetiracetam (mean dose=2,290 mg/day) found significant improvement from baseline of abnormal involuntary movements in 16 patients with TD after 1–3 months (Meco et al. 2006). It has been hypothesized that levetiracetam may improve motor function via free radical oxidative scavenging, enhancement of GABA function, enhancement of nitric oxide production, or reduction of neuronal hypersynchrony in the basal ganglia. Lastly, the hormone melatonin also possesses antioxidant properties; during one 6-week double-blind crossover study in 22 schizophrenia patients with TD, melatonin, dosed nightly (8:00 P.M.) as a single 10-mg tablet, was associated with greater reductions in abnormal involuntary motor movements and high tolerability (Shamir et al. 2001).

Other agents have been studied on the basis of the rationale of presumptive damage to striatal cholinergic neurons associated with TD. Favorable preliminary open-label data have been reported with the procholinergic agent donepezil (5–10 mg/day for 6 weeks) (Caroff et al. 2001), although findings were negative from a larger, controlled trial of the cholinesterase inhibitor galantamine (dosed at 8–24 mg/day for 12 weeks) (Caroff et al. 2007). By contrast, the M_1 selective anticholinergic drug biperiden (2 mg bid) improved both parkinsonian symptoms and abnormal involuntary motor movements better than did placebo during a double-blind crossover study of 32 schizophrenia inpatients with TD (Silver et al. 1995).

Certain dopamine agonists have demonstrated value in treating TD symptoms in patients with schizophrenia. The most notable is amantadine (100 mg bid), which in a study of 32 schizophrenia inpatients with TD yielded better efficacy than placebo and comparable reductions in AIMS scores as compared with biperiden during successive 2-week single-blind randomized crossover trials (Silver et al. 1995).

GABAergic drugs such as baclofen, divalproex, progabide, and tetrahydroisoxazolopyridine also have been studied preliminarily in patients with TD. In a Cochrane Database meta-analysis of eight short-term studies, Alabed et al. (2011) described the evidence for each of these agents as "inconsistent and unconvincing," adding that any potential benefits were typically outweighed by substantial adverse effects involving sedation or the exacerbation of psychotic symptoms.

Eicosapentaenoic acid dosed at 2 g/day was no different from placebo in a study of 84 subjects with schizophrenia or schizoaffective disorder and TD over 12 weeks (Emsley et al. 2006).

Optimistic results were reported from a pilot study of open-label high-dose buspirone (180 mg/day for 12 weeks) in a small group ($N=8$) of schizophrenia patients with TD (Moss et al. 1993), although these findings have not been replicated, and supratherapeutic doses of buspirone have been associated with seizures, gastrointestinal problems, sedation, paresthesias, and blurred vision. Coadministration of buspirone with other serotonergic agents also may increase the risk for serotonin syndrome.

Branched-chain amino acids received interest as a potential strategy for treating TD on the basis of observations that the large neutral amino acid phenylalanine appears to be associated with TD, whereas ingestion of branched-chain amino acids (i.e., valine, leucine, isoleucine) may correspondingly diminish brain phenylalanine availability, which in turn may reduce TD symptoms (Richardson et al. 2003). A proprietary powdered drink mix containing large branched-chain amino acids (Tarvil) became commercially available in 2002, but in 2007 it was discontinued by its manufacturer, Nutricia North America.

A number of studies have examined the potential for some atypical antipsychotics to diminish the symptoms of TD (in contrast to the masking of TD, which can be observed using increased doses of FGAs). Among these drugs, low-dose clozapine has perhaps the most robust evidence, with global improvement rates in TD symptoms reportedly in the range of 70% to 80% over periods of up to 18 weeks (Spivak et al. 1997). Some case reports suggest that the D_2 partial agonist aripiprazole may improve (Karabulut et al. 2008) or cause (Abbasian and Power 2009) TD, and other reports suggest improvement in TD symptoms after quetiapine is substituted for other antipsychotics (Abbasian and Power 2009). The substitution of olanzapine for other atypical antipsychotics or FGAs in schizophrenia patients with TD has been associated with reductions in TD symptoms, with improvements sustained over an 8-month period, and no rebound worsening of TD symptoms during imposed dosage reduction periods (Kinon et al. 2004).

A long-acting form of acamprosate, SNC-102, has been in Phase II development trials as a possible novel TD treatment strategy. Other possible therapeutic treatment options under development for TD include Tardoxal (MC-1; pyridoxal-5'-phosphate), noninvasive transcranial focused ultrasound surgery guided by magnetic resonance imaging (the transcranial ExAblate system [MRgFUS]) and the Activa PC neurostimulator.

In our experience, none of the available pharmacological options to reduce TD symptoms or curtail their progression yield a dramatic or substantial benefit, with the notable exception of valbenazine. TD remains a difficult and often intransigent problem for which there is no reliable or well-proven remedy. Realistic expectations should be established with patients before embarking on experimental strategies such as those described in this section. In some cases, despite the presence of TD, the severity of psychotic symptoms may be sufficiently great to outweigh the risks of potential worsening of TD and warrant continued dopamine antagonist therapy. In such instances, the use of antipsychotic agents with relatively loose D_2 receptor affinities, such as clozapine or quetiapine, may at least theoretically help to minimize the known and sometimes accepted risk for TD worsening.

Withdrawal Dyskinesias

General Recommendations

To minimize the potential for withdrawal dyskinesias, the preferable action is to gradually taper off or cross-taper an existing antipsychotic rather than to abruptly discontinue it.

Abrupt cessation of antipsychotics may provoke motor adverse effects suggestive of a withdrawal dyskinesia. Some clinicians believe this phenomenon to reflect more accurately the unmasking of an underlying tardive movement disorder rather than a true process induced by withdrawal of an antipsychotic. The clinician should consider this possibility as being especially likely with antipsychotics that have short half-lives (cf. aripiprazole [$t_{1/2}$=75 hours] or brexpiprazole [$t_{1/2}$=91 hours]) or agents with especially tight D_2 binding affinities in the basal ganglia (e.g., risperidone, haloperidol). Withdrawal dyskinesias are sometimes self-limited and may require no intervention apart from continued monitoring. If the withdrawal dyskinesia is significantly discomforting, clinicians might 1) reintroduce the discontinued antipsychotic, followed by a slower taper; 2) substitute an alternative antipsychotic with lesser known risk for disturbing extrapyramidal movements; 3) introduce a benzodiazepine; or 4) use adjunctive clonidine on a short-term basis. Withdrawal dyskinesias pose no known increased risk for future development of TD.

Tremor

General Recommendations

Clinicians should properly evaluate the characteristics and likely primary versus secondary etiology of a newly observed tremor, reduce dosages when feasible, and assure the absence of other signs of neurotoxicity. Propranolol begun at 10 mg tid or primidone dosed at 100–300 mg/day (maximum of 750 mg/day) in two or three divided doses may help to reduce or ameliorate a drug-induced tremor.

Tremor is defined as "rhythmical, involuntary oscillatory movement of a body part" (Deuschl et al. 1998, p. 3). It may be caused by numerous psychotropic agents, and its presence should signal the need for careful evaluation before changing treatments or dosages or initiating adjunctive pharmacotherapies. Tremor sometimes is a sign of neurotoxicity that should be evaluated in the context of other features that could suggest supratherapeutic dosing of a given agent (e.g., a coarse postural tremor in the setting of gastrointestinal upset and ataxia would be consistent with probable lithium toxicity). A careful history should include the assessment of caffeine intake, use of sympathomimetic agents, risk for alcohol or benzodiazepine withdrawal, history of familial or essential tremor, and other pertinent factors that may contribute to the emergence of tremor. Physiologic or benign tremors can be exacerbated by some psychotropic agents (e.g., carbamazepine, divalproex, lithium, psychostimulants, SSRIs, tricyclic antidepressants).

The evaluation of a tremor should include 1) localization of affected regions (i.e., upper and/or lower extremities; head and neck or trunk; unilateral or bilateral presence), 2) characteristics (e.g., occurring at rest or with action; qualitative dimensions such as a pill-rolling or parkinsonian tremor vs. resting tremor), 3) pupillary examination and assessment of nystagmus, 4) assessment of deep tendon reflexes, and 5) identification of the presence of cerebellar signs (e.g., ataxia, dysdiadochokinesia, Romberg sign). The differential diagnosis of tremor is vast, and its comprehensive discussion falls beyond the scope of this work.

Tremors are often characterized as occurring at rest (resting tremor) or only during voluntary muscle movement (action tremors). Action tremors are often further subclassified as

- *Postural:* occurring with outstretched hands against gravity.
- *Intention:* occurring when making purposeful movements, such as touching finger to nose.
- *Kinetic:* occurring during any voluntary movement.
- *Isometric:* occurring during a sustained voluntary muscle contraction, such as holding a heavy object.
- *Task-specific:* occurring during repetitive specific motor tasks, such as writing.

Major distinguishing characteristics among tremors that may be useful for the clinician to consider are summarized in Table 17–5.

In the absence of other signs of frank neurotoxicity, tremor can be an otherwise benign but disruptive adverse drug effect that may be remediable either by dosage reductions or by the use of adjunctive medications. β-Blockers that exert peripheral effects such as propranolol likely are the most commonly undertaken medication strategy to counteract drug-induced tremors. Metoprolol, which is moderately lipophilic, also may

TABLE 17–5.   Clinical characteristics of specific drug-induced and noniatrogenic tremors

Suspected cause	Clinical description
Alcohol/benzodiazepine withdrawal	Rapid (>8 Hz) coarse tremor at rest, mainly in hands; coarse tremors in general are more suggestive of toxicity states.
Divalproex	Fine (8–12 Hz) tremor, usually postural but may occur at rest, often affecting limbs as well as head, mouth, and tongue. Incidence ~6%–45% (Rinnerthaler et al. 2005).
Essential tremor	An intention/action tremor varying from 4 to 12 Hz, most often affecting the hands but may also affect head, voice, tongue, legs, and trunk. Tremor is absent during sleep. Onset is usually in mid-adulthood, but treatment-seeking may peak in older adulthood. Course may be progressive. A positive family history can be identified in a majority of individuals.
Lithium	Fine (8–12 Hz) postural tremor (i.e., evident when upper extremities are held forward outstretched against gravity); incidence ~4%–65% (Gelenberg and Jefferson 1995).
SSRIs, TCAs	6–12 Hz postural or action tremor, with incidence up to 20%, typically arising 1–2 months after treatment is started (Morgan and Sethi 2005); may be an early sign of serotonin syndrome during SSRI therapy.
Parkinsonian/ antipsychotic-induced	Bradykinesia; low frequency (3–6 Hz) high-amplitude resting tremor. Tremor in Parkinson's disease is often asymmetric and diminishes with voluntary movement.

Note.   SSRI=selective serotonin reuptake inhibitor; TCA=tricyclic antidepressant.

treat lithium-induced tremor (Gaby et al. 1983). Hydrophilic β-blockers such as atenolol, which do not appreciably cross the blood-brain barrier, also have shown efficacy in treating lithium-induced tremor (Davé 1989).

For tremors caused by lithium, divalproex, or most other psychotropics, propranolol dosing is typically begun at 10 mg bid or tid and may increase to 20–40 mg bid or tid prn, with a maximum reported efficacious dosage of 320 mg/day in a single (long-acting) or divided dosing schedule. Clinicians must monitor for bradycardia and hypotension, although the latter is less common at relatively low doses of propranolol. Long-acting or once-daily preparations of β-blockers such as propranolol (Inderal LA) may sometimes be substituted for the immediate-release formulation, provided that the higher doses in which Inderal LA is formulated pose no risk for hypotension in a given patient. As noted in earlier sections of this chapter, β-blockers are relatively contraindicated in the presence of hypotension, significant bradycardia, sick sinus syndrome, second- or third-degree atrioventricular block, and forms of chronic obstructive pulmonary disease such as asthma.

Alternatively, the pyrimidinedione anticonvulsant primidone is commonly used in off-label fashion for treatment of essential tremor, with efficacy comparable to that with propranolol (Zesiewicz et al. 2005). Dosing is typically begun at 50–100 mg at bedtime for the first few days, and the dosage then increased to 100 mg bid for an additional 2–3 days, and then titrated further upward if necessary (based on response) to 100 mg tid or as high as 250 mg tid. In studies of primidone in essential tremor, high-dose primidone (i.e., 750 mg/day) has not demonstrated superior efficacy to a daily dose of 250 mg (Serrano-Dueñas 2003). Use of primidone as an anecdotal remedy to counteract psychotropic-induced tremor is an extrapolation from data involving its use in essential tremor; formal studies of primidone for this specific purpose have not been reported. One must keep in mind that primidone is a highly potent inducer of CYP3A4 and CYP1A2 isoenzymes and can hasten the metabolism of drugs that are substrates for them (see Chapter 2, Table 2–7).

Other anticonvulsants that have shown at least preliminary value in the treatment of essential tremor include topiramate, gabapentin, levetiracetam, and oxcarbazepine.

The carbonic anhydrase inhibitors acetazolamide (begun at 125 mg/day and increased by 125 mg weekly to a maximum of 500 mg/day; usual mean dose=250–300 mg/day) and methazolamide (begun at 25 mg/day and increased to a maximal dose of about 200 mg/day) have been reported to improve essential tremor (particularly in the presence of head tremor), but the literature contains only a handful of small case reports using these agents to counteract tremor induced by lithium, anticonvulsants (e.g., divalproex), or other agents. Additionally, one may also then need to contend with adverse effects from carbonic anhydrase inhibitors (e.g., headache, paresthesias, sedation). Lastly, open data also support the possible efficacy of vitamin B_6 (900–1,200 mg/day) to reduce lithium tremor, while case reports suggest that amantadine (100 mg bid) may improve divalproex-associated tremor.

Muscle Twitching, Fasciculations, and Myoclonus

General Recommendations

Medication-induced fasciculations or muscle twitches are generally benign phenomena that require no intervention. Clinicians should assure the absence of noniatrogenic and remediable causes of fasciculations (e.g., dehydration, hypomagnesemia, hypocalcemia) that may occur as phenomena that arise coincidentally during pharmacotherapy.

Fasciculations refer to small, involuntary contractions of a skeletal muscle fascicle visible under the skin, whose movement may or may not be rhythmic. Fasciculations that occur in periorbital muscle groups are a focal dystonia described as *blepharospasms.* Although most instances of muscle twitching or fasciculations are benign in nature, they can also result from mineral deficiencies or other medical or neurological causes that may warrant consideration depending on clinical circumstances. Etiologies of particular relevance to psychiatry include dehydration, hypomagnesemia, hypocalcemia, hypoparathyroidism, excessive caffeine intake, benzodiazepine withdrawal, serotonin syndrome, Lyme disease, myasthenia gravis, amyotrophic lateral sclerosis, and lower motor neuron disease (e.g., denervation). Stress or anxiety may exacerbate existing fasciculations. In the case of blepharospasm, fatigue (or poor sleep), dry eyes, and local irritants should be considered during clinical evaluation. Psychotropic medications known to be associated with benign fasciculations include anticholinergic agents, diphenhydramine, amphetamine, dopamine agonists (e.g., ropinirole and similar antiparkinsonian drugs), trazodone, selegiline, phenelzine, tranylcypromine, theophylline, and depolarizing muscle blockers such as succinylcholine (as used during electroconvulsive therapy).

Myoclonic movements are sudden jerklike contractions or twitches of whole muscle groups (e.g., shoulder twitch, elbow flexion, wrist extension) that are usually benign. They may occur during sleep onset (known as hypnic jerks) or while awake, although sometimes they may reflect underlying CNS disease. Myoclonus can arise from numerous causes, including seizures (e.g., myoclonic epilepsy), infection or encephalopathy (e.g., Lyme disease, HIV, syphilis), autoimmune disorders (e.g., systemic lupus erythematosus), metabolic disorders (e.g., hyperthyroidism, hepatic or renal failure), neurodegenerative diseases (e.g., Huntington's disease, multiple sclerosis), drug toxicities, vascular origins (e.g., poststroke), inflammatory processes, and paraneoplastic syndromes. In juvenile myoclonic epilepsy, the anticonvulsant levetiracetam is FDA approved as an adjunctive therapy.

Myoclonus rarely results from psychotropic drugs, apart from its presence as part of serotonin syndrome, or sometimes as an early sign of lithium toxicity. Medications that have been associated with myoclonus include SSRIs, TCAs, morphine, midazolam, and tramadol. Myoclonic jerks that become intrusive or persistent can be treated with clonazepam, baclofen, fluoxetine, and propranolol.

Nystagmus

General Recommendations

Nystagmus may indicate neurotoxicity from a medication. A careful review should be made of all medications, their dosages, and patient adherence, as well as illicit substances. Additionally, the clinician should assess the patient for other neurological or systemic signs of toxicity. Laboratory assessments (e.g., serum drug levels) to determine supratherapeutic doses may sometimes provide corroborative information. When nystagmus is thought to represent neurotoxicity, dosage reductions or the elimination of a suspected causal agent may be necessary.

Nystagmus is a focal neurological sign with a wide differential diagnosis that may include neurotoxicity from a number of psychotropic drugs. It may occur as part of alcohol or benzodiazepine withdrawal or intoxication states, as well as intoxication from phencyclidine, phenobarbital, and organic solvents. Nystagmus can variably be described as downbeat, upbeat, rotary, horizontal, pendular, and gaze evoked. Distinct types of nystagmus may reflect localized CNS lesions: upward nystagmus often reflects cerebellar or medullary disease, whereas horizontal nystagmus is the most common type of drug-induced nystagmus, involving low-amplitude beating with slow-velocity movements.

Drug-related nystagmus may occur without other clinical signs of toxicity. Lithium, for example, has been reported to cause downbeat nystagmus even at dosages producing nontoxic blood levels, and dosage reductions do not necessarily ameliorate or diminish the phenomenon. Other medications known to cause nystagmus include carbamazepine, divalproex, lamotrigine, MAOIs, and propranolol. Gabapentin has been used successfully to treat congenital nystagmus and is not known to cause drug-related nystagmus. Nystagmus may occur as part of serotonin syndrome (but not NMS), although it has not otherwise been described in association with the use of serotonergic antidepressants. It may be a rare adverse effect of SNRIs. Nystagmus has not been reported in conjunction with the use of antipsychotics, apart from one report of coarse horizontal nystagmus after an ultimately fatal overdose of olanzapine.

The presence of nystagmus signals the need for a review of all existing medications and dosages, with an awareness of pertinent pharmacokinetic interactions (e.g., lamotrigine toxicity from unadjusted dosing when coadministered with divalproex). A basic neurological examination should target cranial nerve abnormalities and neurotoxic signs (e.g., slurred speech, tremor, ataxia), and laboratory measures should include a toxicology screen and assessment of pertinent drug levels (see Table 1–2 in Chapter 1, "The Psychiatrist as Physician"). Suspected causal drugs should be discontinued if dosage reductions alone do not resolve symptoms or if other systemic manifestations of toxicity are evident.

Paresthesias and Neuropathies

General Recommendations

Paresthesias attributable to psychotropic medications are usually benign phenomena that may result from drug properties such as carbonic anhydrase inhibition or other direct effects on sensory nerve endings. They generally pose no medical concern and require no intervention, other than the ruling out of other possible etiologies unrelated to a suspected pharmacotherapy. Neuropathies rarely result from psychotropic drugs, benignly arising most often from lithium or phenelzine.

Paresthesias commonly occur during treatment with carbonic anhydrase inhibitors (e.g., topiramate was associated with paresthesias in 35%–49% of migraine patients at doses of 50 mg/day and 200 mg/day, respectively) and are identified in package insert labels as a rare event reported with a wide range of psychotropic drugs, including divalproex,

most SGAs and SSRIs, venlafaxine, desvenlafaxine, duloxetine, mirtazapine, stimulants, and some nonbenzodiazepine sedative-hypnotics.
Other nonpsychotropic medications that are known to cause paresthesias include certain antibiotics (e.g., doxycycline), acetazolamide, antineoplastic agents, and a number of antiretroviral agents, among other
compounds. In addition, potential medical causes of paresthesias include
hyperventilation (e.g., secondary to panic attacks), local trauma or nerve
entrapment (e.g., carpal tunnel syndrome, disk herniation), diabetic
neuropathy, migraine, peripheral vascular disease, vitamin B_{12} deficiency,
toxic exposures, malignancy, infections, or connective tissue diseases.
Withdrawal from SSRIs or SNRIs may be associated with paresthesias,
remediable by undertaking more protracted drug tapers or by allowing
for the passage of time alone, inasmuch as paresthesias in this context
are medically benign. Iatrogenic paresthesias that occur in the absence
of other focal neurological signs require no intervention.

Psychotropic drugs are rarely associated with peripheral neuropathies.
Anticonvulsants other than phenytoin are not known to cause neuropathy
(and in fact are often used in the treatment of diabetic neuropathy or
neuropathic pain). Neuropathy has been reported in connection with
lithium toxicity. The literature contains several dozen case reports of
peripheral or optic neuropathy associated with disulfiram, typically at
doses >250 mg/day, usually (but not always) resolving up to several
months (but as long as 14 months) after drug discontinuation. Antipsychotics are not associated with neuropathy, although some case reports
identify its development in the course of NMS. Antidepressants are not
associated with the development of peripheral neuropathy, with the exception of the MAOI phenelzine—a compound that falls within a chemical class known as hydrazines, which have been shown in preclinical and
human studies to reduce levels of vitamin B_6 (pyridoxine)—which, in
turn, can lead to peripheral neuropathy that may be remediable within several weeks' time by the administration of supplemental pyridoxine dosed
150–300 mg/day (Stewart et al. 1984). Measurement of serum pyridoxine levels is not necessary to justify an empirical trial of supplemental
therapy in this dosing range, which is a relatively benign intervention.

Seizures

General Recommendations

The seizure threshold may be lowered by antidopaminergic drugs
and bupropion, often in dose-related fashion. Coadministration
of anticonvulsants may be advisable in patients for whom high

doses of antipsychotics (particularly clozapine) or bupropion are deemed necessary.

Among antidepressants, seizure risk during FDA registration trials with most SSRIs has been reported as approximately 0.2%, with higher rates associated with TCAs. Risk for seizures with antidepressants in general also appears related to high doses or frank toxicity states. Manufacturer's product information for bupropion identifies a dose-dependent risk for seizures in about 4 in 1,000 patients when bupropion is prescribed up to 450 mg/day. Among anticonvulsants, long-term use raises the seizure threshold, which can, at least in theory, pose an increased risk for seizures following abrupt drug discontinuation. There-fore, anticonvulsant cessation should ideally occur over about a 2-week period. However, rapid anticonvulsant cessation mainly poses a concern for seizure induction in epilepsy patients, and for practical purposes (e.g., prior to ECT initiation), lengthy taper-offs may not always be necessary.

Clozapine-induced seizures (■) are more likely to occur at high clozapine dosages (incidence rate of 5% above 600 mg/day per the manufacturer), during rapid dose increases, during concomitant use of other medications that lower the seizure threshold or inhibit its metabolism, or in patients with a neurological deficit (Toth and Frankenburg 1994). Clinicians sometimes coadminister an anticonvulsant with clozapine when the latter is dosed >500–600 mg/day to help minimize the potential for seizures. (Co-administration of clozapine with lamotrigine represents an especially attractive strategy in that it could simultaneously provide seizure prophylaxis and possible antipsychotic synergy, as has been suggested from several early reports.) All antipsychotics have the potential to lower an individual's seizure threshold, although risks appear highest with clozapine, loxapine, and chlorpromazine, and appear lowest with haloperidol, pimozide, thiothixene, and most SGAs other than clozapine (<1%–2% incidence). Risk factors include a past history of seizures, concomitant medications that also lower the seizure threshold, and rapid dose escalations. Decisions about whether to stop, reduce, or continue an otherwise efficacious drug after seizure occurrence depend on the presence of an underlying seizure diathesis, the risk-benefit analyses for continuing the drug in question, and viable methods to manage the risk for possible subsequent seizures.

Yawning

General Recommendations

Yawning is a generally medically benign, uncommon side effect of some antidepressants. It requires no intervention. It is not clearly dose related. If yawning is sufficiently distressing to the patient, the presumed causal agent might be discontinued and substituted with another medication with a presumptive different mechanism of action (e.g., switching from an SSRI or SNRI to bupropion or a TCA).

Excessive daytime yawning has been described in postmarketing reports with the SSRIs fluoxetine, sertraline, and citalopram, among others, as well as the SNRIs duloxetine and venlafaxine. Yawning has been hypothesized to occur as a reflex that is modulated by catecholaminergic, serotonergic, and other transmitter systems (including cholinergic, glucocorticoids, nitric oxide) in the paraventricular nucleus of the hypothalamus (De Las Cuevas and Sanz 2007) and that may become altered during antidepressant therapy. Usually, yawning is a benign phenomenon, although reports exist that its frequency may occasionally pose a disabling effect (e.g., yawning-associated orgasms during clomipramine therapy [McLean et al. 1983]). Iatrogenic yawning sometimes may be diminished by adjunctive cyproheptadine.

18

Ophthalmological System

Cataracts

General Recommendations

Product labeling for quetiapine includes mention of the potential for development of cataracts, as well as a recommendation for periodic slit-lamp examinations, although no human studies have affirmed a clear distinction between cataracts that develop due to quetiapine and senile cataracts that develop as part of normal aging.

Cataracts normally occur in 0.2% of the general population. They are generally categorized as congenital, age related (i.e., senile cataracts), traumatic, or secondary (e.g., to pharmacotherapies, radiation exposure, or diseases such as diabetes), and are further classified by their degree of opacity and location within the lens. The occurrence of cataracts in animal studies of high-dose quetiapine (specifically, in beagles) led its manufacturer to advise baseline and semiannual slit-lamp ophthalmological examinations. A review of the National Registry of Drug-Induced Ocular Side Effects in 2004 identified 34 spontaneous case reports of cataracts associated with quetiapine use in nonelderly adults, occurring at a mean of 29 weeks after treatment initiation, and leading the author to conclude that quetiapine-induced cataracts were a rare event for which semiannual ophthalmological examinations are probably unnecessary

(Fraunfelder 2004). Another survey of 620,000 adult quetiapine recipients identified an incident risk for cataracts of 0.005%, markedly lower than the base rate in the general population (Shahzad et al. 2002). Complicating the discovery of a relationship between adult human cataracts and quetiapine use is the virtually impossible ability to differentiate between senile cataracts and secondary cataracts. Some FGAs, including phenothiazines and haloperidol, also have been implicated as possible causes of cataracts, although the validity of such associations remains controversial (Shahzad et al. 2002). A study of 2,144 schizophrenia patients taking various atypical antipsychotics found no higher incidence of cataracts than in a matched healthy control sample, but the study did find that physical comorbidities, antidepressant use, and concurrent glaucoma or retinal disorders were significantly related to cataract development (Chou et al. 2016).

TCAs as well as some SSRIs or SNRIs have also been suggested to pose a small but observable increased risk for cataracts. For example, a nested case-control study of 18,784 cases and matched control subjects found 1.2- to 1.4-fold increased risk ratios for cataracts during treatment with fluvoxamine, venlafaxine, or paroxetine, with a mean appearance at about 2 years after treatment initiation (Etminan et al. 2010). Corticosteroids represent another known pharmacological cause of secondary cataracts.

Diplopia, Blurred Vision, and Loss of Vision

General Recommendations

Blurry vision is a common, often dose-related phenomenon caused most often by anticholinergic drugs. When iatrogenic, it is typically nonpermanent, but if time or dosage reductions fail to improve symptoms, patients may prefer to discontinue a causal agent depending on the level of severity and distress. Sudden loss of vision warrants emergent medical evaluation.

Blurry vision commonly results from the anticholinergic action of psychotropic medications on the ciliary muscle of the eye. Indeed, patients who wear corrective lenses or who are planning to have their eyes refracted should be advised that the introduction of some psychotropic medicines may cause blurry vision, which could interfere with the ability to accurately determine visual acuity until the possible effects of a new medication or medication change are fully known.

Sudden loss of vision may occur from a number of underlying medi-cal disorders that predispose to thrombo-embolic phenomena. In particular, a condition known as *nonarteritic anterior ischemic optic neuropathy* (NAION) involves ischemic damage to the optic nerve; it is essentially an optic nerve white matter stroke in which the patient typically presents with painless, sudden onset of unilateral or bilateral hemifield loss. In addition to NAION's potential etiology from cardiovascular risk factors (e.g., hypertension), a risk for NAION of about 2–12 per 100,000 males > age 50 has been linked with the use of PDE inhibitors such as sildenafil and vardenafil.

Glaucoma

General Recommendations

Secondary narrow-angle glaucoma is a rare adverse effect of topiramate, usually occurring in the first few weeks after treatment initiation. Patients who start topiramate should be counseled to be alert to visual changes or eye pain and to seek immediate evaluation should these occur.

Secondary narrow-angle glaucoma due to choroidal effusion and increased intraocular pressure has been reported as a rare event in association with topiramate, leading to a manufacturer's "warning letter" sent to physicians in 2001, followed by an FDA package warning label. Iatrogenic uveitis has also been reported as a possible rare event. A 2004 literature review identified 86 reported glaucoma cases, although an absolute risk estimate is unavailable (Fraunfelder et al. 2004). Narrow-angle glaucoma typically manifests with myopia and blurred vision in the first few weeks after initiation of treatment. Intraocular pressure may not necessarily be elevated. Preexisting demographic or other risk factors have not been identified. The phenomenon has been reported to be reversible within 1 week of drug cessation when recognized early, along with administration of topical atropine 1% solution and topical steroids (e.g., prednisone acetate 1% solution). Pilocarpine is considered *not* an appropriate remedy because it can cause spasm of the ciliary muscle and further narrowing of the angle of the anterior chamber. Because topiramate-associated glaucoma is an idiosyncratic phenomenon, screening for a history of glaucoma appears not to be either useful or necessary for anticipating possible visual changes during treatment with this medication. Topiramate should promptly be discontinued if a patient develops blurry vision, other visual changes, or eye pain, particularly in the first month of treatment.

A number of other psychotropic agents have the potential to exacerbate existing narrow-angle glaucoma, either due to anticholinergic effects or via a mydriatic effect that can interfere with drainage of aqueous humor from the anterior chamber of the eye (e.g., sympathomimetic agents). In addition to obvious anticholinergic drugs (e.g., hydroxyzine, benztropine, low-potency FGAs, tricyclics), case reports cite many other non-antimuscarinic psychotropics (e.g., SSRIs, benzodiazepines, bupropion) as potential aggravators of narrow-angle glaucoma, although often such risks may be more theoretical than probable. Moreover, in modern times, individuals who are identified with narrow angles are often advised to undergo laser iridotomy to prevent narrow-angle closure from glaucoma; in addition, earlier detection and treatment of cataracts also may help to reduce the incidence of narrow-angle closure glaucoma.

Retinopathies

General Recommendations

Clinicians should be aware of the rare and possibly permanent known risk for retinal changes caused by thioridazine and chlorpromazine.

Macular degeneration and retinal pigmentation are both rare complications associated with thioridazine. Although pigmentary changes can continue during ongoing thioridazine exposure, debate exists about whether functional visual changes can be progressive. Cases have been reported of the continued loss of retinal pigment epithelium (presumably because thioridazine remains bound to melanin), as well as diminished visual acuity with normal funduscopic appearance years after drug cessation; however, establishing causality can be difficult in such instances. Risk appears linked to the use of high dosages (i.e., ≥800 mg/day).

Pigmentary retinopathy has been reported with very high dosages of chlorpromazine (e.g., ≥2,400 mg/day) and may be irreversible.

19

Sleep Disturbances

Hypersomnia and Sleep Attacks

General Recommendations

Sleep attacks may occur, although rarely, with several psychotropic agents, most notably certain dopamine agonists (e.g., pramipexole, ropinirole) and MAOIs. Antihistaminergic psychotropic drugs often cause insomnia at treatment initiation, which may or may not diminish with continued use. Consideration should be given to the role of sleep studies to assess excessive daytime sleepiness, particularly if noniatrogenic etiologies (e.g., sleep apnea, narcolepsy) are suspected. Adjunctive stimulants, or wakefulness-promoting agents such as modafinil or armodafinil, may be of value to counteract excessive daytime somnolence or suspected sleep attacks. Persistent symptoms that disrupt or imperil normal daytime functioning may require drug cessation.

Sleep attacks may involve sleep-onset REM periods and may be a manifestation of narcolepsy when accompanied by sleep paralysis upon falling asleep or waking, cataplexy, and hypnagogic hallucinations. Narcolepsy per se affects about 0.02% of the population, usually first arising in adolescence or young adulthood. DQB1*06:02 genotyping is a sensitive but not specific laboratory test to gauge the likelihood of narcolepsy when it is clinically suspected, with the DQB1*06:02 genotype being present in

90% or more of the individuals who manifest both sudden sleep attacks plus cataplexy (but in fewer than half of those with sleep attacks alone).

A limited number of psychotropic drugs have been reported to cause sleep attacks, which may include falling asleep while driving. The most well known among these drugs are dopamine agonists (e.g., pramipexole and ropinirole) when used in patients with Parkinson's disease, producing an approximate 5-fold increased risk for somnolence as compared with placebo across several randomized trials. It is unknown whether this risk similarly pertains to other patient groups (e.g., those with restless legs syndrome or bipolar depression) who may take these medicines. (Notably, patients with restless legs syndrome typically have intrinsic sleep architecture disturbances that neither pramipexole nor ropinirole directly alters, either beneficially or adversely, apart from improving nighttime sleep quantity and adequacy.) In a retrospective review of patients with Parkinson's disease who took dopamine agonists, sleep attacks were identified in 6.6% of patients without significant differences across agents (Homann et al. 2002). It is unknown whether dosage reductions can ameliorate sleep attack events; therefore, caution favors the discontinuation of such agents if sleep attacks cannot otherwise be explained, with caution against driving until sleep attacks fully resolve.

Case reports exist of excessive daytime sleepiness with MAOIs. Traditional psychostimulants such as amphetamine or methylphenidate pose sympathomimetic risks that complicate their use to counteract MAOI-related sedation, although case reports do describe the safe use of carefully monitored amphetamine plus MAOIs without consequent hypertension or hyperthermia. Alternatively, the wakefulness-promoting agent modafinil (or its enantiomer, armodafinil) lacks pressor effects and thus may be more compatible with MAOI treatment.

Modafinil or armodafinil have been used broadly in "off label" fashion to counteract excessive daytime sedation caused by other psychotropic drugs, including FGAs, SGAs, and SSRIs. In the case of clozapine-induced sedation, it is noteworthy that one small ($N=35$) double-blind, placebo-controlled trial failed to demonstrate an advantage for modafinil (up to 300 mg/day) in improving wakefulness/fatigue (Freudenreich et al. 2009). Additionally, modafinil has been reported to increase serum clozapine levels, potentially via its inhibition of CYP2C19, with resultant decreased metabolic clearance of clozapine, leading to paradoxical worsening of sedation, dizziness, and gait unsteadiness (Dequardo 2002).

If amphetamine or methylphenidate is prescribed, in general, clinicians should bear in mind that cessation can sometimes trigger rebound increases in non-REM sleep, which in turn may increase daytime fatigue and somnolence.

Insomnia

General Recommendations

Insomnia, whether arising as a symptom of a psychiatric disorder or as a condition by itself, can be difficult to treat. The clinician must rule out other contributing medical causes (e.g., obstructive sleep apnea, restless legs syndrome, pain, substance withdrawal) or psychiatric etiologies (e.g., mania, depression). Initial conservative approaches for managing simple insomnia caused by psychotropic drugs involve modifying drug dosing schedules and assuring sleep hygiene. Iatrogenic insomnia is often transient but may warrant treatment with sedative-hypnotics or other soporific agents; its persistence, particularly after resolution of other psychiatric symptoms being treated, may signal the presence of an independent sleep disorder that merits independent evaluation.

Insomnia is among the most common phenomena whose etiologies can be difficult to discriminate among iatrogenic or illness-related causes. In the case of depression, for example, initial, middle, or terminal insomnia may be a target symptom of a depressive episode, a treatment-emergent adverse effect, or both. In the treatment of patients with bipolar mania, experts emphasize the importance of differentiating a loss of the need to sleep from difficulty falling or staying asleep with consequent fatigue the following day. A complaint of insomnia must be assessed as the possible manifestation of a more fundamental psychiatric or medical problem, for which proper remediation requires more effective treatment of the underlying cause.

DSM-5 has eliminated the formal distinction between primary and secondary insomnia but does identify "insomnia disorder" as a condition involving trouble falling or staying asleep at least three nights per week for at least 3 months, which must not simply result from the physiological effects of a substance or medication (American Psychiatric Association 2013). Drug-induced insomnia may occur from a wide range of catecholaminergic, indoleaminergic, and sympathomimetic agents that are alerting or stimulating. The degree to which some psychiatric medicines may cause either insomnia or hypersomnia is often unpredictable. For example, package insert descriptions from FDA registration trials of paroxetine for major depression report insomnia as occurring in 13% of patients but somnolence in 23% of patients. Insomnia rates may also vary substantially with the same agent across different disorders; for example, higher rates of insomnia were seen in FDA trials of fluoxetine for bulimia (33%) or obsessive-compulsive disorder (28%) than for major depression (16%).

In the case of sertraline, insomnia rates were highest in obsessive-compulsive disorder (28%) and lowest in major depression (16%).

Depression increases sleep latency, increases waking after sleep onset, decreases REM latency but increases REM density and duration, increases early morning awakenings, decreases stages 3 and 4 (slow-wave) sleep, and shifts REM sleep to earlier in the night. The effects of antidepressants and other psychotropics on sleep architecture vary, as summarized in Tables 19–1 through 19–3. The clinician should be aware of the ways in which the drugs may disrupt sleep latency or continuity, while bearing in mind the effects of depression itself on these sleep parameters. Antihistaminergic drugs generally increase sleep continuity and may have variable effects on other elements of sleep architecture. Anticholinergic drugs as well as many serotonergic, noradrenergic, and dopaminergic binding agents generally suppress REM sleep and increase REM latency. Postsynaptic serotonin type 2A (5-HT$_{2A}$) antagonists (e.g., SGAs) typically increase sleep continuity and increase slow-wave sleep.

Decreases in slow-wave sleep can interfere with patients' feeling rested after waking from sleep. Conflicting data exist on the extent to which disruption of REM sleep may interfere with memory consolidation, as had once been more widely assumed. Most antidepressants (with the notable exceptions of bupropion, mirtazapine, and nefazodone) markedly suppress REM in dose-related fashion (presumably via 5-HT$_{1A}$ stimulation) and yet do not adversely affect learning and memory; paradoxically, SSRI- or SNRI-induced REM suppression may even improve verbal memory (Rasch et al. 2008). Antidepressant cessation initially leads to decreased REM latency and increases the percentage of time spent in REM sleep.

Minimal research has specifically examined strategies to counteract iatrogenic sleep disturbances caused by psychotropic medications, as opposed to adjunctive medications to selectively target poor sleep quality as part of the syndrome of depression. Most pharmacotherapy antidotes to iatrogenic insomnia have been extrapolated from use in primary sleep disorders. Perhaps the most obvious interventions when a medication appears to cause insomnia include altering its dosing schedule (e.g., morning instead of evening administration), determining whether any concomitant medications might better account for iatrogenic insomnia, eliminating other factors that may disrupt sleep (e.g., alcohol or caffeine intake), and assuring normal sleep hygiene. To the extent that some SSRIs such as fluoxetine have been shown to cause significant periodic limb movement disorders during sleep, adjunctive sedative-hypnotics that also diminish restless legs (e.g., clonazepam) may be particularly effective as sleep aids. Moreover, depressed patients who begin fluoxetine treat-

TABLE 19–1. Known effects of antidepressants and anxiolytics on sleep architecture

Agent	REM	REM latency	Slow-wave sleep	Sleep continuity
Benzodiazepines	Suppress	Decrease	Decrease	Increase
Bupropion	Increases	Decreases	No effect	No effect or may impair
Buspirone	No effect	No effect	No effect	No effect
MAOIs	Suppress (virtually abolish)	Increase	No effect	No effect or may impair
Mirtazapine	No suppression or increase	No effect	No effect or may increase	Improves
Nefazodone	Increases	Decreases	No effect	Improves
SNRIs	Decrease	Increase	No effect or may decrease	Impair
SSRIs	Suppress	Increase	No effect or may decrease	No effect or may impair
TCAs	Suppress	Increase	No effect or may increase	No effect or may improve
Trazodone	No effect or may suppress	Increases	No effect or may increase	Improves
Vilazodone	Suppresses	Increases	Increases	Not reported
Vortioxetine	Suppresses	Increases	No effect	May impair

Note. MAOI=monoamine oxidase inhibitor; REM=rapid eye movement; SNRI=serotonin-norepinephrine reuptake inhibitor; SSRI=selective serotonin reuptake inhibitor; TCA=tricyclic antidepressant.

TABLE 19–2.   Known effects of antipsychotics on sleep architecture[a]

Agent	REM	REM latency	Slow-wave sleep	Sleep continuity
Aripiprazole	Not reported	Not reported	Not reported	Not reported
Asenapine	Not reported	Not reported	Not reported	Not reported
Brexpiprazole	No effect	No effect	Decreases[b]	Improves
Cariprazine	Not reported	Not reported	Not reported	Not reported
Clozapine	No effect or suppresses	No effect or increases	No effect or decreases	Improves
Iloperidone	Not reported	Not reported	Not reported	Not reported
Lurasidone	Suppresses	Not reported	Increases	Not reported
Olanzapine	Can either increase or suppress	No effect or increases	No effect or increases	Improves
Paliperidone	Increases	No effect	No effect	Improves
Pimavanserin	Not reported	Not reported	Increases	Improves
Quetiapine	No effect or suppresses	No effect or increases	Increases	Improves
Risperidone	No effect or suppresses	No effect	No effect or increases	Improves
Ziprasidone	Can either increase or suppress	No effect or increases	Increases	Improves

Note.   REM=rapid eye movement.
[a]Based on manufacturers' product information as well as Monti et al. (2017). Effects on sleep architecture may vary across patients versus healthy control subjects.
[b]Brexpiprazole diminishes duration of slow-wave sleep but improves latency to slow-wave sleep (Krystal et al. 2016).

TABLE 19–3. Known effects of anticonvulsants and lithium on sleep architecture

Agent	REM	REM latency	Slow-wave sleep	Sleep continuity
Carbamazepine	Suppresses	Increases	Increases	Increases
Divalproex	Suppresses	Not reported	Increases	Increases
Gabapentin	Increases	Not reported	Increases	Increases
Lamotrigine	Increases	No known effect	Decreases	No known effect
Lithium	Suppresses	Increases	Increases	Increases
Topiramate	Not reported	Not reported	Not reported	Not reported

Note. REM=rapid eye movement.

ment with adjunctive clonazepam develop less treatment-emergent insomnia and anxiety than do those taking fluoxetine alone (Londborg et al. 2000).

Table 19–4 summarizes information on the use and sleep architectural effects of agents that are commonly used to counteract simple insomnia. Often, clinicians find themselves choosing between benzodiazepines and nonbenzodiazepine soporific drugs to counteract insomnia. Nonbenzodiazepine sleep aids increase total sleep time while disrupting sleep architecture less extensively than benzodiazepines. They also generally carry less abuse potential, less often cause rebound insomnia or withdrawal upon cessation, and are often less likely to cause the types of cognitive problems (e.g., retrograde memory impairment) associated with benzodiazepines.

The treatment of apparent iatrogenic insomnia first requires a differential diagnostic assessment. For example, individuals with bipolar disorder who have trouble sleeping require assessment of other possible signs of mania or hypomania, and the use of sedating antidepressants as sleep aids (e.g., trazodone, mirtazapine, TCAs) would be less desirable than nonantidepressant sedative-hypnotics (e.g., benzodiazepines or benzodiazepine agonists) while optimizing patients' fundamental antimanic regimen. Individuals with sleep problems caused by restless legs syndrome may benefit more from a dopamine agonist (e.g., pramipexole, ropinirole) than a dopamine antagonist (e.g., quetiapine). Individuals with sleep apnea likely would be better served by a continuous positive airway pressure (CPAP) device and possible use of modafinil, armodafinil, or sodium oxybate.

Insomnia that results from nonsedating antidepressants (e.g., SSRIs, SNRIs, bupropion) is often an initial, transient phenomenon. Morning rather than evening dosing may help to minimize the potential for interference with normal sleep. Some reports suggest that independent treatment of antidepressant-induced insomnia with a hypnotic agent (e.g., adjunctive benzodiazepine at night) yields better overall outcomes than when antidepressant-associated insomnia receives no independent treatment.

A fundamental issue in choosing from among sedative-hypnotics involves the relative advantages or disadvantages of using a benzodiazepine versus a nonbenzodiazepine. With benzodiazepines, the patient incurs greater potential disruption to sleep architecture, a potential for rebound insomnia and withdrawal, the possibility for developing dependence and tolerance over time, the potential for abuse, a risk for respiratory suppression (particularly among individuals with underlying pulmonary disease), and the risk for daytime cognitive impairment and

TABLE 19–4. **Pharmacological strategies for psychotropic-induced insomnia**

Agent	Comments
Benzodiazepines	Promotes more time in light sleep (stage 2), reduction in slow-wave sleep and REM; potential for tolerance, abuse, and rebound insomnia after cessation
Chloral hydrate	Decreases sleep latency
Eszopiclone	Does not alter slow-wave sleep or REM
Gabapentin	Increases slow-wave sleep
Melatonin	Causes minimal disruption of sleep architecture
Mirtazapine	Decreases sleep latency; increases total sleep time and sleep efficiency; increases time spent in stage 2 sleep, REM sleep, and slow-wave sleep (Schittecatte et al. 2002; Winokur et al. 2000)
Ramelteon	Increases REM and slow-wave sleep; ~10-fold higher binding affinity to M_1 and M_2 melatonin receptors than melatonin itself
Suvorexant	Plasma half-life ~12 hours; increases REM > non-REM sleep
Tasimelteon	Plasma half-life ~1.3 hours; improves sleep latency and sleep efficiency and reduces awakenings after sleep onset
Trazodone	Decreases sleep stages 1 and 2, increases slow-wave sleep, has little effect on REM sleep; few efficacy studies focusing on insomnia, although some suggestion of a lesser reduction in sleep latency than zolpidem for primary insomnia; no known studies on use in counteracting psychotropic-induced insomnia
Zaleplon	Plasma half-life ~1 hour; better for sleep initiation than maintenance
Zolpidem	Preserves slow-wave sleep

Note. REM = rapid eye movement.

retrograde memory impairment; nonbenzodiazepine sedatives, such as zolpidem, zaleplon, ramelteon, and eszopiclone, carry relatively lesser risks in these domains (Wagner and Wagner 2000).

In 2014, the FDA approved suvorexant, a dual orexin receptor antagonist (DORA), for the treatment of initial or middle insomnia dosed at 10, 15, or 20 mg at bedtime. Although not yet formally studied specifically to counteract insomnia caused by psychotropic medications, suvorexant represents a promising alternative to traditional (GABAergic or antihistaminergic) sedative-hypnotics. It is contraindicated in people with narcolepsy because of their preexisting low levels of CNS orexin . Although not known to cause physical dependence, tolerance, or withdrawal, suvorexant is a Schedule IV drug—a decision made by the FDA based mainly on its "likability" among individuals with substance use disorders and consequent potential for abuse.

Nightmares and Vivid Dreams

General Recommendations

Nightmares and vivid dreams may occur at any point during treatment with a variety of antidepressants and other psychotropic drugs. It is unknown whether the phenomenon may be dose related, and presumptive mechanisms are not well understood. Abnormal dreams are medically benign, but if they create substantial distress, then a causal agent may need to be stopped if dosage reductions alone prove ineffective.

Vivid dreams have been reported as a relatively uncommon, medically benign adverse effect associated with dopaminergic agents (including bupropion and antiparkinsonian drugs) and with many serotonergic or serotonergic-noradrenergic antidepressants. Other psychotropic drugs with which vivid or abnormal dreams have been identified as possible adverse effects include lamotrigine, gabapentin, quetiapine (2% incidence in FDA registration trials), and lurasidone (<1% incidence in FDA registration trials).

Serotonergic agents have been shown to suppress REM sleep in a dose-related fashion and, correspondingly, would be expected to diminish (or disrupt) dream activity. Over time, tolerance to antidepressant-associated REM suppression may account for the development of vivid dreams as treatment progresses. Some authors have suggested that $5\text{-}HT_2$ receptor agonism may also lead to vivid dreams or nightmares and noted the potential value of $5\text{-}HT_2$ antagonists (e.g., trazodone, mirtazapine,

SGAs, or cyproheptadine) to counteract nightmares. On the basis of extrapolations from the literature on nightmares associated with posttraumatic stress disorder (PTSD), α_2-adrenergic agonists such as guanfacine (0.5–1 mg at bedtime) or clonidine (0.1–0.3 mg at bedtime), or the α_1-blocking agent prazosin (dosed from 1–4 mg at night, or potentially as high as 10 mg/day as studied in PTSD-related nightmares among combat veterans [Raskind et al. 2003]), may help to diminish nightmares by providing a soporific effect at bedtime as well as by reducing noradrenergic hyperactivity. Blood pressure monitoring by the prescriber is advisable to assure the absence of clinically meaningful hypotension.

Of note, when prescribing prazosin, the clinician must be aware of the potential for orthostatic syncope to occur after an initial first dose. Hence, the recommendation is to begin no higher than 1 mg/night for the first few days, with a subsequent increase to 2 mg/day for several days if necessary; dosing may then be increased to 4 mg/day for 1 week if improvement does not occur, followed by an increase to 6 mg/day after 1 week if necessary. Additional dosage increases (by 2 mg/week) have been described such that 2–4 mg are administered in the afternoon followed by up to 6 mg at bedtime (Raskind et al. 2003). Furthermore, the clinician must be cautious not to abruptly discontinue prazosin or other α_1-blockers (typically, they are tapered off over days to weeks), in order to minimize the potential for rebound hypertension; patients should be counseled about this potential risk if doses are missed.

Other medications that have been described by the Standards of Practice Committee of the American Academy of Sleep Medicine as generally having potential value for the treatment of nightmares include topiramate, low-dose cortisol, fluvoxamine, triazolam and nitrazepam, phenelzine, gabapentin, and TCAs; notably, venlafaxine is considered inadvisable for the treatment of PTSD-associated nightmares (Aurora et al. 2010). Each of these agents would involve extrapolation to use for the treatment of iatrogenic nightmares.

Parasomnias

General Recommendations

Some antidepressants and nonbenzodiazepine hypnotics (e.g., zolpidem, zopiclone, eszopiclone) carry an increased risk for abnormal REM and non-REM sleep behavior disorders (notably, sleepwalking, sleep-driving, and sleep-related eating disorders). Suspected causal agents should be stopped in patients who report such events.

Parasomnias comprise a series of sleep disorders that occur during transitions from wakefulness and REM or non-REM sleep. *REM parasomnias* (often also referred to as REM sleep behavior disorders) involve loss of muscle atonia (i.e., loss of paralysis normally associated with REM sleep) that can manifest as the acting out of dreams through uncoordinated movements (e.g., kicking or punching). *Non-REM parasomnias* occur during slow-wave sleep and involve intact muscle tone, leading to bruxism, restless legs syndrome, and more complex behaviors such as sleepwalking, sleep-related eating disorders, sleep-driving, sexual activity, or conversations. After waking, patients usually are amnestic for parasomnic events. Although parasomnias are not in themselves thought to represent psychopathology, epidemiological studies suggest that they may be more common among people with major depression (but not primary psychotic disorders or bipolar illness) (Lam et al. 2008). Iatrogenic parasomnias most often result from antidepressants or nonbenzodiazepine hypnotics. Antidepressants (notably, fluoxetine, venlafaxine, and TCAs) have been known to induce or worsen preexisting REM sleep behavior disorders (Schenck and Mahowald 2002). Although incidence rates with specific nonbenzodiazepines are not available, manufacturers' product information for zolpidem and eszopiclone warn of the potential for complex hazardous behaviors such as sleep-driving and advise drug discontinuation if patients report such experiences.

A review of parasomnias among 1,235 psychiatric outpatients found that parasomnias among SSRI recipients typically were associated with sleep-related eating disorders and REM sleep behavior disorders, whereas sedating antidepressants (e.g., TCAs, trazodone) more often involved sleepwalking and sleep-related eating disorders (Lam et al. 2008). Among nonbenzodiazepine hypnotics, zolpidem was linked with both sleepwalking and sleep-related eating disorders, whereas zopiclone led only to sleepwalking. Parasomnia risk was higher among regular versus intermittent nonbenzodiazepine hypnotic users. Complex sleep behaviors associated with zolpidem appear to be linked to doses exceeding the manufacturer's maximum (Hwang et al. 2010). Coadministration of benzodiazepine agonists with alcohol or other CNS depressants may also increase the risk for REM sleep behavior disorders. FDA registration trials of suvorexant for treatment of insomnia reported no cases of complex sleep behaviors. Interestingly, antipsychotics may be negatively associated with some parasomnias. Benzodiazepines and mood stabilizers have not been reported to cause parasomnias.

20

Systemic Reactions

Allergic Reactions and Angioedema

General Recommendations

Allergic angioedema is a medical emergency that necessitates airway protection and treatment with antihistamines or possibly steroids. Psychotropic drugs that cause angioedema should be immediately discontinued, and rechallenges generally should not be undertaken.

Adverse cutaneous reactions have been reported to occur in up to 5% of individuals who receive antipsychotic medications. True allergic reactions are IgE–mediated phenomena. Angioedema refers to the relatively rapid development of facial edema with swelling of oropharyngeal mucosal membranes and possible airway constriction. Allergic angioedema is similar to anaphylactic shock and may involve urticarial eruptions. In the presence of stridor or other signs of respiratory distress, allergic angioedema constitutes a medical emergency that may require intubation to maintain an intact airway.

Case reports have described the occurrence of urticaria and angioedema with asenapine, bupropion, lurasidone, oxcarbazepine (oxcar-

---

The symbol ■ is used in this chapter to indicate that the FDA has issued a boxed warning for a prescription medication that may cause serious adverse effects.

bazepine-related angioedema has been determined to arise in 9.8 per 1 million pediatric cases; Knudsen et al. 2007), paroxetine, risperidone (with uneventful rechallenge), and ziprasidone.

Among patients with allergies to sulfonamide antibiotics such as sulfamethoxazole-trimethoprim (so-called sulfa allergies), there has been debate and uncertainty about the potential for allergic cross-reactivity to non-antibiotic sulfonamide drugs, including certain anticonvulsants (e.g., zonisamide) or carbonic anhydrase inhibitors (e.g., topiramate) (Wulf and Matuszewski 2013). Most experts argue that in patients with known sulfa antibiotic allergies, type I immediate hypersensitivity reactions to nonantibiotic sulfonamides would be unlikely because of stereospecific differences in molecular structure between sulfonamide antibiotics and nonantibiotics.

Antiepileptic Hypersensitivity Reactions

General Recommendations

Hypersensitivity reactions should be suspected in anticonvulsant recipients who develop systemic, multiorgan system disturbances, regardless of the presence or absence of a skin rash. Hypersensitivity reactions are potentially life threatening, and the suspected causal agent should be immediately discontinued. Prompt medical attention involves supportive measures and a possible role for steroids. The suspected causal agent should not subsequently be reintroduced.

Certain anticonvulsants (and a select number of other agents) have been associated with rare idiosyncratic hypersensitivity reactions (often referred to in the literature as drug rash [or reaction] with eosinophilia and systemic symptoms [DRESS] syndrome), which have been described most extensively with carbamazepine, lamotrigine, phenytoin, and phenobarbital. Through mechanisms that are not well understood, such reactions are thought to involve an immunological response to toxic effects of the parent compound or a metabolite. When hypersensitivity reactions occur, they usually do so within the first 8 weeks of treatment. Characteristic features involve fever, multiorgan system involvement, and possible skin eruptions. Associated phenomena may include rhabdomyolysis (identifiable by myoglobinuria on urinalysis), which in itself should prompt a review of all medications that are known to cause this phenomenon, including statins and antiparkinsonian agents.

In August 2010, the FDA issued a warning that aseptic meningitis may arise as a type of rare hypersensitivity reaction to lamotrigine, particularly during the first few months after treatment initiation. This warning was based on 40 reported postmarketing cases from December 1994 through November 2009. Symptoms typically arose within days 1–42 after drug initiation (mean=16 days). Accordingly, the onset of meningeal signs (headache, fever, nausea, vomiting, nuchal rigidity, photophobia, and myalgias) during this time frame likely warrants cessation of therapy. Symptoms typically resolve after drug discontinuation.

Body Temperature Dysregulation

General Recommendations

Patients who take FGAs or SGAs should be counseled about the potential disruption to maintaining their core body temperature when they are exposed to ambient extremes.

Both hypo- and hyperthermia can result from the use of FGAs and SGAs, most often arising near the time of treatment initiation or dosage increases. Antipsychotics disrupt the medullary chemoreceptor trigger zone, which among other functions, maintains homeostatic core body temperature. Pharmacological mechanisms thought to impair thermoregulation and thereby cause poikolothermia include the blockade of D_1 and D_2 dopamine receptors, as well as possible disruption of compensatory peripheral vasoconstriction due to α_1-adrenergic blockade by most antipsychotics. Antipsychotic-induced temperature dysregulation may lead to medical hospitalization (nearly 70% of cases) or mortality (~4% of cases) (van Marum et al. 2007).

Patients who take FGAs or SGAs should be warned that their body temperature could rise significantly under conditions such as strenuous exercise or exposure to hot climates and should be instructed to monitor their body temperature periodically in such circumstances, as well as in the setting of infection. Management of hyperthermia typically involves hydration, acetaminophen, and cooling blankets or ice packs if necessary, along with removing the patient from exposure to high ambient temperature. Antipsychotic-induced hypothermia is rare and routine screening is considered unnecessary, although the possible presence of hypothermia should be considered in antipsychotic recipients who develop subjective coldness along with acute mental status changes, bradycardia, fatigue, and focal neurological signs, such as ataxia.

Cancer and Excess Mortality

Several large retrospective studies have drawn media attention after reporting an increased risk for cancer (e.g., Kao et al. 2012) or premature death (odds ratio=3.32 after adjustment for confounding factors; Weich et al. 2014) among patients taking benzodiazepines. In the largest of such studies, Kao et al. (2012) compared a database of 59,647 Taiwanese adults (mean age=48 years) who took benzodiazepines with age-matched controls; an overall 19% increased risk for developing cancer, particularly liver, prostate, bladder, and kidney cancers, was found among benzodiazepine recipients. Despite the fact that confounders such as age, smoking, and medical morbidity were controlled for, it is nevertheless difficult to draw definitive causal inferences from such retrospective database reviews given the inherent increased mortality associated with major psychiatric disorders such as schizophrenia, bipolar disorder, and major depression. In some studies, absence of information about causes of death (e.g., accidents, suicides) further limits the ability to discern plausible mechanistic explanations for increased mortality. Moreover, the nonrandomized designs of such chart reviews preclude knowledge about chronology and causality; in other words, while it is possible that benzodiazepines may cause cancer, it is no less plausible that cancer patients are especially likely to take benzodiazepines.

Discontinuation Syndromes

General Recommendations

Withdrawal symptoms from abrupt cessation of most short-acting SSRIs and all SNRIs warrant gradual tapers that may require many days to weeks. Antidepressant withdrawal symptoms are medically benign but uncomfortable and can be managed either by extending the duration of tapering off the medication or by providing supportive pharmacotherapies as indicated (e.g., trimethobenzamide or promethazine for nausea; acetaminophen or ibuprofen for headaches or myalgias). Augmentation or switching an SNRI or short-acting SSRI to fluoxetine, followed by discontinuation of fluoxetine, may also help diminish the potential for symptoms of discontinuation syndrome.

In the middle to late 1990s, withdrawal syndromes were first described in the setting of abrupt cessation of short-acting SSRIs (see Table 2–2, Chapter 2, "Pharmacokinetics, Pharmacodynamics, and Pharmacogenomics"), with features including dizziness, insomnia, nervousness, nausea, or agitation; fluoxetine, by virtue of the long elimination half-life of its metabolite norfluoxetine, appears significantly less likely to cause this phenomenon than are other SSRIs (Rosenbaum et al. 1998). A review by Fava and colleagues (2015) found high variability in reported incident rates of SSRI discontinuation symptoms ranging from 6% to 47% of patients, with lower frequencies associated with longer-half-life SSRIs such as fluoxetine. No demographic or clinical characteristics appear to predict the likelihood of developing withdrawal symptoms after SSRI discontinuation, and withdrawal phenomena have been reported to persist for up to 3 weeks or longer following drug cessation, although symptoms usually resolve within 24 hours of SSRI resumption. Withdrawal features from the abrupt cessation (or sometimes even a few missed doses) of SNRIs can be even more substantial and protracted than occurs with SSRIs.

Two main strategies are usually advocated for managing SSRI or SNRI discontinuation syndromes. The first involves resuming either a discontinued agent or a dose that had been reduced and then undertaking a protracted taper of the existing antidepressant (per manufacturers' recommendations) — in some instances, over the course of several weeks or longer, with supportive management of emergent withdrawal symptoms using antinausea drugs (e.g., trimethobenzamide, promethazine, prochlorperazine), meclezine for vertigo, and analgesics (e.g., acetaminophen, ibuprofen) as needed for headaches and myalgias. However, Fava and colleagues (2015) observed that gradual SSRI tapers did not reliably diminish the chances for discontinuation symptoms to occur. The second approach is to augment the initial antidepressant with fluoxetine for several days, then discontinue the original antidepressant entirely and capitalize on the long half-life of fluoxetine plus its metabolite, norfluoxetine, and then discontinue fluoxetine after several days with a lesser likelihood of withdrawal phenomena. Conceivably, a similar approach could be taken by switching an existing short $t_{1/2}$ serotonergic antidepressant to vortioxetine, given its relatively long $t_{1/2}$ of 66 hours — although the actual implementation of this strategy has not yet been reported in the literature.

Abrupt cessation of MAOIs has been associated with discontinuation phenomena that may include hallucinations, anxiety, agitation, paranoia, and delirium. It is therefore recommended that MAOIs be tapered over at least several days or more rather than being abruptly stopped, except in the setting of palpitations or frequent headaches that may be thought to reflect a hypertensive crisis.

Drug-Induced Lupus Erythematosus

General Recommendations

Drug-induced lupus erythematosus (DILE) is rarely caused by psychotropic drugs. In suspected cases, symptoms mirror those seen with systemic lupus erythematosus (SLE) and involve flulike symptoms, myalgias, arthralgias, and fever. The causal agent should be discontinued and not subsequently reintroduced. Symptoms typically resolve within 1–2 weeks either spontaneously or with the use of NSAIDs or (more infrequently) oral steroids.

DILE is an autoimmune phenomenon with clinical features and laboratory findings similar to those of SLE. Symptoms may include flulike symptoms, myalgias, arthralgias, and fever. Rashes or other skin lesions (e.g., oral ulcers) are less common with DILE than with SLE. More severe cases of DILE can involve cardiac or pulmonary inflammation. By definition, DILE is triggered by the use of certain medications, including several psychotropic agents—each considered by the Lupus Foundation of America (www.lupus.org) to have a low or very low risk. From among the nearly 40 known drugs associated with DILE, cases most commonly result from the use of procainamide, hydralazine, and quinidine. Psychotropic agents that have rarely been associated with DILE include carbamazepine, oxcarbazepine, lithium, clonidine, pindolol, chlorpromazine, perphenazine, and phenelzine. Limited risk factors have been identified for developing DILE, including chronicity of drug therapy, male sex, age >50, and the presence of the so-called "slow acetylator" phenotype (see the section "Pharmacokinetics and Pharmacodynamics" in Chapter 2, "Pharmacokinetics, Pharmacodynamics, and Pharmacogenomics").

Diagnosis of DILE depends on clinical presentation as well as corroboration from laboratory indices (notably, antinuclear antibody and antihistone antibodies). Treatment involves discontinuing the causal agent alongside supplemental NSAIDs or oral steroids, corticosteroid creams to treat skin rashes, and hydroxychloroquine to treat arthralgias. More rarely, immunosuppressants such as azathioprine or cyclophosphamide are also necessary. Reintroduction of a causal agent is generally not advised. DILE is an iatrogenic phenomenon that is fundamentally different from SLE. Long-term consequences or recurrences of DILE would not be expected unless the suspected causal agent was reintroduced.

Neuroleptic Malignant Syndrome

General Recommendations

NMS can occur with any FGAs or SGAs and should be considered in any patient receiving an antipsychotic who develops a fever. Treatment involves immediate cessation of dopamine antagonists followed by supportive measures (e.g., hydration and autonomic monitoring).

NMS is a relatively rare adverse systemic reaction to any antipsychotic drugs (including antiemetic phenothiazines such as prochlorperazine and related compounds such as metoclopramide) as well as other non-neuroleptic drugs with antidopaminergic effects, such as phenelzine, some TCAs (e.g., desipramine, trimipramine), and lithium. NMS rarely arises beyond 1 month after initiation of an antidopaminergic drug. (Two-thirds of cases occur within the first 7 days of starting an antidopaminergic drug.) Although clear risk factors have not been empirically determined, some authors have observed that NMS may be more likely to occur in patients with psychomotor agitation or dehydration, in those who receive high doses of antipsychotics, and in recipients of frequent intramuscular injections of FGAs. Key symptoms include fever, muscle rigidity, acute mental status changes (e.g., delirium), autonomic instability, elevation of serum CK, tremor, and leukocytosis. Serum CK levels typically exceed 1,000 IU/L and in some cases may be as high as 100,000 IU/L (Levenson 1985). However, NMS is a clinical diagnosis that can manifest in various ways, and no one symptom is pathognomonic. The clinician must also recognize nonpsychotropic drugs that may cause myalgias with possible rhabdomyolysis (e.g., statins), which could be mistaken for the muscle rigidity of NMS. Indeed, it is critical for practitioners to differentiate NMS from other systemic drug reactions (e.g., serotonin syndrome [see the section "Serotonin Syndrome" below] or anticholinergic delirium) as well as other forms of delirium or encephalopathy, infectious etiologies, or heat stroke, and also to avoid mistaking it for manifestations of primary psychopathology (including catatonia).

NMS is a medical emergency. Treatment hinges on the prompt discontinuation of antipsychotics and other potential antidopaminergic drugs, supportive treatment of hyperthermia (e.g., cooling blankets, ice packs), and hydration (usually intravenous, both for circulatory support and to minimize the potential for kidney damage due to myoglobinuria). Intravenous use of the muscle relaxant dantrolene (1–2.5 mg/kg initially, followed by 1 mg/kg every 6 hours) is typically reserved for extreme hyperthermia and the persistent abnormalities of marked vital signs despite supportive care. In patients not responding to the above treatments, electroconvulsive therapy (ECT) is sometimes advised based on the rationale of its known efficacy for malignant catatonia (reviewed by Davis et al. [1991]). A history of prior NMS may increase the likelihood of future episodes of NMS. There is no contraindication to resuming antipsychotic drugs after the resolution of NMS, although recurrence happens in up to 30% of individuals; SGAs are preferred over FGAs, and clinicians should use the lowest possible dosages and monitor carefully for early signs of reemergent NMS.

Serotonin Syndrome

General Recommendations

Serotonin syndrome is a medically emergent toxicity state resulting from excessive serotonergic activity, usually caused by an interaction among drugs that increase serotonin through different mechanisms. Management involves cessation of serotonergic drugs and supportive measures that fundamentally include hydration and airway monitoring and protection.

A constellation of signs and symptoms related to serotonergic hyperstimulation has come to be known as serotonin syndrome, which may be one of a family of CNS toxicity states that also includes NMS. The criteria classically described by Sternbach (1991) for defining serotonin syndrome include the following:

- At least three of the following: agitation, ataxia, diaphoresis, diarrhea, hyperreflexia (particularly in lower extremities), mental status changes (may include hypervigilance, psychosis, confusion, or agitation), myoclonus, shivering, tremor, or hyperthermia
- Emergence of signs and symptoms temporally following either the addition of a serotonergic drug or a dosage increase of an existing serotonergic agent
- No recent addition of an antipsychotic, or dosage increase of an existing antipsychotic
- Features that are not better accounted for by other causes such as infection, intoxication, metabolic derangement, substance abuse, or substance withdrawal

Low specificity of the Sternbach criteria, coupled with observations that clonus appears to be more specific to serotonin syndrome than other drug toxicity states (e.g., NMS, anticholinergic delirium), prompted refinements that led to the Hunter Serotonin Toxicity Criteria (Dunkley et al. 2003), which emphasize the importance of clonus (inducible, spontaneous, or ocular), agitation, diaphoresis, tremor, and hyperreflexia for establishing diagnostic specificity.

Serotonin syndrome typically is associated with drug interactions that increase central serotonergic tone. Drugs that affect serotonin through varied mechanisms of action are thought to incur a greater risk for serotonin syndrome than are drugs with a single mechanism (as in the case of overdosing on a single SSRI; even the combination of an SSRI plus SNRI involves mechanistic redundancy rather than serotonergic novelty, and hence is unlikely to produce serotonin syndrome). Examples of potentially toxic interactions include the following:

- MAOIs+serotonergic antidepressants
- MAOIs+meperidine
- Dextromethorphan (which blocks neuronal serotonin uptake)+MAOIs
- Buspirone+SSRIs or lithium
- Linezolid (synthetic antibiotic that weakly inhibits MAO)+SSRIs or other serotonergic agents
- Triptans+SSRIs or SNRIs (note that in 2006 the FDA issued an alert regarding this combination, although this relative contraindication remains controversial and unnecessarily overconservative in the opinions of some authorities, such as the American Headache Society [Evans et al. 2010])
- MAOIs+amphetamines (which release serotonin)
- 3,4-Methylenedioxymethamphetamine (i.e., Ecstasy)
- Tramadol+SSRIs or SNRIs

Patient-specific risk factors for serotonin syndrome have not been well identified, although some reports suggest that CYP2D6 poor metabolizers may be at greater risk when a second serotonergic drug is added to a first.

Treatment of serotonin syndrome depends on supportive treatment plus cessation of all serotonergic agents. Fundamentally, the condition is self-limited and eventually resolves spontaneously after discontinuation of the offending agent(s). Supportive measures may include intravenous hydration, clonazepam for myoclonus, cooling blankets or ice packs for centrally mediated hyperthermia, and airway protection (with the possible need for mechanical ventilation).

21

Pregnancy and the Puerperium

Psychotropic adverse effects during pregnancy generally do not differ qualitatively from those that may occur at other times, although pregnancy may be a time of increased susceptibility to certain conditions relevant to adverse drug effects (e.g., gestational diabetes and subsequent metabolic dysregulation with SGAs). Pregnancy also may alter drug metabolism in ways that affect both efficacy and tolerability—for example, the third trimester involves both the greatest increase in volume of distribution as well as estrogen-mediated induction of CYP enzymes. Consequently, dosages of SSRIs and other drugs metabolized by CYP isoenzymes may require upward dosing to maintain consistent efficacy, although rapid fluid shifts at the time of delivery may necessitate subsequent dosage reductions to minimize the risk of toxicity.

Teasing apart potential teratogenic effects from base rates of minor or major malformations in the general population is often difficult if not impossible. Complicating the situation further is the need to consider factors such as the adequacy of prenatal care and the possible deleterious effects of undertreated psychopathology on the developing fetus (e.g., the impact of hypercortisolemia in depression on the developing hippocampus).

Breast-Feeding and Teratogenicity

General Recommendations

No absolute contraindications exist to breast-feeding during treatment with any psychotropic drug. Potential benefits of psychotropic drug therapy during breast-feeding must be balanced on a case-by-case basis against the potential for unknown risks. Potential teratogenic risks no longer are described by a letter (A, B, C, D, X) rating system, but rather are delineated by labeling language that summarizes known risks from human and animal data alongside clinical considerations for individual medications, in order to help foster more contextualized decision making about a drug's relative risks versus benefits for a given patient during pregnancy.

Virtually all psychotropic drugs are detectable in breast milk, although the clinical significance of this, if any, is often unknown. Among mood stabilizers, carbamazepine and divalproex are often considered relatively safe during breast-feeding, although case reports exist of infants developing through breast-feeding hepatic dysfunction from exposure to carbamazepine and thrombocytopenia or anemia from exposure to divalproex (Chaudron and Jefferson 2000). Most practitioners advise against breast-feeding during lithium therapy, although it is no longer an absolute contraindication. Serum lithium levels, as well as renal and thyroid function, require monitoring in the newborn during breast-feeding.

Prior to June 30, 2015, the FDA employed a "letter" rating system (A, B, C, D, X) to categorize teratogenic risks associated with pharmaceuticals. That system, deemed overly simplistic, was replaced with the Pregnancy and Lactation Labeling Rule (PLLR) (see https://www.fda.gov/Drugs/DevelopmentApprovalProcess/DevelopmentResources/Labeling/ucm093307.htm). Intended goals of the PLLR include providing more complete safety information about pregnancy and lactation when available, placing animal safety data in the context of human exposure, and contextualizing medical/disease factors as influencing pregnancy outcomes. Central to the PLLR is the establishment of pregnancy exposure registries maintained by industry (i.e., drug manufacturers) and academic institutions (e.g., the Center for Women's Mental Health at the Massachusetts General Hospital) or disease state organizations. While the FDA itself does not develop or maintain such pregnancy registries, it does provide a listing of relevant organizations that do (see https://www.fda.gov/ScienceResearch/SpecialTopics/WomensHealthResearch/ucm134848.htm).

As of June 30, 2015, manufacturer's package insert information must contain pregnancy and lactation "Risk Summary" sections that separately identify human and animal data as well as situations for which no data are available. Revised product labeling also includes a "Clinical Considerations" section with subsections that address the following:

- Disease-associated maternal and/or embryo/fetal risk
- Dose adjustments during pregnancy and the postpartum period
- Maternal adverse reactions
- Fetal/neonatal adverse reactions
- Labor or delivery

A separate product information subsection on lactation also must describe a known risk summary, clinical considerations, and available data to help guide clinical decision making. This includes information on whether a drug is systemically absorbed and its concentration in breast milk, actual or estimated infant daily doses, and effects on breast-fed infants, if known.

A final product labeling change relevant to "Females and Males of Reproductive Potential" includes information about the known roles for pregnancy testing, contraception, and infertility.

Some reasonable guidelines in selecting medications for pregnant women and those planning for pregnancy include the following:

1. Select medications that are likely to benefit the woman following a risk-benefit calculation that includes the risk of mental illness to the woman, because untreated psychiatric disorders are known to increase obstetrical complications and poor neonatal outcomes.
2. Maintain an awareness that the literature regarding pregnancy and psychotropics is evolving and can be difficult to interpret.
3. Consider consultation with perinatal psychiatrists, who specialize in helping women and their providers make educated evidence-based decisions that take into account maternal mental health and reproductive safety of medications.
4. In general, it is best to treat women of reproductive potential with medications that would be reasonable in pregnancy, because many women will require long-term maintenance of psychotropics and will plan pregnancies or become pregnant during their treatment.

A number of psychotropic agents have relatively well-established associations with specific potential adverse effects during pregnancy (either anatomical or behavioral teratogenicity, or gestational complications) that are often small but significant, and that typically represent a topic for risk-benefit discussions to be had between doctor and patient rather than absolute contraindications (Table 21–1).

As a general rule, the clinician should strive during patients' pregnancy to minimize the number of exposures to different drugs, each with their own (often unknown) risks; this principle often favors the retention of an existing psychotropic drug once a pregnancy is confirmed rather than switching to a new drug that introduces additional teratogenic uncertainties. One point of consideration regarding most teratogenic risks is that their relevance often pertains mainly (but not exclusively) to the first trimester, inasmuch as organogenesis is largely completed by the end of the twelfth week of life (cf. the risk for preterm delivery or bleeding diatheses in the newborn due to vitamin K deficiency with third-trimester divalproex exposure). An example of possible teratogenic risk beyond the third trimester is persistent pulmonary hypertension of the newborn (PPHN), a condition typically arising in 1 in 700 live births but found in one study to have an approximate 6-fold increased risk when mothers had been exposed to an SSRI specifically after the twentieth week of gestation (Chambers et al. 2006). Several subsequent studies, however, have failed to support this risk, with most demonstrating no association whatsoever. Therefore, the relationship between PPHN and antidepressants is questionable at this time, but patients must be made aware of this literature and its inconsistent findings. Individual risk-benefit analyses for a given patient must consider the severity of symptoms and the magnitude of response to an SSRI, as well as additional factors that may independently contribute to PPHN (e.g., presence of obesity or diabetes in the mother). Of all the psychotropic medications that have received systematic study in pregnancy, divalproex is the medication most associated with teratogenicity, with a reported rate of 1%–6% of neural tube defects, and long-term neurocognitive deficits demonstrated in exposed 3-year-olds (Meador et al. 2009). In comparison, the risk of cardiovascular anomaly with first-time lithium use is small, less than 1%, and the association between lamotrigine and oral clefting has been only inconsistently observed in registries.

Growth Effects

Conflicting and nonsystematic data exist on the potential relationship between antidepressant exposure during pregnancy and low birth weight or intrauterine growth retardation. Although some studies suggest that antidepressant exposure may lead to lower birth weight and size (e.g.,

TABLE 21–1. Known adverse effects of psychotropic agents during pregnancy

Agent	Adverse effect	Practical implications
Carbamazepine	Neural tube defects, spina bifida, head and facial deformities, cardiac malformations; neonates may have seizures, vomiting, diarrhea, pulmonary problems.	Drug is relatively contraindicated in pregnancy unless benefits are thought to outweigh risks (more often the case in epilepsy than other conditions).
Divalproex	Neural tube defects (■), potential vitamin K deficiency in newborn.	Some clinicians advise supplemental folic acid for divalproex recipients of childbearing potential, although it is not known whether this practice meaningfully counteracts the potential disruption of CNS formation due to first-trimester divalproex exposure.
Lamotrigine	Approximate 10-fold increased risk of cleft lips or palates in infants with first-trimester in utero exposure to lamotrigine compared with nonlamotrigine-exposed deliveries (Holmes et al. 2008).	Patients should be apprised of current information as part of the informed consent process. Most experts and the FDA attach little importance or generalizability to this never-replicated observation from a single-case registry.
Lithium	Approximate 1/1,000 to 1/2,000 risk for Ebstein's anomaly during cardiac development; increased risk for polyhydramnios.	Contemporary perspectives often favor benefits over risk, depending on severity of response to lithium.

TABLE 21–1. Known adverse effects of psychotropic agents during pregnancy *(continued)*

Agent	Adverse effect	Practical implications
Paroxetine	Increased risk for cardiac malformations.	Although paroxetine has become relatively contraindicated in pregnancy, some authorities believe that existing data regarding its possible teratogenicity are too preliminary to draw firm conclusions.
Other SSRIs	As a broad class, may increase risk for preterm labor (specifically, may decrease gestational period by ~7–10 days).	SSRIs, particularly fluoxetine and sertraline, are considered among the safest psychotropic drugs in pregnancy.
Topiramate	Increased incidence of cleft lip or palate (1.4%) relative to other antiepileptic drugs (0.38–0.55%).	Given the minimal psychotropic effects of topiramate, benefits would seldom outweigh risks.

Note. ■=FDA boxed warning; CNS=central nervous system; FDA=U.S. Food and Drug Administration; SSRI=selective serotonin re-uptake inhibitor.

length and head circumference), the potential confounding effects of parental size and metabolic parameters, as well as maternal depression influencing fetal growth and development, often are underappreciated.

Withdrawal in the Newborn

General Recommendations

In general, little rationale exists for stopping or lowering a mother's dosages of antidepressants before delivery during pregnancy. The likelihood of antidepressant discontinuation symptoms in the neonate is low, and if they are suspected, are typically transient and can be managed conservatively with supportive measures. By contrast, the risks for third-trimester or postpartum affective relapse may be considerable and on the whole outweigh the minimal risk for withdrawal phenomena occurring in the newborn.

SSRIs in neonates have been described in case reports to cause possible withdrawal phenomena, comprised of features such as constant crying, shivering, increased muscle tone, and feeding problems. So-called neonatal abstinence syndrome (NAS) has been reported to occur in about 30% of newborns during the first 1–2 weeks of life after maternal exposure to an SSRI; features may include a high-pitched cry, sleep disturbance, difficulty feeding, tachypnea, hyperthermia, frequent yawning, tremors, exaggerated Moro reflex, and hypertonicity or myoclonus (Levinson-Castiel et al. 2006). Phenomena related to NAS are captured and quantified using a measure known as the Finnegan Score (which can be easily determined; see https://www.thecalculator.co/health/Finnegan-Score-For-Neonatal-Abstinence-Syndrome-(NAS)-Calculator-1025.html).

Such phenomena, if they even occur, are typically self-limited and readily managed by supportive care. Furthermore, naturalistic case registry data have shown no significant differences in neonatal health outcomes in pregnant women for whom SSRIs were discontinued versus continued throughout the third trimester (Warburton et al. 2010).

In December 2010, the FDA Center for Drug Evaluation and Research modified the warnings and precautions for all antipsychotics to include a statement identifying the risk for extrapyramidal side effects and withdrawal in neonates. Such occurrences appear to be self-limited and of little medical consequence.

22

Emergency Situations

A number of emergency situations may arise from iatrogenic effects of psychotropic medications. Such situations demand rapid identification. Discontinuation of a suspected causal agent often leads to resolution of many suspected iatrogenic emergencies, although a number of situations require specific forms of medical management. Table 22–1 provides a summary of common adverse psychotropic drug effects that may constitute medical emergencies.

Overdoses of psychotropic medications constitute their own form of medical emergency. Apart from the underlying psychiatric implications of an overdose (e.g., suicide attempts), some agents with relatively wide therapeutic indices may cause little more than an exaggeration of the adverse effects sometimes seen at lower dosages (e.g., sedation, nausea, emesis, headache, tremor). Others may cause more grave end-organ damage that requires vigilant monitoring of cardiovascular status, seizure risk, or renal or CNS sequelae. One must also bear in mind certain drug-specific idiosyncrasies in the setting of overdose: for example, after a toxic overdose of lithium carbonate, high penetration of lithium salts into brain and bone are prone to cause persistent risk for cardiac, renal, or neurotoxic lithium effects for weeks or months after serum lithium levels become undetectable.

Although it is beyond the scope of this summary to provide a comprehensive discussion of emergency medical management and detailed consequences of medication overdoses, Table 22–2 describes common signs and symptoms associated with overdoses of specific psychotropic drugs, as well as basic elements of their management. Notably, however, in the case of toxic overdose ingestions, gastric lavage procedures have generally not shown superior outcomes to the use of activated charcoal alone, and lavage generally is not recommended beyond 60 minutes after an acute ingestion.

TABLE 22–1. Emergency management of serious adverse drug effects

Emergent adverse effect	Clinical description	Associated agents	Management
Cardiovascular			
Hypertensive crisis	Blood pressure exceeding 180/110; may include headache, dyspnea, mental status changes.	MAOIs, SNRIs	Discontinue causal agent.
Cutaneous			
Purpura	Nonblanching hemorrhagic eruptions beneath the skin.	Carbamazepine	Indicative of thrombocytopenia; discontinue likely causal agent and refer for medical management.
Stevens-Johnson syndrome or toxic epidermal necrolysis	Blistering, burnlike lesions on mucocutaneous tissues; facial edema, lymphadenopathy.	Bupropion, carbamazepine, lamotrigine	Discontinue likely causal agent. Steroids may be indicated early in the course of disease but are contraindicated later in course. Do not rechallenge after a serious rash.

TABLE 22–1. Emergency management of serious adverse drug effects (*continued*)

Emergent adverse effect	Clinical description	Associated agents	Management
Gastrointestinal			
Acute pancreatitis	Acute abdominal presentation; diagnose by clinical examination and elevated serum lipase and amylase. A history of pancreatitis unrelated to divalproex is not a known contraindication or predisposing risk factor for developing pancreatitis from divalproex.	Divalproex	Discontinue divalproex and do not reintroduce. Medical management mainly involves taking no food by mouth accompanied by intravenous hydration and rest.
Hematological			
Aplastic anemia	—	Carbamazepine, clozapine	Discontinue offending agent. Monitor for the development of and treat infections (e.g., pharyngitis) that arise in the setting of an immunocompromised state. Bone marrow typically replenishes within 21 days without the need for further intervention.

TABLE 22–1. Emergency management of serious adverse drug effects (continued)			
Emergent adverse effect	Clinical description	Associated agents	Management
Neurological			
Acute dystonia	Markedly increased muscle tone and rigidity in extremities; difficulty swallowing or clearing salivary secretions may indicate laryngospasm	All FGAs, particularly higher-potency agents that lack anticholinergic effects (e.g., haloperidol, fluphenazine)	Administer oral or intramuscular anticholinergic agents (e.g., diphenhydramine or benztropine).
Seizure	—	All FGAs, SGAs, bupropion	Maintain airway and safety; avoid aspiration or head injury.
Systemic			
Aseptic meningitis	Systemic illness involving high fever, nuchal rigidity, nausea, vomiting, photophobia, confusion, depressed sensorium.	Lamotrigine	Discontinue lamotrigine.

TABLE 22–1. Emergency management of serious adverse drug effects (*continued*)

Emergent adverse effect	Clinical description	Associated agents	Management
Systemic (*continued*)			
Neuroleptic malignant syndrome	Fever, abdominal cramping, muscle rigidity; elevated CK (typically >1,000 IU/L).	All antipsychotics	Discontinue the antipsychotic; hydrate; administer dantrolene for marked autonomic instability that does not respond adequately to supportive treatment.
Serotonin syndrome	Clonus	SSRIs, SNRIs, tramadol	Discontinue serotonergic drugs; hydrate, maintain airway, consider cooling blankets.

Note. CK=creatine kinase; FGA=first-generation antipsychotic; MAOI=monoamine oxidase inhibitor; SGA=second-generation antipsychotic; SNRI=serotonin-norepinephrine reuptake inhibitor; SSRI=selective serotonin reuptake inhibitor.

TABLE 22–2. Clinical features associated with medication overdoses, and management[a]

Agent	Maximum reported dose in overdose	Medical consequences	Management
Atomoxetine	1,400 mg	Gastrointestinal symptoms, somnolence, dizziness, tremor, abnormal behavior; reports of seizures, hyperactivity, agitation; rare QTc prolongation, disorientation, hallucinations.	Gastric lavage with administration of activated charcoal if recent ingestion. Monitor cardiac and vital signs.
Buspirone	375 mg	Nausea, vomiting, dizziness, miosis, gastric distress.	Gastric lavage if recent ingestion. Monitor vital signs. No specific management strategies apart from general supportive measures.
Anticonvulsants and lithium			
Carbamazepine	>6,000 mg	Neuromuscular disturbances, irregular breathing, respiratory depression, tachycardia, hyperor hypotension, shock, QRS prolongation and ventricular arrhythmias, impaired level of consciousness (including drowsiness or coma), nystagmus, mydriasis, seizures, nausea, vomiting, anticholinergic effects.	Maintain adequate airway; gastric lavage with activated charcoal may be considered; monitor cardiac rhythm and vital signs.

TABLE 22–2. Clinical features associated with medication overdoses, and management[a] (*continued*)

Agent	Maximum reported dose in overdose	Medical consequences	Management
Anticonvulsants and lithium (*continued*)			
Divalproex	Maximum dose not reported; maximum recommended dose in epilepsy=60 mg/ kg; maximum reported serum valproate level= 2,120 μg/mL	Fever, hallucinations, somnolence (CNS depression at doses > 200 mg/ kg [valproate > 180 μg/mL]), hyperammonemia, tachycardia, heart block, coma; fatalities reported.	Supportive measures, gastric lavage with emesis. Naloxone (0.8–2.0 mg) may reverse the CNS depressant effects of divalproex.
Gabapentin	49,000 mg	Ataxia, labored breathing, ptosis, sedation, hypoactivity, excitation, double vision, slurred speech, drowsiness, lethargy, diarrhea; no fatalities reported.	Supportive care, cardiovascular monitoring, gastric lavage. Gabapentin is dialyzable.
Lamotrigine	15,000 mg (oral LD_{50}=250 mg/kg in rats)	Dizziness, diplopia or blurry vision, rotatory or downbeat nystagmus, truncal ataxia, cognitive disorganization; fatalities reported.	Supportive care, cardiovascular monitoring, induction of emesis, gastric lavage.

TABLE 22–2. Clinical features associated with medication overdoses, and management[a] *(continued)*

Agent	Maximum reported dose in overdose	Medical consequences	Management
Anticonvulsants and lithium *(continued)*			
Lithium	Not reported; serum levels >3 mEq/L may produce seizures, coma, and death; maximum recommended dose = 2,400 mg/day	Neurotoxicity (ataxia, nystagmus, tremor, slow shuffling gait, myoclonic jerks, confusion and disorientation), GI symptoms (nausea, vomiting, abdominal cramps, diarrhea), and cardiac toxicity (including sinus bradycardia and sinoatrial- or atrioventricular block that can produce complete heart block [Serinken et al. 2009]); reports of pulmonary edema; mortality results from CNS toxicity and subsequent cardiovascular collapse.	Consequences of lithium toxicity may persist for weeks or even months after serum lithium levels become undetectable. Following *acute* overdose, measurement of plasma lithium–erythrocyte lithium ratios may reveal higher lithium in plasma than erythrocytes. Management involves hydration, gastric lavage (although activated charcoal does not bind lithium well and tends not to be recommended), and cardiac monitoring; hemodialysis is rarely necessary for serum lithium levels <2.5 mEq/L but is usually required for levels >6 mEq/L, or for lower levels in medically debilitated patients or patients with coma, convulsions, cardiovascular symptoms, or respiratory failure.

TABLE 22–2. Clinical features associated with medication overdoses, and management[a] *(continued)*

Agent	Maximum reported dose in overdose	Medical consequences	Management
Anticonvulsants and lithium *(continued)*			
Oxcarbazepine	24,000 mg	Somnolence, hypotension, tremor, seizures, diplopia, dyspnea, miosis, nystagmus, decreased urine output; no fatalities reported.	Supportive care, gastric lavage with activated charcoal is recommended.
Topiramate	110,000 mg	Stupor or coma, severe metabolic acidosis, convulsions, drowsiness, speech disturbances, blurred vision, diplopia, cognitive impairment, lethargy, abnormal coordination, hypotension, abdominal pain, agitation, dizziness, depression; no reported fatalities.	Gastric lavage or induction of emesis if recent ingestion. Activated charcoal is not thought to absorb topiramate.
Antidepressants			
Bupropion	17,500 mg	Seizure (~1/3 of cases), hallucinations, loss of consciousness, tachycardia.	Maintain adequate airway; cardiac monitoring; gastric lavage if soon after ingestion (but not induction of emesis), with administration of activated charcoal. EEG monitoring is advised for first 48 hours.

TABLE 22–2. Clinical features associated with medication overdoses, and management[a] *(continued)*

Agent	Maximum reported dose in overdose	Medical consequences	Management
Antidepressants *(continued)*			
Citalopram	6,000 mg	Dizziness, sweating, nausea, vomiting, tremor, somnolence, tachycardia; QTc prolongation, nodal rhythms, ventricular arrhythmias, and torsades de pointes reported.	Maintain adequate airway; gastric lavage with activated charcoal may be considered; monitor cardiac rhythm and vital signs.
Desvenlafaxine	>600 mg	Tachycardia, somnolence, mydriasis, seizures, vomiting, hypotension, liver necrosis, rhabdomyolysis, serotorin syndrome; QTc or QRS prolongation and bundle branch block on ECG.	Maintain adequate airway; monitor cardiac rhythm and vital signs; gastric lavage if soon after ingestion.
Escitalopram	>1,000 mg	Seizures, coma, dizziness, hypotension, insomnia, acute renal failure, tachycardia; QTc prolongation and rare torsades de pointes on ECG.	Maintain adequate airway; cardiac monitoring; gastric lavage if soon after ingestion.

TABLE 22–2. Clinical features associated with medication overdoses, and management[a] *(continued)*

Agent	Maximum reported dose in overdose	Medical consequences	Management
Antidepressants *(continued)*			
Fluoxetine	8,000 mg	Variable outcomes (e.g., full recovery) after 8,000-mg ingestion, although 34 fatalities reported by manufacturer following 633 monotherapy overdoses; signs of overdose include seizures, nausea, vomiting, tachycardia, somnolence; more severe overdoses may lead to visual and gait disturbances, confusion, unresponsiveness, nervousness, respiratory distress, tremor, hypertension, impotence, movement disorders, hypomania.	Maintain adequate airway; cardiac rhythm and vital sign monitoring; gastric lavage if soon after ingestion. Do not induce emesis. Beware of coingestion of TCAs and the pharmacokinetic potential for their increased accumulation.

TABLE 22–2. Clinical features associated with medication overdoses, and management[a] *(continued)*

Agent	Maximum reported dose in overdose	Medical consequences	Management
Antidepressants *(continued)*			
Fluvoxamine	12,000 mg	Variable outcomes (e.g., full recovery after 12,000-mg ingestion but lethality after 1,400-mg ingestion); signs of overdose include GI upset, coma, hypokalemia, hypotension, respiratory difficulties, somnolence, tachycardia, bradycardia, QTc prolongation, first-degree AV block and other arrhythmias, seizures, tremor, hyperreflexia.	Maintain adequate airway; cardiac rhythm and vital sign monitoring; gastric lavage if soon after ingestion. Beware of coingestion of TCAs and the pharmacokinetic potential for their increased accumulation.
Levomilnacipran	360 mg	Not described; no fatalities reported.	Supportive care; no specific interventions recommended.
Mirtazapine	975 mg (Fawcett and Barkin 1998)	Disorientation, somnolence, impaired memory, tachycardia; no known potential for seizures or ECG abnormalities; unlikely fatality.	Maintain adequate airway; monitor cardiac rhythm and vital signs. Gastric lavage with activated charcoal if soon after ingestion. Induction of emesis is not recommended.
Nefazodone	11,200 mg	Nausea, vomiting, somnolence; fatalities reported when overdoses occurred in combination with other substances.	Maintain adequate airway; monitor cardiac rhythm and vital signs. Gastric lavage if soon after ingestion. Induction of emesis is not recommended.

TABLE 22–2.   Clinical features associated with medication overdoses, and management[a] (continued)

Agent	Maximum reported dose in overdose	Medical consequences	Management
Antidepressants (continued)			
Paroxetine	2,000 mg	Somnolence, coma, nausea, tremor, tachycardia, confusion, vomiting, dizziness.	Maintain adequate airway; gastric lavage if soon after ingestion (but not induction of emesis), with administration of activated charcoal.
TCAs	Not reported	Drowsiness, lethargy, confusion, tachycardia, hyper- or hypotension, urinary retention with desipramine (highest risk for fatality due to potent sodium channel blockade), nortriptyline, imipramine, amitriptyline, clomipramine, protriptyline, doxepin.	Cardiac monitoring; intravenous hydration (observe for hypotension due to sodium channel blockade); gastric lavage with activated charcoal if within first few hours after ingestion; intravenous administration of sodium bicarbonate (alkalinize urine) if QRS > 100 msec, ventricular arrhythmias; observe for seizure risk (highest in first several hours after ingestion; may require anticonvulsant benzodiazepines, phenobarbital, or other antiseizure therapy). Avoid β-blockers, calcium channel blockers, ipecac syrup.

TABLE 22–2. Clinical features associated with medication overdoses, and management[a] *(continued)*

Agent	Maximum reported dose in overdose	Medical consequences	Management
Antidepressants *(continued)*			
Vilazodone	280 mg	Serotonin syndrome, lethargy, restlessness, hallucinations, disorientation.	Maintain adequate airway; monitor cardiac rhythm and vital signs. Gastric lavage with activated charcoal if soon after ingestion. Induction of emesis is not recommended.
Vortioxetine	75 mg	Nausea, dizziness, diarrhea, abdominal discomfort, pruritis, somnolence, flushing.	Supportive care.
Anxiolytics/Sedative-hypnotics			
Benzodiazepines	Not reported	Somnolence, confusion, coma, hyporeflexia, hypotension, miosis or sluggish/delayed pupillary responses, nystagmus.	Supportive care including cardiovascular monitoring, gastric lavage, and intravenous hydration. Flumazenil may be administered to reverse sedative effects of benzodiazepines.
Buspirone	375 mg	Nausea, vomiting, dizziness, drowsiness, miosis, gastric distress; no fatalities reported.	Supportive care, cardiovascular monitoring.

TABLE 22–2. Clinical features associated with medication overdoses, and management[a] *(continued)*

Agent	Maximum reported dose in overdose	Medical consequences	Management
Anxiolytics/Sedative-hypnotics *(continued)*			
Eszopiclone	270 mg	Somnolence, coma, rare fatalities when combined with other CNS drugs or alcohol.	Immediate gastric lavage where appropriate; IV fluids; flumazenil may be useful; monitor vital signs; general supportive care.
Ramelteon	Not reported	Somnolence.	General supportive care; gastric lavage where appropriate; IV fluids as needed.
Suvorexant	240 mg	Somnolence.	General supportive care; gastric lavage where appropriate; IV fluids as needed.
Tasimelteon	Not available	Somnolence.	General supportive care; gastric lavage where appropriate; IV fluids as needed.
Zaleplon	200 mg	CNS depression, drowsiness, coma, ataxia, hypotonia, hypotension, respiratory depression, rare fatalities.	General supportive care; gastric lavage where appropriate; IV fluids as needed; flumazenil may be appropriate; monitor vital signs.
Zolpidem	Not available	Somnolence, coma, cardiovascular and respiratory compromise, possible fatality.	General supportive care; gastric lavage where appropriate; IV fluids as needed; flumazenil may be useful (but may lead to convulsions); monitor vital signs.

TABLE 22–2. Clinical features associated with medication overdoses, and management[a] *(continued)*

Agent	Maximum reported dose in overdose	Medical consequences	Management
Psychostimulants			
Amphetamine	Deaths reported at dosages > 1.3 mg/kg	Restlessness, tremor, hyperreflexia, tachypnea, confusion, assaultiveness, hallucinations, panic, hyperpyrexia, rhabdomyolysis, convulsions, coma, arrhythmias, hypo- or hypertension, circulatory collapse, nausea, vomiting, diarrhea, abdominal cramps, death.	General supportive care; gastric lavage where appropriate; administration of activated charcoal; IV phentolamine may counteract hypertension, if necessary; chlorpromazine antagonizes the central stimulant effects of amphetamine and may be useful.
Methylphenidate	1,134 mg (Klampfl et al. 2010)	Vomiting, agitation, muscle twitching, seizures, confusion, psychosis, hyperhidrosis, headache, fever, tachycardia, palpitations, rhabdomyolysis, mydriasis, dry mouth, death.	General supportive care; gastric lavage where appropriate; administration of activated charcoal.

TABLE 22–2. Clinical features associated with medication overdoses, and management[a] *(continued)*

Agent	Maximum reported dose in overdose	Medical consequences	Management
Psychostimulants *(continued)*			
Modafinil	12,000 mg	Excitation, agitation, restlessness, insomnia, disorientation, confusion, hallucinations, nausea, diarrhea, tremor, tachycardia, bradycardia, hypertension, chest pain; no fatalities reported.	Supportive care, cardiovascular monitoring, induction of emesis or gastric lavage if not contraindicated.
SGAs			
Aripiprazole	1,260 mg	Vomiting, somnolence, tremor, confusion, bradycardia, tachycardia, QTc prolongation, coma, respiratory failure, seizures.	Supportive care, cardiac monitoring; activated charcoal if given soon after ingestion may reduce serum levels.
Asenapine	400 mg	Agitation, confusion.	Maintain adequate airway; cardiac monitoring. Monitor for possible hypotension and circulatory collapse. Anticholinergic medication should be used if severe EPS occur.

TABLE 22–2. Clinical features associated with medication overdoses, and management[a] *(continued)*

Agent	Maximum reported dose in overdose	Medical consequences	Management
SGAs *(continued)*			
Brexpiprazole	Not available	Not described.	Supportive monitoring; maintenance of airway; administration of activated charcoal if within 4 hours of overdose.
Cariprazine	48 mg	Orthostatic hypotension, sedation.	Supportive monitoring; maintenance of airway; no other specific intervention recommended.
Iloperidone	576 mg	Drowsiness, sedation, tachycardia, hypotension, EPS, QTc prolongation; no fatalities reported.	Maintain adequate airway; cardiac monitoring; gastric lavage if soon after ingestion with activated charcoal plus a laxative should be considered. Cardiac monitoring should include continuous electrocardiography due to the risk for arrhythmias. Monitor for seizure risk and dystonic reactions.

TABLE 22–2. Clinical features associated with medication overdoses, and management[a] (*continued*)

Agent	Maximum reported dose in overdose	Medical consequences	Management
SGAs (*continued*)			
Lurasidone	560 mg	Recovery without medical sequelae.	Avoid α-adrenergic blocking agents or sympathomimetic drugs with β-agonist activity (e.g., epinephrine, dobutamine) to minimize risk for hypotension; avoid disopyramide, procainamide, or quinidine if arrhythmias occur, to minimize additive risk for QTc prolongation. No sequelae following single overdose case of 560 mg/day.
Olanzapine	1,500 mg	Agitation, dysarthria, tachycardia, EPS, reduced level of consciousness or coma; fatality from overdoses of olanzapine alone reported from doses as low as 450 mg.	Maintain adequate airway; cardiac monitoring; gastric lavage if soon after ingestion with activated charcoal plus a laxative should be considered. Cardiac monitoring should include continuous electrocardiography due to the risk for arrhythmias.

TABLE 22–2. Clinical features associated with medication overdoses, and management[a] (continued)

Agent	Maximum reported dose in overdose	Medical consequences	Management
SGAs *(continued)*			
Paliperidone	405 mg	Gait unsteadiness, drowsiness, EPS, seizures, QTc prolongation, tachycardia, hypotension.	Maintain adequate airway; cardiac monitoring; gastric lavage if soon after ingestion. Anticholinergic agents should be used for severe EPS. Intravenous hydration may be necessary to counteract hypotension. Avoid parenteral epinephrine or dopamine because beta stimulation may exacerbate hypotension from paliperidone-induced alpha blockade.
Pimavanserin	Unavailable	Nausea, vomiting, possible QTc prolongation.	Immediate cardiovascular/continuous ECG monitoring; if antiarrhythmics are needed, avoid agents that may further prolong QTc (e.g., procainamide, quinidine, disopyramide).
Quetiapine	9,600 mg	Drowsiness, sedation, tachycardia, hypotension, hypokalemia, first-degree heart block; prolonged delirium described in adolescents.	Maintain adequate airway; cardiac monitoring; gastric lavage with activated charcoal and a laxative if soon after ingestion; continuous ECG monitoring.

TABLE 22–2. Clinical features associated with medication overdoses, and management[a] *(continued)*

Agent	Maximum reported dose in overdose	Medical consequences	Management
SGAs *(continued)*			
Risperidone	360 mg	Drowsiness, sedation, tachycardia, hypotension, EPS, electrolyte abnormalities, seizures, QTc prolongation with QRS widening on ECG.	Maintain adequate airway; cardiac monitoring; gastric lavage with activated charcoal and a laxative if soon after ingestion; continuous ECG monitoring.
Ziprasidone	3,240 mg	Sedation, slurred speech, transient hypertension, EPS, somnolence, tremor, anxiety.	Maintain adequate airway; cardiac monitoring; gastric lavage if soon after ingestion.

Note. AV=atrioventricular; CNS=central nervous system; ECG=electrocardiogram; EEG=electroencephalogram; EPS = extrapyramidal symptoms; GI=gastrointestinal; IV=intravenous; SGA=second-generation antipsychotic; TCA=tricyclic antidepressant.
[a]Information based on manufacturers' package insert materials.

PART III

Summary
Recommendations

23

Summary
Recommendations

Decisions about when to pursue antidotes for adverse psychotropic drug effects versus when to choose alternative pharmacotherapies must be tailored to the needs and circumstances of an individual patient. Risk-benefit analyses usually favor drug retention with active management of adverse effects when efficacy is dramatic and few if any comparable alternatives exist, unless insurmountable hazards exceed potential benefits, or unless the true inability to manage benign but bothersome adverse events would likely cause treatment nonadherence. A goal of this book has been to afford readers a greater awareness of viable options and resources for managing adverse effects than they might have previously realized, and of the circumstances under which the active management of side effects can produce better treatment outcomes. One of the greatest challenges in practicing contemporary psychopharmacology involves recognizing the factors and contexts that comprise risk-benefit analyses while considering the gravity of psychiatric symptoms alongside the manageability and medical dangerousness of adverse psychotropic drug effects.

In some respects, psychiatry has only fairly recently joined the ranks of other medical specialties in which treatment risk-benefit analyses have long been routine. Excess morbidity and mortality attributable to untreated or undertreated psychopathology pose disease risks that have become recognized and quantified in just the past two decades. By contrast, patients and clinicians alike have for centuries been aware of the excess morbidity and mortality associated with primary medical problems such as arrhythmias, infectious diseases, and cancer, yet seldom if ever avoid effective treatments due to safety concerns or the need for careful end-organ monitoring. Drugs such as warfarin, digitalis, amphotericin B, interferon, prednisone, and most antineoplastics all entail substantial (and sometimes life-threatening) adverse effects, yet the potential life-saving benefit of such drugs is seldom accorded secondary importance to their tolerability.

It is particularly striking that mental health professionals may eschew drugs that require end-organ monitoring and have narrow therapeutic indices (e.g., lithium), may be lethal in overdose (e.g., lithium, MAOIs, or TCAs), or carry the potential for metabolic dysregulation (most notably, clozapine) when many of these very agents have been shown to dramatically reduce mortality from suicide (in the case of lithium) or suicide attempts (in the case of clozapine). It is equally disconcerting when clinicians undertake complex combination drug regimens without clearly knowing whether efficacy even exists, or whether benefits do in fact outweigh risks. This is especially worrisome for treatments involving understudied patient groups, such as psychopharmacology for mood and behavior disorders in children younger than age 10 years, or management of agitation and psychosis related to dementia in older adults. When clinical problems outpace the existing evidence-based literature, it becomes all the more vital for practitioners to articulate the thought process behind their decision making and the rationales that lead them to favor one course of action over another.

When psychiatric symptoms are mild, nondisabling, and nonserious, high drug tolerability (i.e., a high NNH) often rightly assumes greater importance than the magnitude of efficacy (i.e., large effect size). Milder forms of psychopathology also may be more responsive to adjunctive psychotherapies, allowing for less exclusive focus on drug efficacy. Successful clinicians who opt for low-efficacy, high-tolerability drugs may underappreciate nonpharmacodynamic aspects of treatment that may be contributing to favorable outcomes, such as "inadvertent" psychotherapy or the importance of the therapeutic alliance in itself. By contrast, with more moderate to severe forms of psychopathology, drugs with more robust effects (large effect sizes, low NNTs) are often necessary to cause meaningful improvement. In such instances, it is often hard to justify the use of high-tolerability (high-NNH) drugs with small effect sizes (or negative efficacy data) when the hazards of undertreated psychopathology are substantial. High tolerability in such settings becomes practically meaningless.

One of the greatest psychotherapeutic challenges during pharmaco-therapy involves helping patients to cope with adverse effects that are bothersome, medically inconsequential, and without viable antidotes. There are unfortunately no panaceas or special strategies to navigate such obstacles, but the sheer avoidance of low-NNH drugs has little merit if efficacy is inconsequential. Sometimes, a useful approach is to coach patients in skills that may help them to better deal with distress. Such efforts obviously require educating patients about adverse effects that are benign but bothersome (e.g., dry mouth, sexual dysfunction, modest weight gain, chronic insomnia, tinnitus), and differentiating those effects from others that may be more easily treated (e.g., nausea, akathisia, tremor) or frankly dangerous (e.g., fever, dystonia, serious rashes). Discussing benign or bothersome versus medically hazardous iatrogenic events can be a formidable task for which a strong therapeutic alliance and sense of partnership are likely necessary prerequisites. As much as most clinicians would probably prefer to avoid discussing or having to deal with adverse effects altogether — and may fear that even mentioning potential side effects serves to invite nonadherence — engaging patients in a dialogue around their reality is fundamental to providing proper care. Such a dialogue involves a number of core principles:

- Encourage an environment that invites open discussion about possible adverse events; normalize the inclination to want to stop a medicine if it causes problems; and empathize with potential hesitation on the part of the patient to raise treatment objections ("I'm committed to helping you the best that I can if a problem comes up; if you're thinking about stopping a medicine because of a side effect, or for any other reason, I hope you'll consider first talking with me about the problem, since we might find the best solution if we work on it together").
- Educate patients about differentiating benign or bothersome versus hazardous adverse drug effects.
- Clarify misconceptions and presumptions about specific types of adverse drug effects.
- Review the risks and benefits of any treatment; explain the rationale for deciding what is the "best" treatment for a given malady and discuss whether or not alternative options are likely to be comparable.
- Recognize the patient's past experiences with adverse events and sensitivities about particular types of adverse drug effects.
- Estimate the likelihood and transience or persistence of a particular adverse effect.

- Project the time course for clinical improvement versus the emergence of adverse events (and their magnitude), and establish benchmarks for periodic reassessments of risk-benefit analyses.
- Provide reassurance that the clinician will monitor adverse effects as well as efficacy, and intervene when necessary to assure medical safety; patients are more apt to trust the treatment if they believe the clinician cares as much about their concerns as they themselves do.

The Future

Research-based strategies to manage the most common and vexing adverse effects of psychotropic drugs lag far behind the pace of efforts to develop novel treatments for psychiatric disorders. We might imagine that as current proprietary formulations of psychotropic drugs lose patent protection with the passage of time, clinician interest will continue to wane in the prescribing of drugs with high side-effect burdens. The development of new psychotropic compounds that provide high-efficacy drugs with few adverse effects has long been an elusive pursuit — a conundrum that has unfortunately prompted a number of prominent pharmaceutical companies to divest their efforts altogether from new CNS drug development. Perhaps a next generation of psychopharmacology progress will involve greater incentives for drug manufacturers to devote greater resources toward developing more effective strategies to counteract common adverse iatrogenic effects.

Until the time arrives when high-efficacy psychotropic drugs that lack adverse effects come into existence, it remains the challenge for mental health practitioners to understand drug efficacy, tolerability, and suitability for a given patient on a case-by-case basis, and — as occurs in all areas of medicine — to engage the patient as a partner in an ongoing process of shared decision making that provides the foundation for a meaningful therapeutic alliance.

APPENDIX 1

Summary of Major Adverse Effects and Monitoring/ Management Considerations

Adverse effect	Known causal drugs	Frequency and timing of occurrence	Known risk factors	Dose-related?	Monitoring and management options
Akathisia	FGAs, SGAs; reports with lithium, SSRIs, mirtazapine	May be immediate or tardive (>1 month after antipsychotic discontinuation)	Possibly older age, female sex, negative symptoms, affective symptoms, cognitive dysfunction; iron deficiency; polyantipsychotic therapy	Yes	Dosage reductions; add centrally acting beta-blocker (e.g., propranolol 30–90 mg/day) or a benzodiazepine; amantadine 100–200 mg/day; gabapentin up to 1,200 mg/day; anticholinergics generally not useful
Alopecia	Divalproex, lithium, carbamazepine, lamotrigine, topiramate, some SSRIs, SNRIs, TCAs, mirtazapine, amphetamine, methylphenidate	Divalproex:12%–14% incidence; lithium: up to 10%; carbamazepine: up to 6%; other agents less well characterized: may occur at any time	Not well identified	Unlikely	Biotin 10,000 µg/day; zinc and selenium supplements; minoxidil topical solution or foam

Adverse effect	Known causal drugs	Frequency and timing of occurrence	Known risk factors	Dose-related?	Monitoring and management options
Antidepressant discontinuation syndrome	Short-half-life serotonergic antidepressants	Typically within 2–4 days of stopping drug, may persist up to 3 weeks	None known	No	If very slow tapers with supportive cotherapies (e.g., antiemetics, meclizine, acetaminophen) are ineffective, consider switch to longer-half-life serotonergic antidepressant (e.g., fluoxetine) for 2 weeks and then discontinue

Adverse effect	Known causal drugs	Frequency and timing of occurrence	Known risk factors	Dose-related?	Monitoring and management options
Bruxism	SSRIs, SNRIs, buspirone, FGAs, SGAs, atomoxetine, stimulants, dopamine agonists	14%–24% during SSRI treatment, at any time	Possibly older age, female sex; smoking; stress (in daytime > sleep bruxing); possible genetic vulnerability	No	Appliance therapy (bite guards); clonazepam 1 mg PO qHS; propranolol 60–160 mg/day (divided dosing in daytime bruxism); buspirone 10 mg bid–tid; L-Dopa 100 mg at bedtime then repeat 4 hours later; anecdotal: cyclobenzaprine 2.5–10 mg qHS, trazodone 150–200 mg qHS, divalproex 500 mg qHS, topiramate 25–100 mg qHS, hydroxyzine 10–25 mg qHS, metoclopramide 10–15 mg qHS, gabapentin 300 mg qHS

Adverse effect	Known causal drugs	Frequency and timing of occurrence	Known risk factors	Dose-related?	Monitoring and management options
Cutaneous reactions	All drugs	Rashes usually but do not necessarily occur early after initial drug exposure; serious rashes associated with lamotrigine typically occur within 2–8 weeks of drug initiation (incidence of 0.08% in clinical trials for bipolar disorder)	Lamotrigine: younger age, rapid dosing, concomitant use of divalproex without lamotrigine dosage reduction; aromatic > nonaromatic anticonvulsants (e.g., phenytoin, carbamazepine, oxcarbazepine)	Likely related to rate of dose escalation	Investigate non-drug-related causes of rash (e.g., contact dermatitis, acne rosacea, psoriasis); benign rashes often may be observed and treated with topical steroid creams and/or oral antihistamines; signs of systemic rash (e.g., fever, exfoliation, lymphadenopathy, blistering lesions) require prompt cessation of the suspected causal drug and dermatological evaluation

Adverse effect	Known causal drugs	Frequency and timing of occurrence	Known risk factors	Dose-related?	Monitoring and management options
Dystonia	FGAs, SGAs	Usually early in treatment	Possibly young age, male sex	No	Parenteral or oral diphenhydramine 50–100 mg; biperiden 1–5 mg IM; benztropine 1–2 mg; parenteral diazepam 5–10 mg
Hyperhidrosis	SSRIs	Up to 20% of patients taking antidepressants; may occur at any time	None known	No	Terazosin 1–2 mg/day; clonidine 0.1 mg/day; glycopyrrolate 1 mg qd–bid; oxybutynin 5–10 mg qd–tid

Adverse effect	Known causal drugs	Frequency and timing of occurrence	Known risk factors	Dose-related?	Monitoring and management options
Hyperpro-lactinemia	FGAs, SGAs; rarely: ramelteon, opiates, TCAs, fluoxetine, paroxetine, venlafaxine	Usually early in treatment	Tight D_2-binding drugs; FGAs>SGAs; women>men; premenopausal>postmenopausal; possibly DRD2*A1 variant of the D_2 receptor gene	Yes	Favor low-liability agents (e.g., aripip-razole, brexpiprazole, lurasidone); consider adjunctive amanta-dine, pramipexole, bromocriptine, ropinirole
Leukopenia	FGAs, SGAs, carbamazepine, divalproex, TCAs	May occur at any time. Reported incident rates: carbamazepine 2.1%; divalproex 0.4%; TCAs 0.3% (Tohen et al. 1995)	Possibly older age	Unknown	Monitor WBC count; discontinue suspected causal agent if deemed clinically significant or approaching neutropenia
Myocarditis	Clozapine	0.015%–0.188% incidence usually occurs within 4–8 weeks of treatment initiation	Rapid dose titration	Possibly	Discontinue suspected causal agent; possible use of beta-blockers, ACE inhibitors, diuretics

Adverse effect	Known causal drugs	Frequency and timing of occurrence	Known risk factors	Dose-related?	Monitoring and management options
Neuroleptic malignant ayndrome (NMS)	FGAs, SGAs; rarely, TCAs, lithium, phenelzine	0.01%–0.02% incidence; usually occurs within 1 week of drug initiation	Prior occurrence of NMS	Possibly	Discontinue suspected causal agent; hydration, cooling blankets, IV dantroline (1–2.5 mg/kg initially, followed by 1 mg/kg every 6 hours) if persistent fever/autonomic instability
Orthostatic hypotension	TCAs, α_1 agonists, FGAs, SGAs, MAOIs	Variable	Not established	MAOIs, some FGAs and SGAs	Assure normovolemia; fludrocortisone 0.1–0.2 mg/day (maximum dose= 0.4–0.6 mg/day); midodrine 5 mg tid

Adverse effect	Known causal drugs	Frequency and timing of occurrence	Known risk factors	Dose-related?	Monitoring and management options
Sedation/ Somnolence	Antihistaminergic agents, α_1 agonists, benzodiazepines, GABAergic anticonvulsants	Usually early in treatment; may not be transient	Varies by degree of antihistaminergic, anticholinergic, or α-agonism drug properties	Likely	Dosage reductions when feasible; minimize use of multiple sedating agents; adjunctive amphetamine, methylphenidate, (ar)modafinil as appropriate
Seizures	Bupropion, clozapine	Bupropion incidence 4/1,000	Bulimia, electrolyte abnormalities	Likely	Evaluate underlying seizure disorder; discontinue causal agent
Serotonin syndrome	Combinations of serotonergic agents	May have rapid onset when multiple serotonergic agents are used	Possibly CYP2D6 PMs	Unknown	Prompt discontinuation of suspected causal agents usually leads to resolution; supportive measures (e.g., hydration, clonazepam for myoclonus, cooling blankets), airway protection

Adverse effect	Known causal drugs	Frequency and timing of occurrence	Known risk factors	Dose-related?	Monitoring and management options
Sexual dysfunction	SSRIs, SNRIs, TCAs, MAOIs, most FGAs and SGAs	Usually early in treatment	Hyperprolactinemia; possibly *GRIA1*, *GRIA2*, *GRIN3A* genotypes	Likely	Assure absence of hyperprolactinemia; favor antidepressants with minimal risk (e.g., bupropion, mirtazapine, vortioxetine); PDE inhibitors, adjunctive bupropion, cyproheptadine, buspirone
SIADH	Serotonergic antidepressants	Reported incident rates of 0.1%–8% depending on agent, serum (Na$^+$) threshold, and age	Older age, women > men, low body weight, smoking, concomitant use of thiazide diuretics, ACE inhibitors, or laxatives	Unlikely	Discontinue serotonergic antidepressants; consider replacement with bupropion or mirtazapine if there is pressing need for an alternative antidepressant

Adverse effect	Known causal drugs	Frequency and timing of occurrence	Known risk factors	Dose-related?	Monitoring and management options
Sialorrhea	Clozapine; less often: olanzapine, risperidone, quetiapine	Occurs in 30%–80% of clozapine recipients	Possibly *DRD4* tandem duplication polymorphism in D$_4$ gene (clozapine-induced)	Unlikely	Sublingual atropine sulfate 1% ophthalmic solution 1–2 drops qhs, may increase to two to three times per day; ipratropium bromide 0.03% nasal spray, 2 sprays administered sublingually qhs, may increase to tid
Tardive dyskinesia	FGAs, SGAs, other antidopaminergics (e.g., prochlorperazine, metoclopramide)	≥3 months' cumulative exposure to antipsychotics or ≥1 month if >age 60 (American Psychiatric Association 2013)	Chronic D$_2$ blockade; age; dose; duration; affective disorder; prior EPS/akathisia; female sex; possibly Ser9Gly variant of the dopamine D$_3$ receptor gene *DRD3*	Likely	Valbenazine 40–80 mg/day; deutetrabenazine 6 mg/day up to 24 mg twice daily

Adverse effect	Known causal drugs	Frequency and timing of occurrence	Known risk factors	Dose-related?	Monitoring and management options
Thrombo-cytopenia	Divalproex, carbamazepine, SSRIs, clonazepam, diazepam	Considered a rare event; can occur at any time, but often within the first 1–3 weeks after drug initiation	Dose, serum (valproate), longer duration of use; may also reflect immune-mediated mechanisms	Yes	Reduce dose if feasible; discontinue if considered hemostatically dangerous
Tics	Psychostimulants; rarely, bupropion, some SSRIs, imipramine, lamotrigine, carbamazepine	Can occur at any time	Unknown	Unclear	Commonly exacerbated by stimulants; eliminating causal agents is preferred, although a modest database supports the use of alpha agonists (e.g., guanfacine 0.5–3.0 mg/day, clonidine 0.1–0.3 mg/day), FGAs and SGAs

Adverse effect	Known causal drugs	Frequency and timing of occurrence	Known risk factors	Dose-related?	Monitoring and management options
Tremor	Lithium, divalproex, SSRIs, TCAs, bupropion	*Lithium:* 4%–65% incidence; may occur immediately or months or years after initiation *Divalproex:* 6%–45% incidence, usually first 3–12 months *SSRIs and TCAs:* approximately 20% of patients, usually within first 1–2 months	Dose; age; male sex; excessive caffeine intake; anxiety; family history of tremor	Yes	Ensure absence of neurotoxicity; propranolol 10 mg bid or tid, increased as needed to maximum of 320 mg/day as tolerated; primidone 50–100 mg at bedtime—may increase as needed in 50- to 100-mg/day increments up to 250–500 mg/day in divided doses

Adverse effect	Known causal drugs	Frequency and timing of occurrence	Known risk factors	Dose-related?	Monitoring and management options
Urinary hesitancy/ retention	SNRIs, amphetamine, (ar)modafinil, α-agonists, dopamine agonists, opiates, benzodiazepines	Usually early in treatment or after dosage increases	Older age	Likely	Bethanechol 10–50 mg tid–qid may sometimes be helpful for urinary hesitancy; dosage reductions are empirically appropriate before discontinuing; acute urinary retention can quickly become a medical emergency requiring catheterization

Adverse effect	Known causal drugs	Frequency and timing of occurrence	Known risk factors	Dose-related?	Monitoring and management options
Weight gain	Some FGAs, most SGAs, lithium, divalproex, most SSRIs, most SNRIs, MAOIs, mirtazapine	SGAs often rapid and may persist for several months; other agents often more insidious	Rapid initial weight gain; younger age; nonwhite; female; low BMI	Likely	Nutriticnal counseling and exercise; weight gain due to appetite stimulation may be tempered via topiramate, zonisamide, amantadine, phentermine, amphetamine, methylphenidate; weight gain arising from insulin resistance (e.g., SGAs) may respond to metformin, liraglutide

Adverse effect	Known causal drugs	Frequency and timing of occurrence	Known risk factors	Dose-related?	Monitoring and management options
Xerostomia	Anticholinergic drugs, lithium	Usually early in treatment	Unknown	Possibly	Sugarless candies and saliva-stimulating glycerate-polymer gels and oral sprays; pilocarpine 5–10 mg one to three times per day; cevimeline 30 mg/day

Note. ACE=angiotensin-converting enzyme; bid=twice daily; BMI=body mass index; EPS=extrapyramidyl symptoms; FGA=first-generation antipsychotic; GABA=γ-aminobutyric acid; IM=intramuscular; IV=intravenous; MAOI=monoamine oxidase inhibitor; qd=once a day; qhs=every night at bedtime; qid=four times daily; PM=poor metabolizer; PO=by mouth; SGA=second-generation antipsychotic; SIADH=syndrome of inappropriate antidiuretic hormone secretion; SNRI=serotonin-norepinephrine reuptake inhibitor; SSRI=selective serotonin reuptake inhibitor; TCA=tricyclic antidepressant; tid=three times daily; WBC=white blood cell count.

APPENDIX 2

Self-Assessment Questions and Answers

Select the single best response for each question.

Questions

1. The rationale for using metformin to counteract psychotropically induced weight gain involves which of the following?

    A. Decreasing insulin sensitivity.
    B. Direct appetite suppression via the hypothalamic satiety center.
    C. Blockade of postsynaptic 5-HT$_{2C}$ receptors.
    D. Agonism of H$_1$ receptors.

2. Which *one* of the following statements about antidepressant-associated hyponatremia is *true*?

    A. Risk appears lower with mirtazapine or tricyclics than with other antidepressants.
    B. Risk appears lower with SNRIs than with SSRIs.
    C. SIADH during antidepressant therapy is more common in men < 65 years old.
    D. Replacement of one SSRI with another is likely to resolve the condition.

3. All of the following have been shown to potentially diminish or help manage SSRI-induced bruxism *except*

    A. Risperidone 0.25–0.5 mg at night.
    B. An acrylic dental bite guard.
    C. Buspirone 10 mg bid or tid.
    D. Clonazepam 1 mg at night.

4. Signs of lamotrigine toxicity include all of the following *except*

    A. Ataxia.
    B. Tremor.
    C. Downbeat nystagmus.
    D. Ventricular arrhythmia.

5. A medically healthy woman successfully treated for major depression with sertraline 150 mg/day complains of anorgasmia. Which of the following would be the most evidence-based intervention to help remedy her SSRI-associated sexual dysfunction?

    A. Adjunctive sildenafil 50–100 mg/day.
    B. Adjunctive buspirone 10 mg tid.
    C. Adjunctive mirtazapine 7.5–15 mg at night.
    D. Adjunctive methylphenidate 5–10 mg before sex.

6. Priapism has been associated with all of the following medications *except*

    A. Citalopram.
    B. Quetiapine.
    C. Divalproex.
    D. Trazodone.

7. A 28-year-old man with bipolar disorder and unintelligible speech presents to the medical emergency department with fever and blisters in his oropharynx and skin exfoliation on his palms and soles. All of the following would be consistent with his history *except*

    A. Presence of the *HLA-B*1502* allele.
    B. Han Chinese ancestry.
    C. Presently taking carbamazepine.
    D. Early age at onset of bipolar disorder.

8. Which of the following adverse drug effects commonly occurs early during treatment with escitalopram but is unlikely to spontaneously remit during continued therapy?

    A. Orgasmic dysfunction.
    B. Headache.
    C. Nausea.
    D. Dizziness.

9. A 32-year-old man with bipolar disorder has been taking topiramate 150 mg/day for 2 months in an effort to counteract a 13.5-kg weight gain caused by psychotropic drugs. He also has been following the Atkins diet, has begun a program of regular exercise, and has lost 5 kg in 3 weeks. He calls to report sharp lower back pain and blood-tinged urine. What is the likely formulation?

    A. Lumbosacral strain and probable myoglobinuria from excessive exercise; he should take an NSAID and, if no better in several days, contact his internist.
    B. Probable nephrolithiasis that may be caused by topiramate, compounded by hypocitraturia and hypercalciuria from his ketogenic diet; he should stop the topiramate and his Atkins diet, hydrate, and be evaluated for renal calculi.
    C. Unclear etiology; discontinue the topiramate and observe for several days.
    D. Likely nephrotic syndrome from possible drug-induced lupus.

10. You newly begin treating a 61-year-old man with bipolar disorder who is on a stable regimen of lithium carbonate 900 mg/day and divalproex 1,500 mg/day. His medical history is notable for asthma and diabetes. You notice a bilateral upper-extremity tremor that appears worse with movement and ask if it is new and whether it has previously been addressed. He remarks that he has noticed it for several years but his prior doctor never suggested any type of treatment. What would be the most appropriate next steps in management?

    A. Ignore the tremor if it does not bother the patient.
    B. Measure serum creatinine, lithium, and divalproex levels to assure that the tremor does not reflect toxicity.
    C. Begin propranolol 10 mg tid.
    D. Begin primidone 100 mg bid or tid.

11. Alopecia has been reported to occur with each of the following medications *except*

    A. Lithium carbonate.
    B. Carbamazepine.
    C. Fluoxetine.
    D. Modafinil.

12. Which of the following would be the most appropriate intervention for lower-extremity edema in an otherwise healthy 31-year-old woman with bipolar disorder who is psychiatrically stable on lithium monotherapy 900 mg/day with a 12-hour serum lithium level of 0.9 mEq/L?

    A. Amiloride 5 mg bid with monitoring of serum potassium.
    B. Hydrochlorothiazide 100 mg/day.
    C. Reduce lithium by 300 mg/day.
    D. Reduce salt intake and increase free water intake.

13. Paresthesias are commonly associated with which of the following anticonvulsants?

    A. Gabapentin.
    B. Topiramate.
    C. Oxcarbazepine.
    D. Lamotrigine.

14. Predictors of more severe adverse effects caused by placebo include all of the following *except*

    A. Hypochondriacal features.
    B. Phobic and obsessive traits.
    C. Severity of depression at baseline.
    D. High suggestibility and expectancy about treatment outcomes.

15. Patients who identify side-effect burden as a reason for poor adherence to psychotropic medications have been shown from research studies to have all of the following characteristics *except*

    A. Female sex.
    B. High baseline somatization.
    C. Psychosis.
    D. Younger age.

16. Interventions that may help to manage dry mouth caused by anticholinergic drugs include all of the following *except*

    A. Glycopyrrolate 1 mg bid.
    B. Pilocarpine 20 mg/day.
    C. Carboxymethyl cellulose solution.
    D. Cevimeline 30 mg/day.

17. A 23-year-old psychotropically naive South African black woman presents for treatment of social anxiety and generalized anxiety disorder. She identifies herself as being "especially sensitive" to side effects in general and asks that you prescribe "the lowest possible dose" of any medication you think appropriate. One week after beginning paroxetine at 10 mg/day, she calls to complain of severe nausea, headaches, and dizziness, and asks for your guidance. What is your impression and recommendation?

    A. Her anxiety is likely exacerbating her sensitivity to side effects; encourage her to stay with the medication at this dose to overcome the very problem for which she is seeking treatment.
    B. Suspect that her adherence is spotty and she is having withdrawal symptoms; emphasize to her the importance of regular daily dosing and full adherence.
    C. Recognize that she has a 1 in 5 likelihood of being a poor CYP2D6 metabolizer and is probably supratherapeutic on a paroxetine dose of 10 mg/day; advise her to lower the dose to 5 mg/day and reassess after several days.
    D. Declare her a "negative therapeutic reactor" and refer her for more intensive psychotherapy.

18. A 24-year-old man with treatment-resistant depression is taking a regimen of pramipexole 2.5 mg/day, lisdexamfetamine 60 mg/day, vortioxetine 10 mg/day, and bupropion XL 300 mg/day. He reports several episodes of almost falling asleep at the wheel while driving. Which of the following would be the *most* appropriate next step in his evaluation and treatment?

    A. Increase his lisdexamfetamine to 70 mg/day.
    B. Add armodafinil 150 mg/day to his regimen.
    C. Discontinue pramipexole.
    D. Measure a serum vortioxetine level to determine if it is supratherapeutic due to a drug interaction with bupropion.

19. In studies of aripiprazole for adults with schizophrenia, which of the following adverse effects demonstrated a dose relationship?

    A. Sedation or somnolence.
    B. Extrapyramidal adverse effects.
    C. Akathisia.
    D. Nausea.

20. All of the following statements regarding skin rashes associated with lamotrigine are true *except*

    A. Rapid dose escalation is a known risk factor for the emergence of serious rashes.
    B. Systemic steroids are sometimes used to treat serious rashes soon after their emergence.
    C. Lamotrigine should always be immediately discontinued whenever any skin rash emerges.
    D. Cotherapy with divalproex may increase the risk of rash because divalproex inhibits the Phase II hepatic metabolism of lamotrigine.

21. Identified risk factors for the development of type 2 diabetes during treatment with SSRIs include which of the following?

    A. High baseline body mass index.
    B. Lengthy exposure and high dosing.
    C. Severity of depression symptoms.
    D. Atypical depressive symptoms.

22. Sexual dysfunction has been shown to be a dose-related phenomenon with all of the following medications *except*

    A. Fluoxetine.
    B. Citalopram.
    C. Venlafaxine.
    D. Risperidone.

23. All of the following are more common in women than men *except*

    A. Higher rates of anorgasmia from SSRIs.
    B. Greater risk for SSRI-associated osteoporosis.

    C. More extensive hyperprolactinemia from antipsychotic med-
       ications.

    D. Higher risk of weight gain from olanzapine or risperidone.

24. Which of the following adverse drug effects is usually a transient
    phenomenon?

    A. Cognitive impairment associated with topiramate.
    B. Tremor associated with divalproex.
    C. Sexual dysfunction during SSRI therapy.
    D. Nausea associated with SSRI initiation.

25. Which of the following physical signs would be useful in differen-
    tiating serotonin syndrome from NMS?

    A. Tremor.
    B. Clonus.
    C. Muscle rigidity.
    D. Fever.

26. Differences between valbenazine and tetrabenazine include all of the
    following *except*

    A. VMAT2 inhibition is irreversible with tetrabenazine but re-
       versible with valbenazine

    B. Tetrabenazine must be dosed more frequently than valbenazine
       because of its shorter half-life.

    C. Valbenazine's predominant metabolite, $[\alpha]$-+-dihydrotetra-
       benazine, has minimal binding affinity at D_1 and D_2 receptors,
       whereas tetrabenazine's multiple active metabolites include
       some with high D_1 and D_2 binding affinities.

    D. Depression and suicidality have not been observed as adverse
       effects in clinical trials of valbenazine, in contrast to tetrabena-
       zine.

27. Which of the following agents has demonstrated over a 5-kg weight
    loss as compared with placebo over 16 weeks in overweight, predia-
    betic patients taking olanzapine or clozapine?

    A. Metformin.
    B. Topiramate.
    C. Liraglutide.
    D. Bupropion.

28. Which of the following statements is *true* for a 38-year-old male non-smoker with schizophrenia who is about to start taking clozapine 200 mg/day and whose pooled cohort risk equation score is 7.5%?

    A. The potential benefits of taking an SGA with high metabolic risk are outweighed by his relatively high risk for a heart attack in the next 10 years.
    B. He has a 92.5% risk of having an MI before age 65.
    C. His score of 7.5% warrants cotherapy with a statin, especially if he is about to begin clozapine.
    D. His risk of a heart attack in the next 10 years is no greater than would be expected for anyone else of his age and sex, posing little increased baseline risk if he begins an SGA that has high metabolic risk.

29. Which of the following SGAs carries the lowest risk for QTc prolongation?

    A. Aripiprazole.
    B. Iloperidone.
    C. Ziprasidone.
    D. Quetiapine.

30. Improvement in dimensions of cognitive functioning in euthymic bipolar disorder patients has been demonstrated in randomized trials with all of the following agents *except*

    A. Lurasidone.
    B. *Withania somnifera.*
    C. Pramipexole.
    D. Divalproex.

31. Logical strategies to manage nausea associated with vortioxetine include all the following *except*

    A. Dosage reductions.
    B. Adjunctive ondansetron 4–8 mg orally once or twice daily as needed.
    C. Adjunctive trimethobenzamide 300 mg orally every 4–6 hours as needed.
    D. Adjunctive prochlorperazine 10 mg orally every 4–6 hours as needed.

32. Evidence-based strategies to minimize the risk for renal insufficiency during long-term lithium therapy include which one of the following?

    A. Once-per-day lithium dosing.
    B. Three-times-per-day lithium dosing.
    C. Use of lithium citrate rather than lithium carbonate.
    D. Favoring serum lithium levels no higher than 0.9 mEq/L when clinically feasible.

33. Pharmacogenetic testing reveals that a 24-year-old white man with major depression and comorbid attention-deficit disorder is a CYP450 2D6 slow metabolizer. Usual maximal dosing should be halved for all of the following drugs *except*

    A. Mixed amphetamine salts.
    B. Citalopram.
    C. Venlafaxine.
    D. Vortioxetine.

34. A 37-year-old man with stable schizoaffective disorder and a history of akathisia on previous low doses of antipsychotics is taking iloperidone 8 mg twice daily, divalproex 1,000 mg/day, vilazodone 40 mg/day, and primidone 100 mg/day for tremor. His internist also prescribes him celecoxib 200 mg/day for chronic back pain as well as hydroxyzine 50 mg/day and medical marijuana (cannabidiol) for anxiety. He has been complaining of palpitations, and his internist obtains an ECG, which shows a QTc of 493 msec. Alarmed, the internist calls you and demands that you immediately stop the patient's iloperidone altogether. Why might this intervention be unnecessary?

    A. The vilazodone is likely raising levels of iloperidone and should be stopped.
    B. The primidone is likely raising levels of iloperidone and should be stopped.
    C. Iloperidone levels could be elevated by celecoxib, hydroxyzine, and cannabidiol, and consideration should be given to stopping those prescriptions if they are not essential.
    D. Divalproex is likely raising levels of iloperidone, and a stat valproic acid level should be checked to rule out valproate toxicity.

35. A 54-year-old African American male with sickle cell trait has been started on escitalopram 10 mg/day for major depression. He complains of anorgasmia and diminished libido. Which one of the following would be the safest evidence-based strategy to counteract this problem?

   A. Add bupropion.
   B. Add sildenafil.
   C. Add trazodone.
   D. Add vardenafil.

36. A 28-year-old married woman with a history of two prior depressive episodes is now 36 weeks pregnant. She had been taking sertraline consistently since it was begun for postpartum depression after the birth of her first child 3 years earlier. Her obstetrician advised her to taper off the medication before delivery in order to avert withdrawal in the newborn. She now seeks a second opinion about her pharmacotherapy. Which one of the following would you likely do?

   A. Agree with her obstetrician that it is wisest to discontinue an SSRI before delivery so as to minimize the risk for neonatal abstinence syndrome.
   B. Tell her that in the unlikely event neonatal abstinence syndrome occurs, it carries a high chance that the baby would require admission to a neonatal intensive care unit and possible endotracheal intubation, but her risk for a recurrence of postpartum depression by stopping sertraline clearly outweighs the possibility of severe withdrawal in the newborn.
   C. Tell her that neonatal abstinence syndrome in the newborn is usually a mild, transient phenomenon occurring only in about a third of women who take an SSRI during pregnancy, but if it occurs it is typically self-limited and requires no special intervention.
   D. Switch the patient's medication now from sertraline to fluoxetine preemptively to minimize the chances of SSRI discontinuation in the newborn.

37. A 41-year-old man with bipolar disorder well controlled on lithium carbonate is training to run a marathon. His primary care doctor noticed that his serum creatinine had recently increased from its usual level of about 0.9 ng/dL to 1.1 ng/dL and is concerned about the rise of

>20% in just 3 months. His lithium level remains steady at 0.7 mEq/L. The patients says he drinks "tons of water." He has now been sent to his psychiatrist with the request that the lithium be stopped and another drug used instead. Which one of the following would be the most appropriate response by the psychiatrist?

A. While preparing for the marathon, advise the patient that he probably is nevertheless dehydrated despite his assumptions to the contrary, and advise him just to increase his fluid intake even further before making any changes to his regimen.

B. Discontinue the lithium over a 2-week period because of the sudden deterioration in his renal function, and cross-taper to divalproex.

C. Measure a serum cystatin C from which to recalculate his estimated glomerular filtration rate (eGFR).

D. Reassure both the patient and the primary care doctor that a serum creatinine of 1.1 ng/dL is still well within the usual normal reference range, and advise just rechecking it again in a month or two.

38. A 29-year-old man with bipolar II disorder and comorbid generalized anxiety disorder takes lithium 900 mg/day and gabapentin 600 mg/day and complains of feeling sedated. His psychotherapist suggested to him that he may have a "slow metabolism" and ought to ask you to please order a phamacogenetic test on him to affirm this. You smile politely and gently state your opinion that pharmacogenetic testing would have no value in this instance. Why?

A. Lithium can cause sedation at a usual dose such as his, and it would be more prudent to check a serum lithium level to make sure that his complaints of sedation do not reflect lithium neurotoxicity.

B. Gabapentin can cause sedation at a usual dose such as his, and one could consider whether a lower dose would be better tolerated.

C. Neither lithium nor gabapentin undergoes hepatic metabolism.

D. All of the above.

39. This same psychotherapist calls you about another female patient with bipolar II disorder on an oral contraceptive who takes lamotrigine 150 mg/day and is clinically stable but feels slight cognitive dulling. The patient obtained pharmacogenetic testing from her current

psychiatrist, who determined that she is a CYP450 2D6 poor metabolizer, and the psychotherapist is concerned the lamotrigine may, for the patient, be supratherapeutically dosed. What would you advise?

A. Suggest measuring a serum lamotrigine level to determine if it is in the toxic range.
B. Obtain neuropsychological testing to document the nature and extent of possible cognitive deficits.
C. Gently state your opinion that the pharmacogenetic testing results are not relevant.
D. Tell her that the oral contraceptive is probably inhibiting the metabolism of lamotrigine and causing a supratherapeutic dosing effect, for which a lower lamotrigine dose may be worth considering.

40. A 44-year-old man with binge-eating disorder, generalized anxiety disorder, obesity, and hypercholesterolemia is taking lisdexamfetamine 60 mg/day, topiramate 100 mg/day, fluoxetine 40 mg/day, and atorvastatin 40 mg/day. He calls to complain of leg pains. He also feels his panic attacks are becoming worse and says he sometimes finds it harder to breathe comfortably. He is afebrile, has a clear sensorium, and denies feeling stiff when asked by telephone. A serum CK level, ordered 2 days earlier by the patient's internist, was 236 IU/L (normal reference range is 60–174 IU/L). BUN and creatinine are within the normal reference range. Which one of the following is the most plausible explanation for his symptom?

A. Statin-induced myositis.
B. Neuroleptic malignant syndrome.
C. Serotonin syndrome.
D. Acute rhabdomyolysis likely secondary to myotoxicity.

41. A patient who demonstrates myoclonic jerking movements would be suspected of having any of the following *except*

A. Serotonin syndrome.
B. Epilepsy.
C. Lithium toxicity.
D. An adverse effect of levetiracetam.

42. An 83-year-old normotensive man with chronic depression that has been well controlled with sertraline 100 mg/day for the past 6 months

presents with somnolence and confusion. He has no recent gastro-intestinal complaints. Which one of the following interventions would be the *most useful* in the diagnosis and management of his acute mental status change?

A. Obtain serum electrolytes.
B. Obtain a serum sertraline level.
C. Switch from generic sertraline to brand name Zoloft.
D. Augment his regimen with a low-dose stimulant to help over-come sedation and possible cognitive dulling from sertraline.

43. A patient with multi-drug-resistant major depression responds well to tranylcypromine 60 mg/day plus aripiprazole 5 mg/day. He complains of dizziness and lightheadedness on standing and has ortho-static blood pressure changes on examination. All of the following interventions would be appropriate *except*

A. Cautiously lower the tranylcypromine dose to see if the anti-depressant response is retained at a lower dose, because or-thostatic hypotension from MAOIs can be dose-dependent.
B. Discontinue the aripiprazole as the probable cause of the or-thostatic hypotension because of its α_1 antagonism.
C. Begin oral midodrine 5 mg three times per day.
D. Begin oral fludrocortisone 0.1 mg/day.

44. The second-generation antipsychotic with the least likelihood for causing weight gain in schizophrenia, based on short-term clinical trials, is which of the following?

A. Ziprasidone.
B. Iloperidone.
C. Asenapine.
D. Lurasidone.

45. A 51-year-old man with schizoaffective disorder has been stabi-lized on clozapine 250 mg/day recently augmented with armodaf-inil 150 mg/day to counteract sedation, sublingual atropine sulfate 1% solution for sialorrhea, and divalproex sodium 500 mg/day tar-geting irritability and affective instability. At routine follow-up, he presents with persistent sedation and new gait instability and dizzi-ness. What is the most likely explanation for these symptoms?

A. Likely additive general side-effect burden of clozapine plus divalproex; check a serum valproate level to ensure it is not toxic and possibly lower the divalproex dose, or else possibly increase the armodafinil dose to promote greater wakefulness effect.

B. Systemic vagolytic effects caused by systemic absorption of sublingual atropine.

C. Increase in serum clozapine levels due to pharmacokinetic inhibition caused by modafinil.

D. Increase in serum clozapine levels due to pharmacokinetic inhibition caused by divalproex.

46. A 24-year-old obese man with major depression has been treated with duloxetine 120 mg/day, lithium carbonate 900 mg/day, and topiramate 100 mg/day. For the past 3 years, he has also used a specially compounded intranasal formulation of ketamine four to five times a week. In the course of his initial evaluation, he mentions having frequent urination, nocturia, and occasional suprapubic pain. Which of the following is the *least likely* iatrogenic explanation for his urinary complaints?

A. Ulcerative cystitis.

B. Nephrogenic diabetes insipidus.

C. Renal calculus.

D. Urinary retention.

47. All of the following medications can be associated with anticholinergic (antimuscarinic or antinicotinic) adverse effects *except*

A. Carbamazepine.

B. Paroxetine.

C. Atomoxetine.

D. Bupropion.

48. A single-agent overdose of which of the following medications would *least expectably* be associated with fatality?

A. 8,000 mg of divalproex in an 84-kg male.

B. 27,000 mg of lithium carbonate in a 75-kg male.

C. 240 mg of dextroamphetamine in an 80-kg male.

D. 49,000 mg of gabapentin in a 62-kg female.

49. A 46-year-old Vietnamese man has for over 3 years been taking lamotrigine 400 mg/day for bipolar II disorder and carbamazepine 600 mg/day for trigeminal neuralgia. He presents with an itchy, tingling, burning, rather linear rash, of 1 week's duration, with some crusting running from below the midline base of his rib cage across his trunk. There is no fever and no oropharyngeal lesions. Which of the following would be the most appropriate next step in his assessment and management?

    A. Obtain pharmacogenetic testing to determine the presence of the DQB1*06:02 gene.
    B. Immediately discontinue both lamotrigine and carbamazepine.
    C. Recommend an as-needed nonsteroidal anti-inflammatory drug for pain but otherwise do nothing.
    D. Recommend an oral antihistamine such as diphenhydramine 50 mg every 6 hours and a topical over-the-counter steroid cream.

50. A 17-year-old male with a suspected drug overdose presents to an emergency department with fever, vomiting, muscle twitching, sweating, tachycardia, and mydriasis. If this presentation occurred from a single-agent toxicity, which of the following would be the *most likely* causal agent?

    A. Lorazepam.
    B. Methylphenidate.
    C. Buspirone.
    D. Mirtazapine.

Answer Guide

1. The rationale for using metformin to counteract psychotropically induced weight gain involves which of the following?

    A. Decreasing insulin sensitivity.
    B. Direct appetite suppression via the hypothalamic satiety center.
    C. Blockade of postsynaptic 5-HT$_{2C}$ receptors.
    D. Agonism of H$_1$ receptors.

The correct response is option A.

Metformin is thought to promote weight loss by decreasing insulin sensitivity. None of the other answers is a correct or plausible explanation for its presumed mechanism of action.

2. Which *one* of the following statements about antidepressant-associated hyponatremia is *true*?

> A. Risk appears lower with mirtazapine or tricyclics than with other antidepressants.
> B. Risk appears lower with SNRIs than with SSRIs.
> C. SIADH during antidepressant therapy is more common in men < 65 years old.
> D. Replacement of one SSRI with another is likely to resolve the condition.

The correct response is option A.

Mirtazapine and tricyclic antidepressants appear to have a somewhat lesser risk for causing hyponatremia or SIADH as compared with other antidepressant classes. Risk appears comparable between SSRIs and SNRIs, and replacing one SSRI with another is unlikely to resolve the abnormality. Age > 65 and female sex are both known risk factors for antidepressant-associated hyponatremia.

3. All of the following have been shown to potentially diminish or help manage SSRI-induced bruxism *except*

> A. Risperidone 0.25–0.5 mg at night.
> B. An acrylic dental bite guard.
> C. Buspirone 10 mg bid or tid.
> D. Clonazepam 1 mg at night.

The correct response is option A.

Risperidone, by virtue of its relatively "tight" binding affinity at the D_2 receptor, carries a substantial risk for movement disorders. Bruxism has been conceptualized within the literature as both a non–rapid-eye-movement sleep disorder as well as a movement disorder and, as such, would likely not be aided by the introduction of a dopamine antagonist. By contrast, each of the remaining choices is an evidence-based strategy used to counteract bruxism.

4. Signs of lamotrigine toxicity include all of the following *except*

    A. Ataxia.
    B. Tremor.
    C. Downbeat nystagmus.
    D. Ventricular arrhythmia.

The correct response is option D.

Lamotrigine toxicity has not been shown to include cardiac arrhythmia, but may include ataxia, tremor, and downbeat nystagmus.

5. A medically healthy woman successfully treated for major depression with sertraline 150 mg/day complains of anorgasmia. Which of the following would be the most evidence-based intervention to help remedy her SSRI-associated sexual dysfunction?

    A. Adjunctive sildenafil 50–100 mg/day.
    B. Adjunctive buspirone 10 mg tid.
    C. Adjunctive mirtazapine 7.5–15 mg at night.
    D. Adjunctive methylphenidate 5–10 mg before sex.

The correct response is option A.

The safety and efficacy of sildenafil for SSRI-induced sexual dysfunction in both men and women is supported by a large-scale randomized placebo-controlled trial, demonstrating significantly improved ability to achieve orgasm and greater quality of orgasm, but no significant improvements in desire, arousal-sensation, or arousal-lubrication (Nurnberg et al. 2008). None of the other agents listed has robust data from placebo-controlled trials involving women.

6. Priapism has been associated with all of the following medications *except*

    A. Citalopram.
    B. Quetiapine.
    C. Divalproex.
    D. Trazodone.

The correct response is option C.

Priapism has rarely been reported in connection with the use of citalopram, quetiapine, and trazodone, but not with divalproex.

7. A 28-year-old man with bipolar disorder and unintelligible speech presents to the medical emergency department with fever and blisters in his oropharynx and skin exfoliation on his palms and soles. All of the following would be consistent with his history *except*

    A. Presence of the *HLA-B*1502* allele.
    B. Han Chinese ancestry.
    C. Presently taking carbamazepine.
    D. Early age at onset of bipolar disorder.

The correct response is option D.

The clinical presentation of a severe cutaneous reaction is most consistent with Stevens-Johnson syndrome due to carbamazepine, with heightened risk in an individual of Han Chinese ancestry who carries the *HLA-B*1502* allele. Indeed, the FDA boxed warning for carbamazepine specifically advises genotyping for the *HLA-B*1502* allelic variant of the *HLA-B* gene among high-risk Asian individuals prior to beginning treatment with carbamazepine, because this risk allele confers increased susceptibility to serious dermatological reactions with carbamazepine. Historical age at onset of bipolar disorder in an adult is extraneous to developing a drug-induced dermatological reaction.

8. Which of the following adverse drug effects commonly occurs early during treatment with escitalopram but is unlikely to spontaneously remit during continued therapy?

    A. Orgasmic dysfunction.
    B. Headache.
    C. Nausea.
    D. Dizziness.

The correct response is option A.

Sexual dysfunction associated with SSRIs has rarely been shown to attenuate with time. By contrast, headache, nausea, and dizziness are common initial adverse effects of SSRIs that usually diminish with time.

9. A 32-year-old man with bipolar disorder has been taking topira-
    mate 150 mg/day for 2 months in an effort to counteract a 13.5-kg
    weight gain caused by psychotropic drugs. He also has been follow-
    ing the Atkins diet, has begun a program of regular exercise, and
    has lost 5 kg in 3 weeks. He calls to report sharp lower back pain and
    blood-tinged urine. What is the likely formulation?

    A. Lumbosacral strain and probable myoglobinuria from exces-
       sive exercise; he should take an NSAID and, if no better in sev-
       eral days, contact his internist.
    B. Probable nephrolithiasis that may be caused by topiramate,
       compounded by hypocitraturia and hypercalciuria from his
       ketogenic diet; he should stop the topiramate and his Atkins
       diet, hydrate, and be evaluated for renal calculi.
    C. Unclear etiology; discontinue the topiramate and observe for
       several days.
    D. Likely nephrotic syndrome from possible drug-induced lupus.

    The correct response is option B.

    Topiramate has an approximate 1% incidence of causing kidney
    stones. A high-protein, ketogenic diet can increase renal calcium
    excretion, further increasing his risk for the formation of calcium
    oxalate renal calculi.

10. You newly begin treating a 61-year-old man with bipolar disorder
    who is on a stable regimen of lithium carbonate 900 mg/day and di-
    valproex 1,500 mg/day. His medical history is notable for asthma and
    diabetes. You notice a bilateral upper-extremity tremor that appears
    worse with movement and ask if it is new and whether it has previ-
    ously been addressed. He remarks that he has noticed it for several
    years but his prior doctor never suggested any type of treatment.
    What would be the most appropriate next steps in management?

    A. Ignore the tremor if it does not bother the patient.
    B. Measure serum creatinine, lithium, and divalproex levels to
       assure that the tremor does not reflect toxicity.
    C. Begin propranolol 10 mg tid.
    D. Begin primidone 100 mg bid or tid.

    The correct response is option B.

Tremors associated with either lithium carbonate or divalproex may be dose-related phenomena; an older adult with diabetes may have decreased renal clearance of both drugs, and the tremor should first be assessed as an indicator of possible toxicity. In the absence of an underlying toxicity, treatment of the tremor with propranolol would be ill advised in the setting of asthma due to the potential for beta blockade to aggravate pulmonary function. Primidone may represent a more viable pharmacological remedy for the tremor, but only after an assessment for neurotoxicity has occurred.

11. Alopecia has been reported to occur with each of the following medications *except*

    A. Lithium carbonate.
    B. Carbamazepine.
    C. Fluoxetine.
    D. Modafinil.

The correct response is option D.

Modafinil has not been associated with alopecia, unlike each of the other choices.

12. Which of the following would be the most appropriate intervention for lower-extremity edema in an otherwise healthy 31-year-old woman with bipolar disorder who is psychiatrically stable on lithium monotherapy 900 mg/day with a 12-hour serum lithium level of 0.9 mEq/L?

    A. Amiloride 5 mg bid with monitoring of serum potassium.
    B. Hydrochlorothiazide 100 mg/day.
    C. Reduce lithium by 300 mg/day.
    D. Reduce salt intake and increase free water intake.

The correct response is option A.

The potassium-sparing diuretic amiloride is often used to treat edema caused by lithium. Hydrochlorothiazide incurs a greater risk for causing elevation of serum lithium levels. Reduction of oral lithium dose is unlikely to alter the presence of peripheral edema. Reduction of salt intake would be expected to cause increased reabsorption of lithium by the kidney, resulting in elevated serum lithium levels without remediation of fluid overload and extravasation of fluid in lower extremities.

13. Paresthesias are commonly associated with which of the following anticonvulsants?

    A. Gabapentin.
    B. Topiramate.
    C. Oxcarbazepine.
    D. Lamotrigine.

The correct response is option B.

Paresthesias occur with topiramate in about one-third to one-half of patients at dosages of 50–200 mg/day. They are not associated with the other drug choices listed.

14. Predictors of more severe adverse effects caused by placebo include all of the following *except*

    A. Hypochondriacal features.
    B. Phobic and obsessive traits.
    C. Severity of depression at baseline.
    D. High suggestibility and expectancy about treatment outcomes.

The correct response is option C.

Greater severity of depression at baseline is typically associated with a *lower* rate of either benefits or adverse effects with placebo, whereas each of the other choices has been linked with a higher incidence of nocebo effects.

15. Patients who identify side-effect burden as a reason for poor adherence to psychotropic medications have been shown from research studies to have all of the following characteristics *except*

    A. Female sex.
    B. High baseline somatization.
    C. Psychosis.
    D. Younger age.

The correct response is option A.

Gender has not been implicated as a contributor to the link between medication adherence and drug side-effect burden. In the 2000 British National Psychiatric Morbidity Survey, individuals who linked treatment adherence with medication side-effect burden were of younger age, had a history of psychosis, and had lower intellectual functioning. Other reports have found that depressed patients who have prematurely dropped out of antidepressant clinical trials due to perceived adverse effects were more likely to have baseline somatic preoccupations.

16. Interventions that may help to manage dry mouth caused by anticholinergic drugs include all of the following *except*

  A. Glycopyrrolate 1 mg bid.
  B. Pilocarpine 20 mg/day.
  C. Carboxymethyl cellulose solution.
  D. Cevimeline 30 mg/day.

The correct response is option A.

Glycopyrrolate 1 mg bid has been shown to improve sialorrhea (not xerostomia) caused by several SGAs. Each of the other interventions has been reported as a potential remedy for dry mouth caused by anticholinergic drugs.

17. A 23-year-old psychotropically naive South African black woman presents for treatment of social anxiety and generalized anxiety disorder. She identifies herself as being "especially sensitive" to side effects in general and asks that you prescribe "the lowest possible dose" of any medication you think appropriate. One week after beginning paroxetine at 10 mg/day, she calls to complain of severe nausea, headaches, and dizziness, and asks for your guidance. What is your impression and recommendation?

  A. Her anxiety is likely exacerbating her sensitivity to side effects; encourage her to stay with the medication at this dose to overcome the very problem for which she is seeking treatment.
  B. Suspect that her adherence is spotty and she is having withdrawal symptoms; emphasize to her the importance of regular daily dosing and full adherence.
  C. Recognize that she has a 1 in 5 likelihood of being a poor CYP2D6 metabolizer and is probably supratherapeutic on a

paroxetine dose of 10 mg/day; advise her to lower the dose to 5 mg/day and reassess after several days.

   D. Declare her a "negative therapeutic reactor" and refer her for more intensive psychotherapy.

The correct response is option C.

South African blacks have a high incidence of the CYP2D6 poor metabolizer genotype (~29%) and therefore may be especially sensitive to adverse effects of drugs that are substrates for this enzyme (which include many psychotropic medications, including paroxetine).

18. A 24-year-old man with treatment-resistant depression is taking a regimen of pramipexole 2.5 mg/day, lisdexamfetamine 60 mg/day, vortioxetine 10 mg/day, and bupropion XL 300 mg/day. He reports several episodes of almost falling asleep at the wheel while driving. Which of the following would be the *most* appropriate next step in his evaluation and treatment?

   A. Increase his lisdexamfetamine to 70 mg/day.
   B. Add armodafinil 150 mg/day to his regimen.
   C. Discontinue pramipexole.
   D. Measure a serum vortioxetine level to determine if it is supratherapeutic due to a drug interaction with bupropion.

The correct response is option C.

An argument could be made to pursue any of the listed choices; however, because pramipexole can idiosyncratically cause sleep attacks at any time and without a clear dose-response relationship, its discontinuation is the safest and wisest immediate next step. Increasing the patient's dose of lisdexamfetamine and/or augmenting with armodafinil might help to counter iatrogenic sedation or somnolence, but such an approach is not established to prevent sleep attacks. Bupropion could increase serum vortioxetine levels by virtue of CYP2D6 inhibition; however, vortioxetine toxicity would more expectably result in gastrointestinal symptoms and general CNS depression rather than sudden sleep attacks. Moreover, in the setting of CYP2D6 inhibition (either due to coadministration with a CYP2D6 inhibitor such as bupropion or when the patient is a CYP2D6 poor metabolizer), the manufacturer advises maximal dosing of 5–10 mg/day—hence, supratherapeutic effects of vortioxetine in the present case would be unexpected.

19. In studies of aripiprazole for adults with schizophrenia, which of the following adverse effects demonstrated a dose relationship?

    A. Sedation or somnolence.
    B. Extrapyramidal adverse effects.
    C. Akathisia.
    D. Nausea.

The correct response is option A.

In both adult and pediatric trials of aripiprazole for schizophrenia (as well as adult trials in acute bipolar mania), sedation or somnolence was more prominent at higher than lower doses. No other adverse effects showed a dose relationship in adult schizophrenia studies. Extrapyramidal side effects and akathisia appeared to be dose related in registration trials of aripiprazole in patients with acute bipolar mania and in adolescents with schizophrenia.

20. All of the following statements regarding skin rashes associated with lamotrigine are true *except*

    A. Rapid dose escalation is a known risk factor for the emergence of serious rashes.
    B. Systemic steroids are sometimes used to treat serious rashes soon after their emergence.
    C. Lamotrigine should always be immediately discontinued whenever any skin rash emerges.
    D. Cotherapy with divalproex may increase the risk of rash because divalproex inhibits the Phase II hepatic metabolism of lamotrigine.

The correct response is option C.

Rashes that arise during treatment with lamotrigine, as well as other anticonvulsants, should be carefully evaluated. Serious rashes are most likely to occur between weeks 2–8 of treatment and are associated with rapid dose escalations, coadministration with divalproex, and use in children and adolescents (although the latter two parameters are not contraindications to lamotrigine therapy). Rashes that cannot likely be explained by other causes (e.g., acne rosacea, contact dermatitis) or those that involve soft mucocutaneous tissues generally should prompt immediate discontinuation of the drug. Prescribers

should exercise clinical judgment, which may include dermatological consultation, when deciding about the clinical significance of a
rash, its likely association with lamotrigine or other etiologies, and
the necessity of drug cessation.

21. Identified risk factors for the development of type 2 diabetes during
    treatment with SSRIs include which of the following?

    A. High baseline body mass index.
    B. Lengthy exposure and high dosing.
    C. Severity of depression symptoms.
    D. Atypical depressive symptoms.

    The correct response is option B.

    Studies of relative risk for developing type 2 diabetes in association
    with SSRI use have found a lower risk in patients with shorter drug
    exposure and the use of lower doses. None of the other characteris-
    tics listed has been linked with SSRI-associated type 2 diabetes.

22. Sexual dysfunction has been shown to be a dose-related phenome-
    non with all of the following medications *except*

    A. Fluoxetine.
    B. Citalopram.
    C. Venlafaxine.
    D. Risperidone.

    The correct response is option A.

    No clear dose relationship has been found between sexual drug side
    effects and fluoxetine, in contrast to demonstrated dose-related sex-
    ual dysfunction with citalopram, venlafaxine, and risperidone.

23. All of the following are more common in women than men *except*

    A. Higher rates of anorgasmia from SSRIs.
    B. Greater risk for SSRI-associated osteoporosis.
    C. More extensive hyperprolactinemia from antipsychotic med-
       ications.
    D. Higher risk of weight gain from olanzapine or risperidone.

    The correct response is option B.

The potential for bone demineralization and osteoporosis attributable to SSRIs appears to be similar in men and women. Each of the other statements regarding gender differences is true.

24. Which of the following adverse drug effects is usually a transient phenomenon?

    A. Cognitive impairment associated with topiramate.
    B. Tremor associated with divalproex.
    C. Sexual dysfunction during SSRI therapy.
    D. Nausea associated with SSRI initiation.

The correct response is option D.

Nausea is a common, typically transient occurrence after beginning treatment with an SSRI. Adverse cognitive effects associated with topiramate are diverse and may include attentional deficits, memory impairment, word-finding difficulties, impaired verbal and nonverbal fluency, psychomotor slowing, and delayed processing speed, sometimes thought to be dose dependent, and usually persistent until treatment is discontinued. Tremor is often a dose-related phenomenon associated with the use of divalproex.

25. Which of the following physical signs would be useful in differentiating serotonin syndrome from NMS?

    A. Tremor.
    B. Clonus.
    C. Muscle rigidity.
    D. Fever.

The correct response is option B.

Clonus is associated with serotonin syndrome but not NMS. Muscle rigidity, fever, and tremor may occur in either syndrome.

26. Differences between valbenazine and tetrabenazine include all of the following *except*

    A. VMAT2 inhibition is irreversible with tetrabenazine but reversible with valbenazine.
    B. Tetrabenazine must be dosed more frequently than valbenazine because of its shorter half-life.

    C. Valbenazine's predominant metabolite, $[\alpha]$-+-dihydrotetra-
       benazine, has minimal binding affinity at D_1 and D_2 receptors,
       whereas tetrabenazine's multiple active metabolites include
       some with high D_1 and D_2 binding affinities.
    D. Depression and suicidality have not been observed as adverse
       effects in clinical trials of valbenazine, in contrast to tetra-
       benazine.

The correct response is option A.

Both tetrabenazine and valbenazine (as well as deutetrabenazine)
are reversible VMAT2 inhibitors. Reserpine, by contrast, irreversibly
inhibits VMAT2. The other responses are all correct. Tetrabenazine
carries a boxed warning in the manufacturer's package insert for
depression and suicidality in patients with Huntington's disease.

27. Which of the following agents has demonstrated over a 5-kg weight
loss as compared with placebo over 16 weeks in overweight, prediabetic patients taking olanzapine or clozapine?

    A. Metformin.
    B. Topiramate.
    C. Liraglutide.
    D. Bupropion.

The correct response is option C.

Over a 16-week randomized trial, liraglutide (injected subcutaneously once daily) was superior to placebo for counteracting metabolic
dysregulation among olanzapine- or clozapine-treated prediabetic
schizophrenia spectrum patients; active drug recipients lost a mean
of 5.3 kg as well as significantly greater reductions in waist circumference, systolic blood pressure, visceral fat, and LDL cholesterol.
Significant, but more modest, weight loss has been reported during
trials with metformin or topiramate in overweight patients taking
second-generation antipsychotics. Bupropion has weight loss properties but has not been studied in randomized trials to counteract antipsychotic-associated weight gain.

28. Which of the following statements is *true* for a 38-year-old male
nonsmoker with schizophrenia who is about to start taking clozapine
200 mg/day and whose pooled cohort risk equation score is 7.5%?

A. The potential benefits of taking an SGA with high metabolic risk are outweighed by his relatively high risk for a heart attack in the next 10 years.
B. He has a 92.5% risk of having an MI before age 65.
C. His score of 7.5% warrants cotherapy with a statin, especially if he is about to begin clozapine.
D. His risk of a heart attack in the next 10 years is no greater than would be expected for anyone else of his age and sex, posing little increased baseline risk if he begins an SGA that has high metabolic risk.

The correct response is option D.

The pooled cohort risk equation calculates the probability of having an MI in the coming 10 years, based on age, sex, race, total cholesterol, HDL cholesterol, systolic blood pressure, presence of diabetes, and smoking status. An increased risk is considered to be present if the pooled cohort equation value is >7.5%. This patient has no appreciably increased risk for an MI above that of the baseline population, which may help to inform a more favorable risk-benefit ratio when considering the potential psychotropic value of clozapine for his condition.

29. Which of the following SGAs carries the lowest risk for QTc prolongation?

    A. Aripiprazole.
    B. Iloperidone.
    C. Ziprasidone.
    D. Quetiapine.

The correct response is option A.

A meta-analysis by Leucht et al. (2013) identified aripiprazole, lurasidone, and paliperidone as having the lowest relative risks among 15 studied FGAs and SGAs (including iloperidone, ziprasidone, and quetiapine) across 212 trials involving over 43,000 participants.

30. Improvement in dimensions of cognitive functioning in euthymic bipolar disorder patients has been demonstrated in randomized trials with all of the following agents *except*

  A. Lurasidone.
  B. *Withania somnifera*.
  C. Pramipexole.
  D. Divalproex.

The correct response is option D.

Divalproex has not been demonstrated to improve cognitive performance in patients with bipolar disorder. By contrast, each of the other listed options has at least one placebo-controlled trial demonstrating efficacy for improving cognitive dysfunction in bipolar disorder patients.

31. Logical strategies to manage nausea associated with vortioxetine include all the following *except*

  A. Dosage reductions.
  B. Adjunctive ondansetron 4–8 mg orally once or twice daily as needed.
  C. Adjunctive trimethobenzamide 300 mg orally every 4–6 hours as needed.
  D. Adjunctive prochlorperazine 10 mg orally every 4–6 hours as needed.

The correct response is option B.

Ondansetron is thought to exert its antiemetic effects via 5-HT$_3$ antagonism, a mechanism that it shares in common with vortioxetine. Nausea associated with vortioxetine is thought to be a dose-related phenomenon that reflects its 5-HT$_{1A}$ agonist properties. Adjunctive trimethobenzamide or prochlorperazine both would be reasonable adjunctive anti-nausea options that are mechanistically nonredundant with 5-HT$_3$ receptor effects.

32. Evidence-based strategies to minimize the risk for renal insufficiency during long-term lithium therapy include which one of the following?

  A. Once-per-day lithium dosing.
  B. Three-times-per-day lithium dosing.
  C. Use of lithium citrate rather than lithium carbonate.
  D. Favoring serum lithium levels no higher than 0.9 mEq/L when clinically feasible.

The correct response is option A.

Once-daily dosing has been demonstrated to be less likely than multiple daily-dosed lithium carbonate to cause glomerulosclerosis and eventual renal insufficiency during long-term treatment. Lithium levels < 6 mEq/L also may confer additional protection against long-term renal insufficiency. Differences in possible nephrotoxicity between lithium carbonate and lithium citrate have not been demonstrated.

33. Pharmacogenetic testing reveals that a 24-year-old white man with major depression and comorbid attention-deficit disorder is a CYP450 2D6 slow metabolizer. Usual maximal dosing should be halved for all of the following drugs *except*

    A. Mixed amphetamine salts.
    B. Citalopram.
    C. Venlafaxine.
    D. Vortioxetine.

The correct response is option B.

Citalopram is metabolized by CYP3A4 and CYP2C19, but not by CYP2D6. A CYP2D6 poor metabolizer phenotype would not be relevant to the dosing of citalopram. Each of the other choices is a substrate for CYP2D6.

34. A 37-year-old man with stable schizoaffective disorder and a history of akathisia on previous low doses of antipsychotics is taking iloperidone 8 mg twice daily, divalproex 1,000 mg/day, vilazodone 40 mg/day, and primidone 100 mg/day for tremor. His internist also prescribes him celecoxib 200 mg/day for chronic back pain as well as hydroxyzine 50 mg/day and medical marijuana (cannabidiol) for anxiety. He has been complaining of palpitations, and his internist obtains an ECG, which shows a QTc of 493 msec. Alarmed, the internist calls you and demands that you immediately stop the patient's iloperidone altogether. Why might this intervention be unnecessary?

    A. The vilazodone is likely raising levels of iloperidone and should be stopped.
    B. The primidone is likely raising levels of iloperidone and should be stopped.

C. Iloperidone levels could be elevated by celecoxib, hydroxy-zine, and cannabidiol, and consideration should be given to stopping those prescriptions if they are not essential.
D. Divalproex is likely raising levels of iloperidone, and a stat val-proic acid level should be checked to rule out valproate toxicity.

The correct response is option C.

Iloperidone is metabolized by CYP2D6, for which celecoxib, hydrox-yzine, and cannabidiol are all inhibitors. CYP2D6 inhibition can raise serum iloperidone levels, which could in turn increase the QTc in-terval on ECG. Although reducing the dose of iloperidone might be one option to consider, eliminating nonessential cotherapies that are potent CYP2D6 inhibitors might normalize the QTc interval. Given the patient's history of akathisia, continued use of iloperidone (which has among the lowest incident rates of akathisia among SGAs) would be preferable to stopping it altogether, if possible. Primidone induces, rather than inhibits, CYP2D6 and as such would more likely decrease, rather than increase, iloperidone levels. Vortioxe-tine neither inhibits CYP2D6 nor contributes directly to QTc prolon-gation. Divalproex does not affect either the QTc interval or the me-tabolism of iloperidone.

35. A 54-year-old African American male with sickle cell trait has been started on escitalopram 10 mg/day for major depression. He com-plains of anorgasmia and diminished libido. Which one of the follow-ing would be the safest evidence-based strategy to counteract this problem?

A. Add bupropion.
B. Add sildenafil.
C. Add trazodone.
D. Add vardenafil.

The correct response is option A.

Men over age 50 with predisposing risk factors for priapism, such as sickle cell disease or trait, have a significantly greater potential for developing priapism due to phosphodiesterase inhibitors.

36. A 28-year-old married woman with a history of two prior depressive episodes is now 36 weeks pregnant. She had been taking sertraline consistently since it was begun for postpartum depression after the birth of her first child 3 years earlier. Her obstetrician advised her to taper off the medication before delivery in order to avert withdrawal in the newborn. She now seeks a second opinion about her pharmacotherapy. Which one of the following would you likely do?

    A. Agree with her obstetrician that it is wisest to discontinue an SSRI before delivery so as to minimize the risk for neonatal abstinence syndrome.
    B. Tell her that in the unlikely event neonatal abstinence syndrome occurs, it carries a high chance that the baby would require admission to a neonatal intensive care unit and possible endotracheal intubation, but her risk for a recurrence of postpartum depression by stopping sertraline clearly outweighs the possibility of severe withdrawal in the newborn.
    C. Tell her that neonatal abstinence syndrome in the newborn is usually a mild, transient phenomenon occurring only in about a third of women who take an SSRI during pregnancy, but if it occurs it is typically self-limited and requires no special intervention.
    D. Switch the patient's medication now from sertraline to fluoxetine preemptively to minimize the chances of SSRI discontinuation in the newborn.

The correct response is option C.

Neonatal abstinence syndrome from SSRIs occurs in about 30% of live births usually during the first 2 weeks of delivery among women exposed to SSRIs during pregnancy. It usually involves mild symptoms (e.g., jitteriness, irritability, abnormal crying) that resolve spontaneously. Case reports exist of infants exposed in utero to SSRIs who postnatally manifest problems with feeding, seizures, or respiratory distress, although such occurrences are highly uncommon.

37. A 41-year-old man with bipolar disorder well controlled on lithium carbonate is training to run a marathon. His primary care doctor noticed that his serum creatinine had recently increased from its usual level of about 0.9 ng/dL to 1.1 ng/dL and is concerned about the rise of >20% in just 3 months. His lithium level remains steady at 0.7 mEq/L. The patient says he drinks "tons of water." He has now been sent to

his psychiatrist with the request that the lithium be stopped and another drug used instead. Which one of the following would be the most appropriate response by the psychiatrist?

A. While preparing for the marathon, advise the patient that he probably is nevertheless dehydrated despite his assumptions to the contrary, and advise him just to increase his fluid intake even further before making any changes to his regimen.

B. Discontinue the lithium over a 2-week period because of the sudden deterioration in his renal function, and cross-taper to divalproex.

C. Measure a serum cystatin C from which to recalculate his estimated glomerular filtration rate (eGFR).

D. Reassure both the patient and the primary care doctor that a serum creatinine of 1.1 ng/dL is still well within the usual normal reference range, and advise just rechecking it again in a month or two.

The correct response is option C.

Serum creatinine is the most commonly used biomarker for estimating GFR, but it can vary with muscle mass, and its accuracy may be poor in the setting of mild chronic kidney disease. Measurement of serum cystatin C has been described as a more accurate estimate of GFR that is not influenced by muscle mass, this value may be a better measure for predicting the likelihood of developing more advanced chronic kidney disease. Excessive loss of fluids and salt during marathon training could cause lithium levels to rise (in turn placing added stress on kidney function), but this is not evident in the current case. There is no need to reflexively discontinue lithium in the present scenario. More frequent periodic monitoring of renal function may be helpful, but reliance on serum creatinine for estimating GFR still would not address its potential inaccuracy in the setting of heavy exercise.

38. A 29-year-old man with bipolar II disorder and comorbid generalized anxiety disorder takes lithium 900 mg/day and gabapentin 600 mg/day and complains of feeling sedated. His psychotherapist suggested to him that he may have a "slow metabolism" and ought to ask you to please order a phamacogenetic test on him to affirm this. You smile politely and gently state your opinion that pharmacogenetic testing would have no value in this instance. Why?

    A. Lithium can cause sedation at a usual dose such as his, and it would be more prudent to check a serum lithium level to make sure that his complaints of sedation do not reflect lithium neurotoxicity.

    B. Gabapentin can cause sedation at a usual dose such as his, and one could consider whether a lower dose would be better tolerated.

    C. Neither lithium nor gabapentin undergoes hepatic metabolism.

    D. All of the above.

The correct response is option C.

Because both lithium and gabapentin are eliminated without undergoing hepatic metabolism, pharmacogenetic testing of pharmacokinetic enzymes would not be relevant to the effects of either drug.

39. This same psychotherapist calls you about another female patient with bipolar II disorder on an oral contraceptive who takes lamotrigine 150 mg/day and is clinically stable but feels slight cognitive dulling. The patient obtained pharmacogenetic testing from her current psychiatrist, who determined that she is a CYP450 2D6 poor metabolizer, and the psychotherapist is concerned the lamotrigine may, for the patient, be supratherapeutically dosed. What would you advise?

    A. Suggest measuring a serum lamotrigine level to determine if it is in the toxic range.

    B. Obtain neuropsychological testing to document the nature and extent of possible cognitive deficits.

    C. Gently state your opinion that the pharmacogenetic testing results are not relevant.

    D. Tell her that the oral contraceptive is probably inhibiting the metabolism of lamotrigine and causing a supratherapeutic dosing effect, for which a lower lamotrigine dose may be worth considering.

The correct response is option C.

Lamotrigine is metabolized by UDP glucuronidation, not by CYP450 2D6. It would be clinically unlikely for a patient taking 150 mg/day of lamotrigine to develop toxicity, particularly while also taking an oral contraceptive, inasmuch as estrogen-containing contraceptives typically reduce lamotrigine plasma levels by 50% or more.

40. A 44-year-old man with binge-eating disorder, generalized anxiety disorder, obesity, and hypercholesterolemia is taking lisdexamfetamine 60 mg/day, topiramate 100 mg/day, fluoxetine 40 mg/day, and atorvastatin 40 mg/day. He calls to complain of leg pains. He also feels his panic attacks are becoming worse and says he sometimes finds it harder to breathe comfortably. He is afebrile, has a clear sensorium, and denies feeling stiff when asked by telephone. A serum CK level, ordered 2 days earlier by the patient's internist, was 236 IU/L (normal reference range is 60–174 IU/L). BUN and creatinine are within the normal reference range. Which one of the following is the most plausible explanation for his symptom?

    A. Statin-induced myositis.
    B. Neuroleptic malignant syndrome.
    C. Serotonin syndrome.
    D. Acute rhabdomyolysis likely secondary to myotoxicity.

The correct response is option A.

Statins may cause myotoxicity (myalgias) in 5%–20% of individuals, characterized as a relatively benign condition when serum CK levels are < 10 times the upper limit of normal (ULN), as described in the current case. Neuroleptic malignant syndrome can vary in its presentation, but traditional major manifestations include fever, muscle rigidity, and elevated serum CK levels (usually >1,000 IU/L), none of which were features present in the current case. Similarly, serotonin syndrome would likely involve additional systemic features such as clonus, tremor, hyperthermia, and diaphoresis, none of which are described in this case. Acute rhabdomyolysis entails a serum CK level that exceeds 10 times ULN in conjunction with signs of renal failure or else at least 50 times ULN in the absence of renal impairment.

41. A patient who demonstrates myoclonic jerking movements would be suspected of having any of the following *except*

    A. Serotonin syndrome.
    B. Epilepsy.
    C. Lithium toxicity.
    D. An adverse effect of levetiracetam.

The correct response is option D.

Myoclonic jerks carry a wide differential diagnosis that can include serotonin syndrome, myoclonic epilepsy, and an early sign of lithium toxicity. It is not typically associated with the use of levetiracetam.

42. An 83-year-old normotensive man with chronic depression that has been well controlled with sertraline 100 mg/day for the past 6 months presents with somnolence and confusion. He has no recent gastrointestinal complaints. Which one of the following interventions would be the *most useful* in the diagnosis and management of his acute mental status change?

   A. Obtain serum electrolytes.
   B. Obtain a serum sertraline level.
   C. Switch from generic sertraline to brand name Zoloft.
   D. Augment his regimen with a low-dose stimulant to help overcome sedation and possible cognitive dulling from sertraline.

The correct response is option A.

Elderly patients are at especially high risk for hyponatremia and SIADH due to serotonergic antidepressants. The acute change in sensorium for the patient described warrants a medical evaluation that should include serum electrolytes to rule in or rule out hyponatremia and possible SIADH. Serum sertraline levels likely would be uninformative in the current setting, in part because the absence of gastrointestinal signs and symptoms would make sertraline toxicity (e.g., overdose) a somewhat less likely cause. Generic versus brand-name SSRI formulations may sometimes lead to greater gastrointestinal or other problems with tolerability but would not be expected to cause an acute mental status change as described here. The addition of a psychostimulant to overcome presumed iatrogenic "sedation" in this instance could be a grave error if one failed to recognize the acute mental status change as the more probable sign of a potentially ominous underlying medical complication.

43. A patient with multi-drug-resistant major depression responds well to tranylcypromine 60 mg/day plus aripiprazole 5 mg/day. He complains of dizziness and lightheadedness on standing and has orthostatic blood pressure changes on examination. All of the following interventions would be appropriate *except*

A. Cautiously lower the tranylcypromine dose to see if the antidepressant response is retained at a lower dose, because orthostatic hypotension from MAOIs can be dose-dependent.
B. Discontinue the aripiprazole as the probable cause of the orthostatic hypotension because of its α_1 antagonism.
C. Begin oral midodrine 5 mg three times per day.
D. Begin oral fludrocortisone 0.1 mg/day.

The correct response is option B.

Orthostatic hypotension is a known dose-related adverse effect of MAOIs. Midodrine and fludrocortisone are both appropriate antidote strategies for managing MAOI-associated hypotension. Although aripiprazole can, in principle, cause orthostatic hypotension because of its α_1-blocking effects, incident rates of this occurring in randomized clinical trials were no different from those with placebo (<1%), making this a much less likely contributing factor to the clinical presentation described.

44. The second-generation antipsychotic with the least likelihood for causing weight gain in schizophrenia, based on short-term clinical trials, is which of the following?

A. Ziprasidone.
B. Iloperidone.
C. Asenapine.
D. Lurasidone.

The correct response is option D.

In acute schizophrenia trials, the NNH for weight gain with lurasidone was 67. NNH for weight gain was lower (i.e., a higher risk for weight gain) with ziprasidone (16), iloperidone (10), and asenapine (35).

45. A 51-year-old man with schizoaffective disorder has been stabilized on clozapine 250 mg/day recently augmented with armodafinil 150 mg/day to counteract sedation, sublingual atropine sulfate 1% solution for sialorrhea, and divalproex sodium 500 mg/day targeting irritability and affective instability. At routine follow-up, he presents with persistent sedation and new gait instability and dizziness. What is the most likely explanation for these symptoms?

A. Likely additive general side-effect burden of clozapine plus divalproex; check a serum valproate level to ensure it is not toxic and possibly lower the divalproex dose, or else possibly increase the armodafinil dose to promote greater wakefulness effect.
B. Systemic vagolytic effects caused by systemic absorption of sublingual atropine.
C. Increase in serum clozapine levels due to pharmacokinetic inhibition caused by modafinil.
D. Increase in serum clozapine levels due to pharmacokinetic inhibition caused by divalproex.

The correct response is option C.

Modafinil has been reported to increase serum clozapine levels, presumably via its inhibition of CYP2C19.

46. A 24-year-old obese man with major depression has been treated with duloxetine 120 mg/day, lithium carbonate 900 mg/day, and topiramate 100 mg/day. For the past 3 years, he has also used a specially compounded intranasal formulation of ketamine four to five times a week. In the course of his initial evaluation, he mentions having frequent urination, nocturia, and occasional suprapubic pain. Which of the following is the *least likely* iatrogenic explanation for his urinary complaints?

    A. Ulcerative cystitis.
    B. Nephrogenic diabetes insipidus.
    C. Renal calculus.
    D. Urinary retention.

The correct response is option D.

Urinary retention or obstructive voiding symptoms occur rarely with duloxetine (approximately 1% in randomized trials), usually within the first few weeks of treatment initiation. Suprapubic pain can occur because of urinary retention, but that would be unlikely in the setting of urinary frequency. Urinary frequency or nocturia have not been described in connection with duloxetine. By contrast, ulcerative cystitis is a recognized adverse effect associated with chronic ketamine use and may present with the symptoms described in the current case. Lithium-associated nephrogenic diabetes insipidus also can present with urinary frequency and nocturia, although it is generally not painful in the absence of a concurrent urinary tract infection. Topiramate carries approximately a 1% risk of causing renal calculi and may present with urinary frequency and renal colic pain that could radiate to the groin. Lower ureteric stones are prone to cause irritative bladder symptoms such as urinary frequency and urgency.

47. All of the following medications can be associated with anticholinergic (antimuscarinic or antinicotinic) adverse effects *except*

    A. Carbamazepine.
    B. Paroxetine.
    C. Atomoxetine.
    D. Bupropion.

The correct response is option C.

Atomoxetine has no known anticholinergic effects, whereas carbamazepine and paroxetine both exert antimuscarinic effects, and bupropion has antinicotinic effects.

48. A single-agent overdose of which of the following medications would *least expectably* be associated with fatality?

    A. 8,000 mg of divalproex in an 84-kg male.
    B. 27,000 mg of lithium carbonate in a 75 kg male.
    C. 240 mg of dextroamphetamine in an 80-kg male.
    D. 49,000 mg of gabapentin in a 62-kg female.

The correct response is option D.

Gabapentin overdoses as high as 49,000 mg have been reported without consequent fatality. Fatalities have been reported with divalproex dosed above 60 mg/kg, amphetamine dosed above 1.3 mg/kg, and lithium carbonate at dosages producing serum lithium levels > 3.0 mEq/L (lithium dosages exceeding 40 mg/kg would expectably produce serum levels > 1.2 mEq/L).

49. A 46-year-old Vietnamese man has for over 3 years been taking lamotrigine 400 mg/day for bipolar II disorder and carbamazepine 600 mg/day for trigeminal neuralgia. He presents with an itchy, tingling, burning, rather linear rash, of 1 week's duration, with some

crusting along his trunk running from below the midline base of his rib cage across his trunk. There is no fever and no oropharyngeal lesions. Which of the following would be the most appropriate next step in his assessment and management?

A. Obtain pharmacogenetic testing to determine the presence of the DQB1*06:02 gene.
B. Immediately discontinue both lamotrigine and carbamazepine.
C. Recommend an as-needed nonsteroidal anti-inflammatory drug for pain but otherwise do nothing.
D. Recommend an oral antihistamine such as diphenhydramine 50 mg every 6 hours and a topical over-the-counter steroid cream.

The correct response is option C.

The clinical description of a painful, itchy, linear truncal rash that does not cross the midline and has begun to crust after a week is a classical description of herpes zoster, or shingles, for which conservative treatment (e.g., NSAIDs) is generally most appropriate. The value of antiviral therapies such as acyclovir has not been well demonstrated when begun more than 72 hours after an acute outbreak, and especially after crusting has begun. Carbamazepine and lamotrigine can both cause Stevens-Johnson syndrome (SJS); however, the description of the rash is not suggestive of a systemic phenomenon such as SJS, and the likelihood of its new development more than 3 years after the start of either of these drugs is remote. The DQB1*06:02 gene has been described in connection with the risk for narcolepsy, rather than severe cutaneous reactions. In patients of Southeast Asian descent, pharmacogenetic testing for HLA-B*1502 *before* (rather than *after*) starting carbamazepine is considered mandatory to gauge risk for developing SJS. Antihistamines and topical over-the-counter steroid creams would be more appropriate for a suspected contact dermatitis than for treatment of zoster.

50. A 17-year-old male with a suspected drug overdose presents to an emergency department with fever, vomiting, muscle twitching, sweating, tachycardia, and mydriasis. If this presentation occurred from a single-agent toxicity, which of the following would be the *most likely* causal agent?

A. Lorazepam.
B. Methylphenidate.
C. Buspirone.
D. Mirtazapine.

The correct response is option B.

Sympathomimetic effects along with the described neurological and systemic symptoms would be most consistent with an overdose of methylphenidate. Lorazepam or other benzodiazepines in overdose are more typically associated with miosis (rather than mydriasis), somnolence, confusion, CNS depression, and hypotension. Mirtazapine in overdose would likely be associated with somnolence, confusion, and tachycardia but no other cardiovascular or systemic manifestations. Overdosages of buspirone can be associated with nausea, vomiting, dizziness, and miosis (rather than mydriasis).

APPENDIX 3

Resources for Practitioners

Summary of Commonly Reported Adverse Effects of Psychotropic Agents

Common Psychotropic Drug Interactions

Useful Web Sites

Rating Scales for Measuring Adverse Drug Effects

Summary of commonly reported adverse effects of psychotropic agents[a]

Agent	Agitation	Anxiety	Appetite ↓	Appetite ↑	Asthenia	Ataxia	Blurry vision	Constipation	Diarrhea	Dizziness	Dry mouth	EPS and akathisia	Gastrointestinal upset	Headache	Insomnia	Nausea	Sedation, somnolence, or fatigue	Sexual dysfunction	Sweating	Tachycardia	Tremor	Weight gain	Weight loss
Atomoxetine	✓			✓							✓		✓	✓	✓	✓	✓						
Buspirone										✓							✓						
Antidepressants																							
Bupropion	✓			✓			✓	✓		✓	✓			✓	✓	✓	✓		✓	✓	✓	✓	✓
Citalopram															✓	✓	✓		✓				
Desvenlafaxine				✓				✓	✓		✓					✓	✓						
Duloxetine								✓		✓					✓	✓	✓						
Escitalopram														✓	✓	✓	✓	✓					
Fluoxetine		✓		✓	✓				✓		✓				✓	✓	✓	✓					
Fluvoxamine													✓	✓		✓					✓		
Levomilnacipran																		✓					

Summary of commonly reported adverse effects of psychotropic agents[a] *(continued)*

Agent	Agitation	Anxiety	Appetite ↓	Appetite ↑	Asthenia	Ataxia	Blurry vision	Constipation	Diarrhea	Dizziness	Dry mouth	EPS and akathisia	Gastrointestinal upset	Headache	Insomnia	Nausea	Sedation, somnolence, or fatigue	Sexual dysfunction	Sweating	Tachycardia	Tremor	Weight gain	Weight loss
Antidepressants *(continued)*																							
Mirtazapine			✓					✓			✓						✓					✓	
Nefazodone								✓		✓				✓	✓	✓	✓						
Paroxetine					✓			✓	✓	✓	✓			✓	✓	✓	✓	✓	✓				
Sertraline									✓	✓	✓			✓	✓	✓	✓	✓					
Transdermal selegiline														✓	✓								
Venlafaxine XR		✓			✓					✓	✓				✓	✓	✓	✓	✓				
Vilazodone									✓							✓							
Vortioxetine									✓							✓		✓b					

Summary of commonly reported adverse effects of psychotropic agents[a] (continued)

Agent	Agitation	Anxiety	Appetite ↓	Appetite ↑	Asthenia	Ataxia	Blurry vision	Constipation	Diarrhea	Dizziness	Dry mouth	EPS and akathisia	Gastrointestinal upset	Headache	Insomnia	Nausea	Sedation, somnolence, or fatigue	Sexual dysfunction	Sweating	Tachycardia	Tremor	Weight gain	Weight loss
Anticonvulsants																							
Carbamazepine										✓						✓	✓						
Divalproex[c]					✓				✓	✓			✓			✓	✓						
Gabapentin						✓				✓							✓						
Lamotrigine															✓	✓							
Oxcarbazepine							✓			✓				✓		✓	✓						
Topiramate		✓		✓		✓				✓						✓	✓						
SGAs																							
Aripiprazole		✓						✓		✓		✓		✓	✓	✓	✓						
Asenapine															✓		✓						
Brexpiprazole												✓											
Cariprazine								✓				✓		✓	✓	✓	✓						

Summary of commonly reported adverse effects of psychotropic agents[a] (continued)

Agent	Agitation	Anxiety	Appetite ↓	Appetite ↑	Asthenia	Ataxia	Blurry vision	Constipation	Diarrhea	Dizziness	Dry mouth	EPS and akathisia	Gastrointestinal upset	Headache	Insomnia	Nausea	Sedation, somnolence, or fatigue	Sexual dysfunction	Sweating	Tachycardia	Tremor	Weight gain	Weight loss
SGAs *(continued)*																							
Clozapine								✓		✓							✓			✓			
Iloperidone										✓	✓					✓	✓			✓			
Lurasidone																✓	✓						
Olanzapine					✓			✓		✓	✓	✓	✓				✓						
Paliperidone												✓		✓	✓		✓			✓			
Pimavanserin[d]			✓[e]																				
Quetiapine								✓		✓	✓						✓						
Risperidone										✓		✓	✓				✓						
Ziprasidone												✓				✓	✓						

Summary of commonly reported adverse effects of psychotropic agents[a] (continued)

Agent	Agitation	Anxiety	Appetite ↓	Appetite ↑	Asthenia	Ataxia	Blurry vision	Constipation	Diarrhea	Dizziness	Dry mouth	EPS and akathisia	Gastrointestinal upset	Headache	Insomnia	Nausea	Sedation, somnolence, or fatigue	Sexual dysfunction	Sweating	Tachycardia	Tremor	Weight gain	Weight loss
Psychostimulants																							
Armodafinil														✓									
Lisdexamfetamine				✓											✓								
Methylphenidate[f]																							
Mixed amphetamine salts				✓							✓		✓	✓									
Modafinil														✓		✓							
Sedative-hypnotics																							
Eszopiclone														✓			✓						
Suvorexant[d]																							
Tasimelteon														✓									
Zaleplon														✓									
Zolpidem[d]																							

Summary of commonly reported adverse effects of psychotropic agents[a] *(continued)*

Agent	Agitation	Anxiety	Appetite ↓	Appetite ↑	Asthenia	Ataxia	Blurry vision	Constipation	Diarrhea	Dizziness	Dry mouth	EPS and akathisia	Gastrointestinal upset	Headache	Insomnia	Nausea	Sedation, somnolence, or fatigue	Sexual dysfunction	Sweating	Tachycardia	Tremor	Weight gain	Weight loss
Other CNS drugs																							
Deutetrabenazine																	✓						
Valbenazine																	✓						

Note. CNS=central nervous system; EPS=extrapyramidal symptoms; FDA=U.S. Food and Drug Administration; SGA=second-generation antipsychotic; XR = extended release.

[a] As reported in ≥10% of subjects in adult FDA registration trials. Data based on manufacturers' product information, collectively for all FDA-approved indications.

[b] Sexual dysfunction > placebo at vortioxetine doses > 10 mg/day.

[c] Based on adverse effects reported for divalproex in acute mania.

[d] No adverse effects occurred with incident rates > 10% in FDA registration trials.

[e] Increased appetite ≥10% observed only with quetiapine in 8-week trials for acute bipolar depression.

[f] Incidence rates are not reported by the manufacturer for adverse events with methylphenidate in FDA registration trials, although nervousness and insomnia are identified as the most common adverse reactions. In pediatric studies of Focalin XR or Concerta, most common adverse effects were anxiety, insomnia, dry mouth, headache, and loss of appetite, as well as nonspecific gastrointestinal complaints.

Common psychotropic drug interactions

Drug	Clinical effect
Buprenorphine	
+benzodiazepines	Postmarketing reports of coma and death.
Carbamazepine	
+cimetidine, erythromycin, clarithromycin, or fluconazole	Increased carbamazepine levels.
Fluvoxamine	
+alprazolam or diazepam	Approximate doubling of alprazolam or diazepam levels.
+clozapine	Fluvoxamine may cause up to a 500% rise in serum clozapine levels, increasing risk for toxicity and seizures.
+pimozide	Increased risk of QTc prolongation.
+ramelteon	Marked increase in Cmax and serum levels of ramelteon; ramelteon and fluvoxamine should not be coprescribed.
Lamotrigine	
+carbamazepine	Carbamazepine induces Phase II hepatic glucuronidation, effectively halving the bioavailability of lamotrigine; lamotrigine dosing must therefore be doubled during carbamazepine cotherapy.
+divalproex	Divalproex inhibits Phase II hepatic glucuronidation, effectively doubling the bioavailability of lamotrigine and consequently increasing the risk for serious drug rashes; lamotrigine dosing must therefore be halved during divalproex cotherapy.
+oral contraceptives	Estrogen-containing oral contraceptives can reduce serum lamotrigine levels by ~50%; lamotrigine dosages may need to be increased by as much as 2-fold during oral contraceptive coadministration; downward dosing adjustments are generally not recommended during the "placebo" week of an oral birth control regimen.

Common psychotropic drug interactions *(continued)*

Drug	Clinical effect
Lithium	
+ACE inhibitors (e.g., ramipril, lisinopril, enalapril)	May decrease lithium elimination (causing increased lithium levels) due to decreased glomerular perfusion pressure.
+β-blockers	May decrease lithium elimination (causing increased lithium levels) due to decreased glomerular perfusion pressure.
+excessive caffeine	May increase renal lithium elimination (causing decreased lithium levels) due to increased glomerular perfusion.
+first-generation antipsychotics	Reports of encephalopathy.
+nifedipine or isradipine	Coadministration may increase renal lithium elimination (causing decreased lithium levels) by altering glomerular perfusion or reducing proximal tubular reabsorption of lithium.
+NSAIDs	Can increase serum lithium levels by ~20% due to increased distal tubule reabsorption; frequent or long-term use may warrant reducing lithium dosages accordingly.
+theophylline	May increase renal lithium elimination (causing decreased lithium levels) due to increased glomerular perfusion.
+thiazide diuretics	May increase serum lithium levels.
+topiramate	Topiramate may increase serum lithium levels; may pertain mainly to topiramate dosages >200 mg/day.
+verapamil	May decrease lithium elimination (causing increased lithium levels) due to decreased glomerular perfusion pressure.

Common psychotropic drug interactions *(continued)*

Drug	Clinical effect
MAOIs	
+buspirone	Risk for serotonin syndrome.
+carbamazepine or oxcarbazepine	Because the tricyclic ring structure of carbamazepine or oxcarbazepine resembles a TCA, there is a theoretical (but undemonstrated) potential to induce a serotonergic or pressor effect; most practitioners view this as clinically unlikely and not relevant. An older literature identified isoniazid-induced elevation of carbamazepine levels, but this has not been demonstrated with other MAOIs.
+general anesthesia	Case reports of excitatory reactions (e.g., hypertension, hyperreflexia) or increased CNS depression; however, most anesthesiologists consider it unnecessary to discontinue MAOIs before elective surgery.
+noradrenergic agents	Increased risk for hypertensive crisis.
+opiates	Additive potential for sedation; contraindicated in manufacturer's product information materials.
+SSRIs	Risk for serotonin syndrome.
Mirtazapine	
+clonidine	Possible opposing actions (clonidine agonizes presynaptic α_2 autoreceptors, while mirtazapine antagonizes those receptors); reports of hypertensive urgency when mirtazapine is added to clonidine.
Olanzapine	
Intramuscular olanzapine +intramuscular benzodiazepine	Reports of excessive sedation, cardiopulmonary depression, and death.

Common psychotropic drug interactions *(continued)*

Drug	Clinical effect
Quetiapine	
+other drugs that can prolong QTc (e.g., Class IA antiarrhythmics [e.g., quinidine], Class III antiarrhythmics [e.g., amiodarone], fluoroquinolone antibiotics, methadone, certain other antipsychotics [e.g., ziprasidone, thioridazine])	Additive risk for QTc prolongation and torsades de pointes.
SSRIs	
+NSAIDs, aspirin, antiplatelet drugs	May increase risk for upper GI bleeding by 8- to 28-fold (Dall et al. 2009).
+TCAs	SSRIs may increase tricyclic blood levels.
+tramadol	Increased risk for seizures, serotonin syndrome.
+triptans	Increased risk for serotonin syndrome.

Note. ACE=angiotensin-converting enzyme; Cmax=maximal drug plasma concentration; CNS=central nervous system; GI=gastrointestinal; MAOI= monoamine oxidase inhibitor; NSAID=nonsteroidal anti-inflammatory drug; SSRI=selective serotonin reuptake inhibitor; TCA=tricyclic antidepressant

Useful Web sites

Topic	Source	Site
Bioequivalence of brand versus generic drug formulations	U.S. Food and Drug Administration's "Orange Book: Approved Drug Products With Therapeutic Equivalence Evaluations"	www.accessdata.fda.gov/scripts/cder/ob/default.cfm
Cardiovascular disease	Framingham Risk Calculator	http://cvdrisk.nhlbi.nih.gov/
Drug interactions	Indiana University School of Medicine, Division of Clinical Pharmacology, "Drug Interactions" (table of CYP drug interactions)	www.medicine.iupui.edu/clinpharm/DDIs
General drug information, dosing, interactions	Thomson Reuters Micromedex	www.micromedex.com www.crediblemeds.org/healthcare/providers/
Pharmacy tools (renal dosing protocols, laboratory reference ranges, medical calculators)	GlobalRPh	www.globalrph.com
Pregnancy (environmental hazards)	REPROTOX information system (developed by the Reproductive Toxicology Center)	www.reprotox.org
	Developmental and Reproductive Toxicology Database (DART)	http://toxnet.nlm.nih.gov/cgi-bin/sis/htmlgen?DARTETIC
Pregnancy (lactation)	United States National Library of Medicine, TOXNET Toxicology Data Network, Drugs and Lactation Database (LactMed)	http://toxnet.nlm.nih.gov/cgi-bin/sis/htmlgen?LACT
Pregnancy (teratology information)	Organization of Teratology Information Specialists (OTIS)	www.otispregnancy.org

Rating scales for measuring adverse drug effects

Phenomenon	Scale	Description
Akathisia	Barnes Akathisia Scale (Barnes 1989)	4-item clinician-rated scale assessing objective and subjective awareness of restlessness, related distress, and global assessment
	Simpson-Angus Extrapyramidal Side Effects Scale (Simpson and Angus 1970; www.outcometracker.org/library/SAS.pdf	10-item clinician-rated assessment of gait; arm drop; stiffness of shoulder, elbow, and wrist; leg swing; head drop; glabellar tap; tremor; and hypersalivation
Antidepressant side effects	Toronto Side Effects Scale (Vanderkooy et al. 2002)	29-item self-reported symptom inventory rating frequency and severity on individual 5-point subscales
	Frequency, Intensity, and Burden of Side Effects Rating (FIBSER) Scale (Wisniewski et al. 2006) www.outcometracker.org/library/FIBSER.pdf	3-item self-report measure of side effects in three domains: frequency, intensity, and side effect burden.
Involuntary movements (including, but not exclusively, tardive dyskinesia)	Abnormal Involuntary Movement Scale (AIMS; Munetz and Benjamin 1988)	12-item clinician-rated scale assessing orofacial movements, extremity and truncal dyskinesias, global severity, incapacitation, patient awareness of movements and distress associated with them, and problems with teeth or dentures

Rating scales for measuring adverse drug effects *(continued)*

Phenomenon	Scale	Description
Sexual dysfunction	Arizona Sexual Experiences Scale (ASEX; McGahuey et al. 2000) www.mirecc.va.gov/visn22/Arizona_Sexual_Experiences_Scale.pdf	5-point self-administered scale with each item ranging from 1 (high) to 6 (none) assessing strength of sex drive, sexual arousal, penile erections or vaginal lubrication, ease of orgasm, and orgasmic satisfaction
	Changes in Sexual Functioning Questionnaire (CSFQ; Clayton et al. 1997)	36- or 35-item (male or female, respectively) semistructured interview or self-report rating assessing sexual desire/frequency; sexual desire/interest; sexual pleasure, arousal/excitement, and orgasm/completion rated via 5-point Likert scale items
	Psychotropic-Related Sexual Dysfunction Questionnaire (PRSexDQ; Montejo and Rico-Villademoros 2008)	7-item self-report measure assessing loss of libido, delayed orgasm or ejaculation, lack of orgasm or ejaculation, erectile dysfunction or vaginal lubrication dysfunction, and tolerance of sexual dysfunction, with individual items scored from 0 (lowest) to 3 (highest) and total scores ranging from 0 to 15

References

Abbasian C, Power P: A case of aripiprazole and tardive dyskinesia. J Psycho-pharmacol 23:214–215, 2009

Adler CM, Fleck DE, Brecher M, et al: Safety and tolerability of quetiapine in the treatment of acute mania in bipolar disorder. J Affect Disord 100:S15–S22, 2007

Adler LA, Rotrosen J, Edson R, et al: Vitamin E treatment for tardive dyskinesia. Veterans Affairs Cooperative Study #394 Study Group. Arch Gen Psychiatry 56:836–841, 1999

Agosti V, Quitkin FM, Stewart JW, et al: Somatization as a predictor of medication discontinuation due to adverse events. Int J Psychopharmacol 17:311–314, 2002

Aiken CB, Orr C: Rechallenge with lamotrigine after a rash: a prospective case series and review of the literature. Psychiatry (Edgmont) 7:27–32, 2010

Aizenberg D, Zemishlany Z, Weizman A: Cyproheptadine treatment of sexual dysfunction induced by serotonin reuptake inhibitors. Clin Neuropharmacol 18:320–324, 1995

Alabed S, Latifeh Y, Mohammad HA, et al: Gamma-aminobutyric acid agonists for neuroleptic-induced tardive dyskinesia. Cochrane Database of Systematic Reviews 2011, Issue 4. Art. No.: CD000203. DOI: 10.1002/14651858.CD000203.pub3.

Alam MY, Jacobsen PL, Chen Y, et al: Safety, tolerability, and efficacy of vortioxetine (Lu AA21004) in major depressive disorder: results of an open-label, flexible-dose, 52-week extension study. Int Clin Psychopharmacol 29:36–44, 2014

Albanese A, Bhatia K, Bressman SB, et al: Phenomenology and classification of dystonia: a consensus update. Mov Disord 28:863–873, 2013

Albert U, De Cori D, Aguglia A, et al: Lithium-associated hyperparathyroidism and hypercalcaemia: a case-control cross-sectional study. J Affect Disord 151:786–790, 2013

Albu S, Chirles F: Intratympanic dexamethasone plus melatonin versus melatonin only in the treatment of unilateral acute idiopathic tinnitus. Am J Otolaryngol 35:615–622, 2014

Alfirevic A, Neely D, Armitage J, et al: Phenotype standardization for statin-induced myotoxicity. Clin Pharmacol Ther 96:470-476, 2014

Allison DB, Mentore JL, Heo M, et al: Antipsychotic-induced weight gain: a comprehensive research synthesis. Am J Psychiatry 156:1686–1696, 1999

Alvestad S, Lydersen S, Brodtkorb E: Cross-sensitivity pattern of rash from current aromatic antiepileptic drugs. Epilepsy Res 80:194–200, 2008

American Diabetes Association: Diagnosis and classification of diabetes mellitus. Diabetes Care 33 (suppl 1):S62–S69, 2010

American Diabetes Association, American Psychiatric Association, American Association of Clinical Endocrinologists, et al: Consensus development conference on antipsychotic drugs and obesity and diabetes. J Clin Psychiatry 65:267–272, 2004

American Psychiatric Association: Diagnostic and Statistical Manual of Mental Disorders, 5th Edition. Arlington, VA, American Psychiatric Association, 2013

Amiaz R, Pope HG Jr, Mahne T, et al: Testosterone gel replacement improves sexual function in depressed men taking serotonergic antidepressants: a randomized, placebo-controlled clinical trial. J Sex Marital Ther 37:243–254, 2011

Amir I, Hermesh H, Gavish A: Bruxism secondary to antipsychotic drug exposure: a positive response to propranolol. Clin Neuropharmacol 20:86–89, 1997

Amsterdam JD, Fawcett J, Quitkin FM, et al: Fluoxetine and norfluoxetine plasma concentrations in major depression: a multicenter study. Am J Psychiatry 154:963–969, 1997

Anand E, Berggren L, Deix C, et al: A 6-year open-label study of the efficacy and safety of olanzapine long-acting injectable in patients with schizophrenia: a post hoc analysis based on the European label recommendation. Neuropsychiatr Dis Treat 11:1349–1357, 2015

Andersohn F, Schade R, Suissa S, et al: Long-term use of antidepressants for depressive disorders and the risk of diabetes mellitus. Am J Psychiatry 166:591–598, 2009

Andersohn F, Schmedt N, Weinmann S, et al: Priapism associated with antipsychotics: role of alpha$_1$ adrenoreceptor affinity. J Clin Psychopharmacol 30:68–71, 2010

Anderson JW, Greenway FL, Fujioka K, et al: Bupropion SR enhances weight loss: a 48-week double-blind, placebo-controlled trial. Obes Res 10:633–641, 2002

Anderson KE, Stamler D, Davis MD, et al: Deutetrabenazine for treatment of involuntary movements in patients with tardive dyskinesia (AIM-TD): a double-blind, randomised, placebo-controlled phase 3 trial. Lancet Psychiatry 4(8):595–604, 2017

Andrade C, Sandarsh S, Chethan KB, et al: Serotonin reuptake inhibitor antidepressants and abnormal bleeding: a review for clinicians and a reconsideration of mechanisms. J Clin Psychiatry 71:1565–1575, 2010

Arana A, Wentworth CE, Ayuso-Mateos JL, et al: Suicide-related events in patients treated with antiepileptic drugs. N Engl J Med 363:542–551, 2010

Aronoff GR, Berns JS, Brier ME, et al (eds): Drug Prescribing in Renal Failure: Dosing Guidelines for Adults, 4th Edition. Philadelphia, PA, American College of Physicians–American Society of Internal Medicine, 1999

Arranz B, San L, Dueñas RM, et al: Lower weight gain with the orally disintegrating olanzapine than with standard tablets in first-episode never-treated psychotic patients. Hum Psychopharmacol 22:11–15, 2007

Ascaso JF, Pardo S, Real JT, et al: Diagnosing insulin resistance by simple quantitative methods in subjects with normal glucose metabolism. Diabetes Care 26:3320–3325, 2003

Ashton AK, Rosen RC: Bupropion as an antidote for serotonin reuptake inhibitor-induced sexual dysfunction. J Clin Psychiatry 59:112–115, 1998

Asnis GS, Bose A, Gommoll CP, et al: Efficacy and safety of levomilnacipran sustained release 40 mg, 80 mg, or 120 mg in major depressive disorder: a phase 3, randomized, double-blind, placebo-controlled study. J Clin Psyhiatry 74:242–248, 2013

Atmaca M, Kuloglu M, Tezcan E, et al: Weight gain and serum leptin levels in patients on lithium treatment. Neuropsychobiology 46:67–69, 2002

Atmaca M, Kuloglu M, Tezcan E, et al: Serum leptin and triglyceride levels in patients on treatment with atypical antipsychotics. J Clin Psychiatry 64: 598–604, 2003

Atmaca M, Kuloglu M, Tezcan E, et al: Nizatidine for the treatment of patients with quetiapine-induced weight gain. Hum Psychopharmacol 19:37–40, 2004

Aubert G, Mansuy V, Voirol MJ, et al: The anorexigenic effects of metformin involve increases in hypothalamic leptin receptor expression. Metabolism 60:327–334, 2011

Aurora RN, Zak RS, Auerbach SH, et al: Best practice guide for the treatment of nightmare disorder in adults. J Clin Sleep Med 6:389–401, 2010

Babu S, Li Y: Statin induced necrotizing autoimmune myopathy. J Neurol Sci 351(1–2):13–17, 2015

Bai YM, Lin CC, Chen JY, et al: Therapeutic effect of pirenzepine for clozapine-induced hypersalivation: a randomized, double-blind, placebo-controlled, crossover study. J Clin Psychopharmacol 21:608–611, 2001

Bai YM, Lin CC, Chen JY, et al: Association of initial antipsychotic response to clozapine and long-term weight gain. Am J Psychiatry 163:1276–1279, 2006

Baldessarini RJ, Tondo L, Ghiani C, et al: Discontinuation rate vs. recurrence risk following long-term antidepressant treatment in major depressive disorder patients. Am J Psychiatry 167:934–941, 2010

Balogh S, Hendricks SE, Kang J: Treatment of fluoxetine-induced anorgasmia with amantadine. J Clin Psychiatry 53:212–213, 1992

Balon R: Intermittent amantadine for fluoxetine-induced anorgasmia. J Sex Marital Ther 22:290–292, 1996

Baptista T, Martínez J, Lacruz A, et al: Metformin for prevention of weight gain and insulin resistance with olanzapine: a double-blind placebo-controlled trial. Can J Psychiatry 51:192–196, 2006

Baptista T, Rangel N, El Fakih Y, et al: Rosiglitazone in the assistance of metabolic control during olanzapine administration in schizophrenia: a pilot double-blind, placebo-controlled, 12-week trial. Pharmacopsychiatry 42:14–19, 2009

Barbhaiya RH, Shukla UA, Chaikin P, et al: Nefazodone pharmacokinetics: assessment of nonlinearity, intrasubject variability and time to attain steady-state plasma concentrations after dose escalation and de-escalation. Eur J Clin Pharmacol 50:101–107, 1996

Bardai A, Blom MT, van Noord C, et al: Sudden cardiac death is associated with both epilepsy and with use of antiepileptic medications. Heart 101:17–22, 2015

Barnes TR: A rating scale for drug-induced akathisia. Br J Psychiatry 154:672–676, 1989

Barnhart WJ, Makela EH, Latocha MJ: SSRI-induced apathy syndrome: a clinical review. J Psychiatr Pract 10:196–199, 2004

Basson BR, Kinon BJ, Taylor CC, et al: Factors influencing acute weight change in patients with schizophrenia treated with olanzapine, haloperidol, or risperidone. J Clin Psychiatry 62:231–238, 2001

Bauer M, Glenn T, Grof P, et al: The association between concurrent psychotropic medications and self-reported adherence with taking a mood stabilizer in bipolar disorder. Hum Psychopharmacol 25:47–54, 2010

Beaugerie L, Pardi DS: Review article: drug-induced microscopic colitis — proposal for a scoring system and review of the literature. Aliment Pharmacol Ther 22:277–284, 2005

Bent S, Padula A, Neuhaus J: Safety and efficacy of citrus aurantium for weight loss. Am J Cardiol 94:1359–1361, 2004

Berigan T: Antidepressant-induced sexual dysfunction treated with vardenafil. Can J Psychiatry 49:643, 2004

Berna F, Misdrahi D, Boyer L, et al: Akathisia: prevalence and risk factors in a community-dwelling sample of patients with schizophrenia: results from the FACE-SZ dataset. Schizophr Res 169(1–3):255–261, 2015

Bernard S, Neville KA, Nguyen AT, et al: Interethnic differences in genetic polymorphisms of CYP2D6 in the US population: clinical implications. Oncologist 11:126–135, 2006

Berner MM, Hagen M, Kriston L, et al: Management of sexual dysfunction due to antipsychotic drug therapy. Cochrane Database of Systematic Reviews 2007, Issue 1. Art. No.: CD003546. DOI: 10.1002/14651858.CD003546.pub2.

Bertilsson L: Geographical/interracial differences in polymorphic drug oxidation. Current state of knowledge of cytochromes P450 (CYP) 2D6 and 2C19. Clin Pharmacokinet 29:192–209, 1995

Biliotti de Gage S, Béquad B, Bazin F, et al: Benzodiazepine use and risk of dementia: prospective population based study. BMJ 345:e6231, 2012

Blouin M, Binet M, Bouchard R-H, et al: Improvement of metabolic risk profile under second-generation antipsychotics: a pilot intervention study. Can J Psychiatry 54:275–279, 2009

Bocchetta A, Ardau R, Fanni T, et al: Renal function during long-term lithium treatment: a cross-sectional and longitudinal study. BMC Med 13:12, 2015

Bodmer M, Meier C, Krähenbühl S, et al: Metformin, sulfonylureas, or other antidiabetes drugs and the risk of lactic acidosis or hypoglycemia: a nested case-control analysis. Diabetes Care 31:2086–2091, 2008

Bond DJ, Torres IJ, Lee SS, et al: Lower cognitive functioning as a predictor of weight gain in bipolar disorder: a 12-month study. Acta Psychiatr Scand 135:239–249, 2017

Borgheini G: The bioequivalence and therapeutic efficacy of generic versus brand-name psychoactive drugs. Clin Ther 25:1578–1592, 2003

Boston Collaborative Drug Surveillance Program: Acute adverse reactions to prednisone in relation to dosage. Clin Pharmacol Ther 13:694–698, 1972

Bostwick JM, Jaffee MS: Buspirone as an antidote to SSRI-induced bruxism in 4 cases. J Clin Psychiatry 60:857–860, 1999

Bouman WP, Pinner G, Johnson H: Cognitive impairment associated with lamotrigine. Br J Psychiatry 170:388–389, 1997

Bowden CL, Calabrese JR, McElroy SL, et al: A randomized, placebo-controlled 12-month trial of divalproex and lithium in treatment of outpatients with bipolar I disorder. Divalproex Maintenance Study Group. Arch Gen Psychiatry 57:481–489, 2000

Bowden CL, Calabrese JR, Ketter TA, et al: Impact of lamotrigine and lithium on weight in obese and nonobese patients with bipolar I disorder. Am J Psychiatry 163:1199–1201, 2006a

Bowden CL, Swann AC, Calabrese JR, et al: A randomized, placebo-controlled, multicenter study of divalproex sodium extended release in the treatment of acute mania. J Clin Psychiatry 67:1501–1510, 2006b

Bowskill R, Clatworthy J, Parham R, et al: Patients' perceptions of information received about medication prescribed for bipolar disorder: implications for informed choice. J Affect Disord 100:253–257, 2007

Brojmohun A, Lou JY, Zardkoohi O, et al: Protected from torsades de pointes? What psychiatrists need to know about pacemakers and defibrillators. Psychosomatics 54:407–417, 2013

Brown ES, Hong SC: Antidepressant-induced bruxism successfully treated with gabapentin. J Am Dent Assoc 130:1467–1469, 1999

Brunswick DJ, Amsterdam JD, Fawcett J, et al: Fluoxetine and norfluoxetine plasma concentrations during relapse-prevention treatment. J Affect Disord 68:243–249, 2002

Buffett-Jerrott SE, Stewart SH: Cognitive and sedative effects of benzodiazepine use. Curr Pharm Des 8:45–58, 2002

Burdick KE, Braga RJ, Nnadi CU, et al: Placebo-controlled adjunctive trial of pramipexole in patients with bipolar disorder: targeting cognitive dysfunction. J Clin Psychiatry 2011 Nov 29. [Epub ahead of print]

Calabrese JR, Keck PE Jr, Macfadden W, et al: A randomized, double-blind, placebo-controlled trial of quetiapine in the treatment of bipolar I or II depression. Am J Psychiatry 162:1351–1360, 2005

Calabrese JR, Sanchez R, Jin N, et al: Efficacy and safety of aripiprazole once-monthly in the maintenance treatment of bipolar I disorder: a double-blind, placebo-controlled, 52-week randomized withdrawal study. J Clin Psychiatry 78:324–331, 2017

Cantiano RN, Alvarenga ME, Garcia-Alcaraz M: Effect of omega-3 fatty acids on the lipid profile of patients taking clozapine. Aust N Z J Psychiatry 40:691–697, 2006

Cantú TG, Korek J: Monoamine oxidase inhibitors and weight gain. Clin Pharmacol 22:755–759, 1988

Canuso CM, Dirks B, Carothers J, et al: Randomized, double-blind, placebo-controlled study of paliperidone extended release and quetiapine in inpatients with recently exacerbated schizophrenia. Am J Psychiatry 166:691–701, 2009

Carbon M, Hsieh CH, Kane JM, et al: Tardive dyskinesia prevalence in the period of second-generation antipsychotic use: a meta-analysis. J Clin Psychiatry 78:e264–e278, 2017

Caroff S, Campbell EC, Havey J, et al: Treatment of tardive dyskinesia with do-
    nepezil: a pilot study. J Clin Psychiatry 62:772–775, 2001
Caroff S, Walker P, Campbell C, et al: Treatment of tardive dyskinesia with ga-
    lantamine: a randomized controlled crossover trial. J Clin Psychiatry 68:
    410–415, 2007
Castro VM, Roberson AM, McCoy TH, et al: Stratifying risk for renal insuffi-
    ciency among lithium-treated patients: an electronic health record study.
    Neuropsychopharmacology 41:1138–1143, 2016
Cates ME, Feldman JM, Boggs AA, et al: Efficacy of add-on topiramate therapy
    in psychiatric patients with weight gain. Ann Pharmacother 42:505–510,
    2008
Cavazzoni P, Tanaka Y, Roychowdhury SM, et al: Nizatadine for prevention of
    weight gain with olanzapine: a double-blind placebo-controlled trial. Eur
    Neuropsychopharmacol 13:81–85, 2003
Centorrino F, Wurtman JJ, Duca KA, et al: Weight loss in overweight patients
    maintained on atypical antipsychotic agents. Int J Obes (Lond) 30:1011–
    1016, 2006
Cephalon: Modafinil (CEP-1538) tablets supplemental NDA 20-717/S-019
    ADHD indication: briefing document for Psychopharmacologic Drugs Ad-
    visory Committee Meeting. Frazer, PA, Cephalon, March 23, 2006
Chambers CD, Hernandez-Diaz S, Van Marter LJ, et al: Selective serotonin-
    reuptake inhibitors and risk of persistent pulmonary hypertension of the
    newborn, N Engl J Med 354:579–587, 2006
Charlier C, Pinto E, Ansseau M, et al: Venlafaxine: the relationship between
    dose, plasma concentration and clinical response in depressive patients.
    J Psychopharmacol 16:369–372, 2002
Chaudron LH, Jefferson JW: Mood stabilizers during breastfeeding: a review.
    J Clin Psychiatry 61:79–90, 2000
Chawla B, Luxton-Andrew H: Long-term weight loss observed with olanzapine
    orally disintegrating tablets in overweight patients with chronic schizo-
    phrenia: a 1 year open-label, prospective trial. Hum Psychopharmacol Clin
    Exp 23:211–216, 2008
Chen CK, Chen YC, Huang YS: Effects of a 10-week weight control program on
    obese patients with schizophrenia or schizoaffective disorder: a 12-month
    follow up. Psychiatry Clin Neurosci 63:17–22, 2009
Chen YW, Dilsaver SC: Comorbidity of panic disorder in bipolar illness: evi-
    dence from the Epidemiologic Catchment Area Survey. Am J Psychiatry
    152:280–282, 1995
Chengappa KN, Rathore D, Levine J, et al: Topiramate as add-on treatment for
    patients with bipolar mania. Bipolar Disord 1:42–53, 1999
Chengappa KNR, Bowie CR, Schlicht PJ, et al: Randomized placebo-controlled
    adjunctive study of an extract of withania somnifera for cognitive dysfunc-
    tion in bipolar disorder. J Clin Psychiatry 74:1076–1083, 2013
Chengappa KNR, Perkins KA, Brar JS, et al: Varenicline for smoking cessation
    in bipolar disorder: a randomized. double-blind, placebo-controlled study.
    J Clin Psychiatry 75:765–772, 2014
Chintoh AF, Mann SW, Lam L, et al: Insulin resistance and decreased glucose-
    stimulated insulin secretion after acute olanzapine administration. J Clin
    Psychopharmacol 28:494–499, 2008

Chintoh AF, Mann SW, Lam L, et al: Insulin resistance and secretion in vivo: effects of different antipsychotics in an animal model. Schizophr Res 108: 127–133, 2009

Chou PH, Chu CS, Lin CH, et al: Use of atypical antipsychotics and risks of cataract development in patients with schizophrenia: a population-based, nested case-control study. Schizophr Res 174(1–3):137–143, 2016

Chung AK, Chua SE: Effects on prolongation of Bazett's corrected QT interval of seven second-generation antipsychotics in the treatment of schizophrenia: a meta-analysis. J Psychopharmacol 25:646–666, 2011

Citrome L: Current guidelines and their recommendations for prolactin monitoring in psychosis. J Psychopharmacol 22(suppl):90–97, 2008

Citrome L: Quantifying risk: the role of absolute and relative measures in interpreting risk of adverse reactions from product labels of antipsychotic medicines. Curr Drug Safety 4:229–237, 2009a

Citrome L: Iloperidone for schizophrenia: a review of the efficacy and safety profile for this newly commercialised second-generation antipsychotic. Int J Clin Practice 63:1237–1248, 2009b

Citrome L: Adjunctive aripiprazole, olanzapine, or quetiapine for major depressive disorder: an analysis of number needed to treat, number needed to harm, and likelihood to be helped or harmed. Postgrad Med 122:39–48, 2010

Citrome L: Number needed to treat: what it is and what it isn't, and why every clinician should know how to calculate it. J Clin Psychiatry 72:412–413, 2011a

Citrome L: Olanzapine-fluoxetine combination for the treatment of bipolar depression. Exp Opin Pharmacotherapy 12:2751–2758, 2011b

Citrome L: Levomilnacipran for major depressive disorder: a systematic review of the efficacy and safety profile for this newly approved antidepressant—what is the number needed to treat, number needed to harm and likelihood to be helped or harmed? Int J Clin Pract 67:1089–1104, 2013a

Citrome L: Cariprazine in bipolar disorder: clinical efficacy, tolerability, and place in therapy. Adv Ther 30:102–113, 2013b

Citrome L: Treatment of bipolar depression: making sensible decisions. CNS Spectr 19(suppl 1):4–11, 2014

Citrome L: The ABC's of dopamine receptor partial agonists—aripiprazole, brexpiprazole and cariprazine: the 15-min challenge to sort these agents out. Int J Clin Pract 69:1211–1220, 2015

Citrome L: Deutetrabenazine for tardive dyskinesia: a systematic review of the efficacy and safety profile for this newly approved novel medication—what is the number needed to treat, number needed to harm and likelihood to be helped or harmed? Int J Clin Pract 71(11), November 2017 (Epub)

Clayton AH, McGarvey EL, Clavet GJ: The Changes in Sexual Functioning Questionnaire (CSFQ): development, reliability, and validity. Psychopharmacol Bull 33:731–745, 1997

Clayton AH, Pradko JF, Croft HA, et al: Prevalence of sexual dysfunction among newer antidepressants. J Clin Psychiatry 63:357–366, 2002

Clayton AH, Keller A, McGarvey EL: Burden of phase-specific sexual dysfunction with SSRIs. J Affect Disord 91:27–32, 2006

Clayton AH, Kornstein S, Prakash A, et al: Changes in sexual functioning associated with duloxetine, escitalopram, and placebo in the treatment of patients with major depressive disorder. J Sex Med 4:917–929, 2007

Clos S, Rauchhaus P, Severn A, et al: Long-term effect of lithium maintenance therapy on estimated glomerular filtration rate in patients with affective disorders: a population-based cohort study. Lancet Psychiatry 2(12):1075–1083, 2015

Cohen J: A power primer. Psychol Bull 112:155–159, 1992

Cohen AJ, Bartlik B: Gingko biloba for antidepressant-induced sexual dysfunction. J Sex Marital Ther 24:139–143, 1998

Cohen LM, Tessier EG, Germain MJ, et al: Update on psychotropic medication use in renal disease. Psychosomatics 45:34–48, 2004

Cooper C, Bebbington P, King M, et al: Why people do not take their psychotropic drugs as prescribed: results of the 2000 National Psychiatric Morbidity Survey. Acta Psychiatr Scand 116:47–53, 2007

Correll CU, Leucht S, Kane JM: Lower risk for tardive dyskinesia associated with second-generation antipsychotics: a systematic review of 1-year studies. Am J Psychiatry 161:414–425, 2004

Correll CU, Manu P, Olshshanskiy V, et al: Cardiometabolic risk of second-generation antipsychotic medications during first-time use in children and adolescents. JAMA 302:1765–1773, 2009

Correll CU, Skuban A, Hobart M, et al: Efficacy of brexpiprazole in patients with acute schizophrenia: review of three randomized, double-blind, placebo-controlled studies. Schizophr Res 174(1–3):82–92, 2016

Dall M, Schaffalitzky de Muckadell OB, Lassen AT, et al: An association between selective serotonin reuptake inhibitor use and serious upper gastrointestinal bleeding. Clin Gastroenterol Hepatol 7:1314–1321, 2009

Dall M, Schaffalitzky de Muckadell OB, Lassen AT, et al: There is an association between selective serotonin reuptake inhibitor use and uncomplicated peptic ulcers: a population-based case-control study. Aliment Pharmacol Ther 32:1383–1391, 2010

Davé M: Treatment of lithium-induced tremor with atenolol. Can J Psychiatry 34:132–133, 1989

Davidson JR, Bose A, Wang Q: Safety and efficacy of escitalopram in the long-term treatment of generalized anxiety disorder. J Clin Psychiatry 66:1441–1446, 2005

Davis JM, Janicak PG, Sakkas P, et al: Electroconvulsive therapy in the treatment of the neuroleptic malignant syndrome. Convuls Ther 7:111–120, 1991

DeBattista C, Solvason B, Poirier J, et al: A placebo-controlled, randomized, double-blind study of adjunctive bupropion sustained release in the treatment of SSRI-induced sexual dysfunction. J Clin Psychiatry 66:844–848, 2005

Deberdt W, Winokur A, Cavazzoni PA, et al: Amantadine for weight gain associated with olanzapine treatment. Eur Neuropsychopharmacol 15:13–21, 2005

De Las Cuevas C, Sanz EJ: Duloxetine-induced excessive disturbing and disabling yawning. J Clin Psychopharmacol 27:106–107, 2007

Delgado PL, Brannan SK, Mallinkrodt CH, et al: Sexual functioning assessed in 4 double-blind placebo- and paroxetine-controlled trials of duloxetine for major depressive disorder. J Clin Psychiatry 66:686–692, 2005

Demyttenaere K, Albert A, Masters P, et al: What happens with adverse events during 6 months of treatment with selective serotonin reuptake inhibitors? J Clin Psychiatry 66:859–863, 2005

De Picker L, Van Dan Eede F, Dumont G, et al: Antidepressants and the risk of hyponatremia: a class-by-class review of the literature. Psychosomatics 55:536–547, 2014

Dequardo JR: Modafinil-associated clozapine toxicity. Am J Psychiatry 159:1243–1244, 2002

de Silva VA, Suraweera C, Ratnatunga SS, et al: Metformin in prevention and treatment of antipsychotic induced weight gain: a systematic review and meta-analysis. BMC Psychiatry 16:341, 2016

DeToledo JC, Toledo C, DeCerce J, et al: Changes in body weight with chronic, high-dose gabapentin therapy. Ther Drug Monit 19:394–396, 1997

Deuschl G, Bain P, Brin M: Consensus statement of the Movement Disorder Society on Tremor: Ad hoc Scientific Committee. Move Disord 13 (suppl 3):2–23, 1998

Diaz FJ, Meary A, Arranz MJ, et al: Acetyl-coenzyme A carboxylase alpha gene variations may be associated with the direct effects of some antipsychotics on triglyceride levels. Schizophr Res 115:136–140, 2009

Dodd S, Schacht A, Kelin K, et al: Nocebo effects in treatment of major depression: results from an individual study participant–level meta-analysis of the placebo arm of duloxetine clinical trials. J Clin Psychiatry 76:702–711, 2015

Doering BK, Nestoriuc Y, Barsky AJ, et al: Is somatosensory amplification a risk factor for an increased report of side effects? Reference data from the German general population. J Psychosom Res 79:492–497, 2015

Dording CM, Fisher L, Papakostas G, et al: A double-blind, randomized, pilot dose-finding study of maca root (L. meyenii) for the management of SSRI-induced sexual dysfunction. CNS Neurosci Ther 14:182–191, 2008

Dumon JP, Catteau J, Lanvin F, et al: Randomized, double-blind, crossover, placebo-controlled comparison of propranolol and betaxolol in the treatment of neuroleptic-induced akathisia. Am J Psychiatry 149:647–650, 1992

Dunkley EJ, Isbister GK, Sibbritt D, et al: The Hunter Serotonin Toxicity Criteria: simple and accurate diagnostic decision rules for serotonin toxicity. QJM 96:635–642, 2003

Dupuis B, Catteau J, Dumon JP, et al: Comparison of propranolol, sotalol, and betaxolol in the treatment of neuroleptic-induced akathisia. Am J Psychiatry 144:802–805, 1987

Durgam S, Earley W, Lipschitz A, et al: An 8-week randomized, double-blind, placebo-controlled evaluation of the safety and efficacy of cariprazine in patients with bipolar I depression. Am J Psychiatry 173:271–281, 2016

Earley W, Durgam S, Lu K, et al: Safety and tolerability of cariprazine in patients with acute exacerbation of schizophrenia: a pooled analysis of four phase II/III randomized, double-blind, placebo-controlled studies. Int Clin Psychopharmacol 32:319–328, 2017a

Earley W, Durgam S, Lu K, et al: Tolerability of cariprazine in the treatment of acute bipolar I mania: a pooled post-hoc analysis of 3 phase II/III studies. J Affect Disord 215:205–212, 2017b

Edwards J, Sperry V, Adams MH, et al: Vilazodone lacks proarrhythmogenic potential in healthy participants: a thorough ECG study. Int J Clin Pharmacol Ther 51:456–465, 2013

Ehret M, Goethe J, Lanosa M, et al: The effect of metformin on anthropometrics and insulin resistance in patients receiving atypical agents: a meta-analysis. J Clin Psychiatry 71:1286–1292, 2010

El-Ganzouri AR, Ivankovich AD, Braverman B, et al: Monoamine oxidase inhibitors: should they be discontinued preoperatively? Anesth Analg 64: 592–596, 1985

Elnazer HY, Sampson A, Baldwin D: Lithium and sexual dysfunction: an under-researched area. Hum Psychopharmacol 30:66–69, 2015

Emiliano ABF, Fudge JL: From galactorrhea to osteopenia: rethinking serotonin-prolactin interactions. Neuropsychopharmacology 29:833–846, 2004

Emsley R, Niehaus DJ, Koen L, et al: The effects of eicosapentanoic acid in tardive dyskinesia: a randomized, placebo-controlled trial. Schiz Res 84:112–120, 2006

English BA, Still DJ, Harper J: Failure of tolterodine to treat clozapine-induced nocturnal enuresis. Ann Pharmacother 35:867–869, 2001

English PJ, Ashcroft A, Patterson M, et al: Metformin prolongs the postprandial fall in plasma ghrelin concentrations in type II diabetes. Diabetes Metab Res Rev 23:299–303, 2007

Ernst CL, Goldberg JF: The reproductive safety profile of mood stabilizers, atypical antipsychotics, and broad-spectrum psychotropics. J Clin Psychiatry 63 (suppl 4):42–55, 2002

Esen-Danaci A, Sarandöl A, Taneli F, et al: Effects of second generation antipsychotics on leptin and ghrelin. Prog Neuropsychopharm Biol Psychiatry 32:1434–1438, 2008

Etminan M, Mikelberg FS, Brophy JM: Selective serotonin reuptake inhibitors and the risk of cataracts: a nested case-control study. Ophthalmology 117: 1251–1255, 2010

Evans RW, Tepper SJ, Shapiro RE, et al: The FDA alert on serotonin syndrome with use of triptans combined with selective serotonin reuptake inhibitors or selective serotonin norepinephrine reuptake inhibitors: American headache Society position paper. Headache 50:1089–1099, 2010

Evins AE, Cather C, Pratt SA, et al: Maintenance treatment with varenicline for smoking cessation in patients with schizophrenia or bipolar disorder: a randomized clinical trial. JAMA 311:145–154, 2014

Faasse K, Grey A, Horne R, et al: High perceived sensitivity to medicines is associated with higher medical care utilisation, increased symptom reporting and greater information-seeking about medication. Pharmacoepidemiol Drug Saf 24:592–596, 2015

Faedda GL, Tondo L, Baldessarini RJ, et al: Outcome after rapid versus gradual discontinuation of lithium treatment in bipolar disorders. Arch Gen Psychiatry 50:448–455, 1993

Fallon BA, Petkova E, Skritskaya N, et al: A double-masked, placebo-controlled study of fluoxetine for hypochondriasis. J Clin Psychopharmacol 28:638–645, 2008

Fava M, Nurnberg HG, Seidman SN, et al: Efficacy and safety of sildenafil in men with serotonergic antidepressant-associated erectile dysfunction: results from a randomized, double-blind, placebo-controlled trial. J Clin Psychiatry 67:240–246, 2006

Fava M, Wisniewski SR, Thase ME, et al: Metabolic assessment of aripiprazole as adjunctive therapy in major depressive disorder: a pooled analysis of 2 studies. J Clin Psychopharmacol 29:362–367, 2009

Fava GA, Gatti A, Belaise L, et al: Withdrawal symptoms after selective serotonin reuptake inhibitor discontinuation: a systematic review. Psychother Psychosom 84:72–81, 2015

Fawcett J, Barkin RL: Review of the results from clinical studies on the efficacy, safety and tolerability of mirtazapine for the treatment of patients with major depression. J Affect Disord 51:267–285, 1998

Fernandez HH, Factor SA, Hauser RA, et al: Randomized controlled trial of deutetrabenazine for tardive dyskinesia: the ARM-TD study. Neurology 88(21):2003–2010, 2017

Finch CK, Kelley KW, Williams RB: Treatment of lithium-induced diabetes insipidus with amiloride. Pharmacotherapy 23:546–550, 2003

Focosi D, Azzarà A, Kast RE, et al: Lithium and hematology: established and proposed uses. J Leukoc Biol 85:20–28, 2009

Fooladi E, Bell RJ, Jane F, et al: Testosterone improves antidepressant-emergent loss of libido in women: findings from a randomized, double-blind, placebo-controlled trial. J Sex Med 11:831–839, 2014

Fraguas D, Correll CU, Merchán-Naranjo J, et al: Efficacy and safety of second-generation antipsychotics in children and adolescents with psychotic and bipolar spectrum disorders: comprehensive review of prospective head-to-head and placebo-controlled comparisons. Eur Neuropsychopharmacol 21:621–645, 2011

Fraunfelder FW: Twice-yearly exams unnecessary for patients taking quetiapine. Am J Ophthalmol 138:870–871, 2004

Fraunfelder FW, Fraunfelder FT, Keates EU: Topiramate-associated acute, bilateral, secondary angle-closure glaucoma. Ophthalmology 111:109–111, 2004

Freeman DJ, Oyewumi LK: Will routine therapeutic drug monitoring have a place in clozapine therapy? Clin Pharmacokinet 32:93–100, 1997

Freudenreich O, Henderson DC, Macklin EA, et al: Modafinil for clozapine-treated schizophrenia patients: a double-blind, placebo-controlled pilot trial. J Clin Psychiatry 70:1674–1680, 2009

Gaby NS, Lefkowitz DS, Israel JR: Treatment of lithium tremor with metoprolol. Am J Psychiatry 140:593–595, 1983

Gadde KM, Franciscy DM, Wagner HR 2nd, et al: Zonisamide for weight loss in obese adults: a randomized controlled trial. JAMA 289:1820–1825, 2003

Gadde KM, Zhang W, Foust MS: Bupropion treatment of olanzapine-associated weight gain: an open-label, prospective trial. J Clin Psychopharmacol 26:409–413, 2006

Gadde KM, Yonish GM, Foust MS, et al: Combination therapy of zonisamide and bupropion for weight reduction in obese women: a preliminary, randomized, open-label study. J Clin Psychiatry 68:1226–1229, 2007

Gadde KM, Allison DB, Ryan DH, et al: Effects of low-dose, controlled-release, phentermine plus topiramate combination on weight and associated co-morbidities in overweight and obese adults (CONQUER): a randomised, placebo-controlled, phase 3 trial. Lancet 377:1341–1352, 2011

Galvão-de Almeida A, Guindalini C, Batista-Neves S, et al: Can antidepressants prevent interferon-alpha-induced depression? A review of the literature. Gen Hosp Psychiatry 32:401–405, 2010

Gao K, Kemp DE, Fein E, et al: Number needed to treat to harm for discontinuation due to adverse events in the treatment of bipolar depression, major depressive disorder, and generalized anxiety disorder with atypical antipsychotics. J Clin Psychiatry 72:1063–1071, 2011

Garza D, Murphy M, Tseng LJ, et al: A double-blind randomized placebo-controlled pilot study of neuropsychiatric adverse events in abstinent smokers treated with varenicline or placebo. Biol Psychiatry 69:1075–1082, 2011

Gebhardt S, Haberhausen M, Heinzel-Gutenbrunner M, et al: Antipsychotic-induced body weight gain: predictors and a systematic categorization of the long-term weight course. J Psychiatr Res 43:620–626, 2009

Gelenberg AJ, Jefferson JW: Lithium tremor. J Clin Psychiatry 56:283–287, 1995

Gelenberg AJ, Kane JM, Keller MB, et al: Comparison of standard and low serum levels of lithium for maintenance treatment of bipolar disorder. N Engl J Med 321:1489–1493, 1989

Gerstner T, Büsing D, Bell N, et al: Valproic acid-induced pancreatitis: 16 new cases and a review of the literature. J Gastroenterol 42:39–48, 2007

Gex-Fabry M, Balant-Gorgia AE, Balant LP, et al: Time course of clinical response to venlafaxine: relevance of plasma level and chirality. Eur J Clin Pharmacol 59:883–891, 2004

Ghadirian AM, Annable L, Bélanger MC: Lithium, benzodiazepines, and sexual function in bipolar patients. Am J Psychiatry 149:801–805, 1992

Ghanizadeh A, Nikseresht MS, Sachraian A: The effect of zonisamide on antipsychotic-associated weight gain in patients with schizophrenia: a randomized, double-blind, placebo-controlled trial. Schizophr Res 147:110–115, 2013

Gibbons RD, Hur K, Bhaumik DK, et al: The relationship between antidepressant use and rate of suicide. Arch Gen Psychiatry 62:165–172, 2005

Gibbons RD, Hur K, Brown CH, et al: Relationship between antiepileptic drugs and suicide attempts in patients with bipolar disorder. Arch Gen Psychiatry 66:1354–1360, 2009

Gidal BE, Maly MM, Budde J, et al: Effect of a high-protein meal on gabapentin pharmacokinetics. Epilepsy Res 23:71–76, 1996

Gitlin M: Lithium-induced renal insufficiency. J Clin Psychopharmacol 13:276–279, 1993

Gitlin M: Lithium and the kidney—an updated review. Drug Saf 20:231–243, 1999

Glassman AH, Bigger JT Jr: Antipsychotic drugs: prolonged QTc interval, torsade de pointes, and sudden death. Am J Psychiatry 158:1774–1782, 2001

Goldberg JF: Adverse cognitive effects of psychotropic medications, in Cognitive Dysfunction in Bipolar Disorder: A Guide for Clinicians. Edited by Goldberg JF, Burdick K. Washington, DC, American Psychiatric Publishing, 2008, pp 137–158

Goldberg JF: Antidepressants in bipolar disorder: seven myths and realities. Curr Psychiatry 9:41–49, 2010

Goldstein TR, Frye MA, Denicoff KD, et al: Antidepressant discontinuation-related mania: critical prospective observation and theoretical implications in bipolar disorder. J Clin Psychiatry 60:563–567, 1999

Goodnick PJ: Blood levels and acute response to bupropion. Am J Psychiatry 149:399–400, 1992

Gopalakrishnan R, Jacob KS, Kuruvilla A, et al: Sildenafil in the treatment of antipsychotic-induced erectile dysfunction: a randomized, double-blind, placebo-controlled, flexible–dose, two-way crossover trial. Am J Psychiatry 163:494–499, 2006

Graham KA, Hongbin G, Lieberman JA, et al: Double-blind, placebo-controlled investigation of amantadine for weight loss in subjects who gained weight with olanzapine. Am J Psychiatry 162:1744–1746, 2005

Gray SL, Anderson ML, Dublin S, et al: Cumulative use of strong anticholinergics and incident dementia: a prospective cohort study. JAMA Intern Med 175:401–407, 2015

Gray SL, Dublin S, Yu O, et al: Benzodiazepine use and risk of incident dementia or cognitive decline: prospective population based study. BMJ 352:i90, 2016

Green CA, Yarborough BH, Leo MC, et al: The STRIDE weight loss and lifestyle intervention for individuals taking antipsychotic medications: a randomized trial. Am J Psychiatry 172:71–81, 2015

Greenway FL, Fujioka K, Plodowski RA, et al: Effect of naltrexone plus bupropion on weight loss in overweight and obese adults (COR-I): a multicentre, randomised, double-blind, placebo-controlled, phase 3 trial. Lancet 376: 595–605, 2010

Grigoriadis DE, Smith E, Hoare SRJ, et al: Pharmacologic characterization of valbenazine (NBI-98854) and its metabolites. J Pharmacol Exper Ther 361:454–461, 2017

Gross MD: Reversal by bethanechol of sexual dysfunction caused by anticholinergic antidepressants. Am J Psychiatry 139:1193–1194, 1982

Grossman E, Messerli FH, Grodzicki T, et al: Should a moratorium be placed on sublingual nifedipine capsules given for hypertensive emergencies and pseudoemergencies? JAMA 276:1328–1331, 1996

Grunebaum MF, Ellis SP, Li S, et al: Antidepressants and suicide risk in the United States, 1985–1999. J Clin Psychiatry 65:1456–1462, 2004

Grünfeld J-P, Rossier BC: Lithium nephrotoxicity revisited. Nat Rev Nephrol 5:270–276, 2009

Guay DR: Are there alternatives to the use of quinine to treat nocturnal leg cramps? Consult Pharm 23:141–156, 2008

Guille C, Sachs G: Clinical outcome of adjunctive topiramate treatment in a sample of refractory bipolar patients with comorbid conditions. Prog Neuropsychopharmacol Biol Psychiatry 26:1035–1039, 2002

Gunnell D, Irvine D, Wise L, et al: Varenicline and suicidal behaviour: a cohort study based on data from the General Practice Research database. BMJ 339:B3805, 2009

Gutgesell H, Atkins D, Barst R, et al: Cardiovascular monitoring of children and adolescents receiving psychotropic drugs. A statement for healthcare professionals from the Committee on Congenital Cardiac Defects, Council on Cardiovascular Disease in the Young, American Heart Association. Circulation 99:979–982, 1999

Hackam DG, Mrkobrada M: Selective serotonin reuptake inhibitors and brain hemorrhage: a meta-analysis. Neurology 79(18):1862–1865, 2012

Hamner N: The effects of atypical antipsychotics on serum prolactin levels. Ann Clin Psychiatry 14:163–173, 2002

Hampton LM, Daubresse M, Chang HY, et al: Emergency department visits by adults for psychiatric medication adverse events. JAMA Psychiatry 71:1006–1014, 2014

Hanssens L, L'Italien G, Loze JY, et al: The effect of antipsychotic medication on sexual function and serum prolactin levels in community treated schizophrenic patients: results from the Schizophreni Trial of Aripiprazole (STAR) study (NCT00237913). BMC Psychiatry 8:95, 2008

Harth Y, Rapoport M: Photosensitivity associated with antipsychotics, antidepressants and anxiolytics. Drug Saf 14:252–259, 1996

Hasani-Ranjbar S, Nayebi N, Larijani B, et al: A systematic review of the efficacy and safety of herbal medicines used in the treatment of obesity. World J Gastroenterol 15:3073–3085, 2009

Hasani-Ranjbar S, Vahidi H, Taslimi S, et al: A systematic review on the efficacy of herbal medicines in the management of human drug-induced hyperprolactinemia; potential sources for the development of novel drugs. Int J Pharmacol 6:691–695, 2010

Henderson DC, Fan X, Copeland PM, et al: Aripiprazole added to overweight and obese olanzapine-treated schizophrenia patients. J Clin Psychopharmacol 29:165–169, 2009a

Henderson DC, Fan X, Sharma B, et al: A double-blind, placebo-controlled trial of rosiglitazone for clozapine-induced glucose metabolism impairment in patients with schizophrenia. Acta Psychiatr Scand 119:457–465, 2009b

Hennen J, Perlis RH, Sachs G, et al: Weight gain during treatment of bipolar I patients with olanzapine. J Clin Psychiatry 65:1679–1687, 2004

Hetmar O, Povlsen UJ, Ladefoged J, et al: Lithium: long-term effects on the kidney: a prospective follow-up study ten years after kidney biopsy. Br J Psychiatry 158:53–58, 1991

Hirsch LJ, Weintraub DB, Du Y, et al: Correlating lamotrigine serum concentrations with tolerability in patients with epilepsy. Neurol 28:1022–1026, 2004

Hirsch LJ, Weintraub DB, Buchsbaum R, et al: Predictors of lamotrigine-associated rash. Epilepsia 47:318–322, 2006

Hollander E, McCarley A: Yohimbine treatment of sexual side effects induced by serotonin reuptake blockers. J Clin Psychiatry 53:207–209, 1992

Holmes LB, Baldwin EJ, Smith CR, et al: Increased frequency of isolated cleft palate in infants exposed to lamotrigine during pregnancy. Neurology 70:2152–2158, 2008

Homann CK, Wenzel K, Suppan K, et al: Sleep attacks in patients taking dopamine agonists: a review. BMJ 324:1483–1487, 2002

Hori A, Kataoka S, Sakai K, et al: Valproic acid-induced hearing loss and tinnitus. Intern Med 42:1153–1154, 2003

Horiguchi J, Inami Y: Effect of clonazepam on neuroleptic-induced oculogyric crisis. Acta Psychiatr Scand 80:521–523, 1989

Hosojima H, Togo T, Odawara T, et al: Early effects of olanzapine on serum levels of ghrelin, adiponectin and leptin in patients with schizophrenia. J Psychopharmacol 20:75–79, 2006

Hough D, Gopal S, Vijapurkar U, et al: Paliperidone palmitate maintenance treatment in delaying the time-to-relapse in patients with schizophrenia: a randomized, double-blind, placebo-controlled study. Schizophr Res 116(2–3):107–117, 2010

Houston JP, Kohler J, Bishop JR, et al: Pharmacogenetic associations with weight gain in olanzapine treatment of patients without schizophrenia. J Clin Psychiatry 73:1077–1086, 2012

Hu XH, Bull SA, Hunkeler EM, et al: Incidence and duration of side effects and those rated as bothersome with selective serotonin reuptake inhibitor treatment for depression: patient report versus physician estimate. J Clin Psychiatry 65:959–965, 2004

Hwang TJ, Ni HC, Chen HC, et al: Risk predictors for hypnosedative-related complex sleep behaviors: a retrospective, cross-sectional pilot study. J Clin Psychiatry 71:1331–1335, 2010

Isbister GK, Bowe SJ, Dawson A, et al: Relative toxicity of selective serotonin reuptake inhibitors (SSRIs) in overdose. J Toxicol Clin Toxicol 42:277–285, 2004

Ishøy PL, Knop FK, Broberg BV, et al: Effect of GLP-1 receptor agonist treatment on body weight in obese antipsychotic-treated patients with schizophrenia: a randomized, placebo-controlled trial. Diabetes Obes Metab 19:162–171, 2017

Isojärvi JI, Laatikainen TJ, Pakarinen J, et al: Polycystic ovaries and hyperandrogenism in women taking valproate for epilepsy. N Engl J Med 329:1383–1388, 1993

Jacobsen FM: Fluoxetine-induced sexual dysfunction and an open trial of yohimbine. J Clin Psychiatry 53:119–122, 1992

Jacobson PL, Mahableshwarkar AR, Chen Y, et al: Effect of vortioxetine vs. escitalopram on sexual functioning in adults with well-treated major depressive disorder experiencing SSRI-induced sexual dysfunction. J Sex Med 12:2036–2048, 2015

Jacobson PL, Mahableshwarkar AR, Palo WA, et al: Treatment-emergent sexual dysfunction in randomized trials of vortioxetine for major depressive disorder or generalized anxiety disorder: a pooled analysis. CNS Spectr 21:357–378, 2016

Jaffee MS, Bostwick JM: Buspirone as an antidote to venlafaxine-induced bruxism. Psychosomatics 41:535–536, 2000

Jain AK, Kaplan RA, Gadde KM, et al: Bupropion SR vs. placebo for weight loss in obese patients with depressive symptoms. Obes Res 10:1049–1056, 2002

Jefferson JW: A clinician's guide to monitoring kidney function in lithium-treated patients. J Clin Psychiatry 71:1153–1157, 2010

Jefferson JW, Kalin NH: Serum lithium levels and long-term diuretic use. JAMA 241:1134–1136, 1979

Joffe G, Takala P, Tchoukhine E, et al: Orlistat in clozapine- or olanzapine-treated patients with overweight or obesity: a 16-week randomized, double-blind, placebo-controlled trial. J Clin Psychiatry 69:706–711, 2008

Joffe H, Cohen LS, Suppes T, et al: Valproate is associated with new-onset oligoamenorrhea with hyperandrogenism in women with bipolar disorder. Biol Psychiatry 59:1078–1086, 2006

Kane JM, Osuntokun O, Krzhanovskaya LA, et al: A 28-week, randomized, double-blind study of olanzapine versus aripiprazole in the treatment of schizophrenia. J Clin Psychiatry 70:572–581, 2009

Kane JM, Detke HC, Naber D, et al: Olanzapine long-acting injection: a 24-week, randomized, double-blind trial of maintenance treatment in patients with schizophrenia. Am J Psychiatry 167:181–189, 2010

Kane JM, Mackle M, Snow-Adami L, et al: A randomized placebo-controlled trial of asenapine for the prevention of relapse of schizophrenia after long-term treatment. J Clin Psychiatry 72:349–355, 2011

Kane JM, Sanchez R, Perry PP, et al: Aripiprazole intramuscular depot as maintenance treatment in patients with schizophrenia: a 52-week, multi-center, randomized, double-blind, placebo-controlled study. J Clin Psychiatry 73:617–624, 2012

Kane JM, Peters-Strickland T, Baker RA, et al: Aripiprazole once-monthly in the acute treatment of schizophrenia: findings from a 12-week, randomized, double-blind, placebo-controlled study. J Clin Psychiatry 75(11):1254–1260, 2014

Kang BJ, Lee SJ, Kim MD, et al: A placebo-controlled, double-blind trial of gingko biloba for antidepressant-induced sexual dysfunction. Hum Psychopharmacol 17:279–284, 2002

Kao CH, Sun LM, Su KP, et al: Benzodiazepine use possibly increases cancer risk: a population-based retrospective cohort study in Taiwan. J Clin Psychiatry 73:e555–e560, 2012

Kapur S, Seeman P: Does fast dissociation from the dopamine d(2) receptor explain the action of atypical antipsychotics? A new hypothesis. Am J Psychiatry 158:360–369, 2001

Kapur S, Langlois X, Vinken P, et al: The differential effects of atypical antipsychotics in prolactin elevation are explained by their differential blood-brain disposition: a pharmacological analysis in rats. J Pharmacol Exp Ther 302:1129–1134, 2002

Karabulut V, Gonenli S, Yumrukcal H, et al: Aripiprazole improves neuroleptic-associated tardive dyskinesia, but it does not ameliorate psychotic symptoms. Prog Neuropsychopharmacol Biol Psychiatr 32:1342–1343, 2008

Karagianis J, Hoffman VP, Arranz B, et al: Orally disintegrating olanzapine and potential differences in treatment-emergent weight gain. Hum Psychopharmacol 23:275–281, 2008

Karagianis J, Grossman L, Landry J, et al: A randomized controlled trial of the effect of sublingual orally disintegrating olanzapine versus oral olanzapine on body mass index: the PLATYPUS Study. Schizophr Res 113:41–48, 2009

Kashani L, Raisi F, Saroukhani S, et al: Saffron for treatment of fluoxetine-induced sexual dysfunction in women: randomized double-blind placebo-controlled study. Hum Psychopharmacol 28:54–60, 2013

Keck PE Jr, Marcus R, Tourkodimitris S, et al: A placebo-controlled, double-blind study of the efficacy and safety of aripiprazole in patients with acute bipolar mania. Am J Psychiatry 160:1651–1658, 2003

Keck PE Jr, Perlis RH, Otto MW, et al: The Expert Consensus Guidelines: Treatment of Bipolar Disorder 2004. A Postgraduate Medicine Special Report. Minneapolis, MN, McGraw-Hill, 2004, pp 1–120

Kelly DL, Conley RR: Thyroid function in treatment-resistant schizophrenia patients treated with quetiapine, risperidone, or fluphenazine. J Clin Psychiatry 66:80–84, 2005

Kelly KV: Parallel treatment: therapy with one clinician and medication with another. Hosp Commun Psychiatr 43:778–780, 1992

Kelly S, Davies E, Fearns S, et al: Effects of oral contraceptives containing ethinylestradiol with either drospirenone or levonorgestrel on various parameters associated with well-being in healthy women: a randomized, single-blind, parallel-group, multicentre study. Clin Drug Investig 30:325–336, 2010

Kennedy SH, Rizvi S: Sexual dysfunction, depression, and the impact of antidepressants. J Clin Psychopharmacol 29:157–164, 2009

Kennedy SH, Eisfeld BS, Dickens SE, et al: Antidepressant-induced sexual dysfunction during treatment with moclobemide, paroxetine, sertraline, and venlafaxine. J Clin Psychiatry 61:276–281, 2000

Kessler RC, Stang PE, Wittchen HU, et al: Lifetime panic-depression comorbidity in the National Comorbidity Survey. Arch Gen Psychiatry 55:801–808, 1998

Ketter TA, Kalali AH, Weisler RH, et al: A 6-month, multicenter, open-label evaluation of beaded, extended-release carbamazepine capsule monotherapy in bipolar disorder patients with manic or mixed episodes. J Clin Psychiatry 65:668–673, 2004

Ketter TA, Sachs GS, Durgam S, et al: The safety and tolerability of cariprazine in patients with manic or mixed episodes associated with bipolar I disorder: a 16-week open-label study. J Affect Disord 225:350–356, 2018

Kim BJ, Sohn JW, Park CS, et al: Body weight and plasma levels of ghrelin and leptin during treatment with olanzapine. J Korean Med Sci 23:685–690, 2008

Kim NW, Song YM, Kim E, et al: Adjunctive alpha-lipoic acid reduces weight gain compared with placebo at 12 weeks in schizophrenic patients treated with atypical antipsychotics: a double-blind, randomized, placebo-controlled study. Int Clin Psychopharmacol 31:265–274, 2016

Kim SW, Shin IS, Kim JM, et al: Factors potentiating the risk of mirtazapine-associated restless legs syndrome. Hum Psychopharmacol 23:615–620, 2008

Kinahan JC, NiChorcorian A, Cunningham S, et al.: Risk factors for polyuria in a cross-section of community psychiatric lithium-treated patients. Bipolar Disord 17:15–62, 2015

Kinon BJ, Basson BR, Gilmore JA, et al: Long-term olanzapine treatment: weight change and weight-related health factors in schizophrenia. J Clin Psychiatry 62:92–100, 2001

Kinon BJ, Gilmore JA, Liu H, et al: Prevalence of hyperprolactinemia in schizophrenic patients treated with conventional antipsychotic medications or risperidone. Psychoneuroendocrinology 28 (suppl 2):55–68, 2003

Kinon BJ, Jeste DV, Kollack-Walker S, et al: Olanzapine treatment for tardive dyskinesia in schizophrenia patients: a prospective clinical trial with patients randomized to blinded dose reduction periods. Prog Neuropsychopharmacol Biol Psychiatry 28:985–996, 2004

Kirov G, Tredget J: Add-on topiramate reduces weight in overweight patients with affective disorders: a clinical case series. BMC Psychiatry 5:19, 2005

Kishi T, Fujita N, Eguchi T, et al: Mechanism for reduction of serum folate by antiepileptic drugs during prolonged therapy. J Neurol Sci 145:109–112, 1997

Klampfl K, Quattländer A, Burger R, et al: Case report: intoxication with high dose of long-acting methylphenidate (Concerta(®)) in a suicidal 14 year-old girl. Atten Defic Hyperact Disord 2:221–224, 2010

Klein DJ, Cottingham EM, Sorter M, et al: A randomized, double-blind, placebo-controlled trial of metformin treatment of weight gain associated with initiation of atypical antipsychotic therapy in children and adolescents. Am J Psychiatry 163:2072–2079, 2006

Knudsen JF, Flowers CM, Kortepeter C, et al: Clinical profile of oxcarbazepine-related angioneurotic edema: case report and review. Pediatr Neurol 37:134–137, 2007

Ko DT, Herbert PR, Coffey CS, et al: Beta-blocker therapy and symptoms of depression, fatigue and sexual dysfunction. JAMA 288:351–357, 2002

Kontaxakis VP, Karaiskos D, Havaki-Kontaxaki BJ, et al: Can quetiapine-induced hypothyroidism be reversible without quetiapine discontinuation? Clin Neuropharmacol 32:295–296, 2009

Kraszewska A, Chlopocka-Wozniak M, Abramowicz M, et al: A cross-sectional study of thyroid function in 66 patients with bipolar disorder receiving lithium for 10-44 years. Bipolar Disord 17:375–380, 2016

Kraus MR, Schäfer A, Schöttker A, et al: Therapy of interferon-induced depression in chronic hepatitis C with citalopram: a randomised, double-blind, placebo-controlled study. Gut 57:531–536, 2008

Krauthammer C, Klerman GL: Secondary mania. Manic syndromes associated with antecedent physical illness or drugs. Arch Gen Psychiatry 35:1333–1339, 1978

Kreinin A, Miodownik C, Mirkin V, et al: Double-blind, randomized, placebo-controlled trial of metoclopramide for hypersalivation associated with clozapine. J Clin Psychopharmacol 36:200–205, 2016

Kristiana I, Sharpe LJ, Catts VS, et al: Antipsychotic drugs upregulate lipogenic gene expression by disrupting intracellular trafficking of lipoprotein-derived cholesterol. Pharmacogenomics J 10:396–407, 2010

Krystal AD, Mittoux A, Meisels P, et al: Effects of adjunctive brexpiprazole on sleep disturbances in patients with major depressive disorder: an open-label, flexible-dose, exploratory study. Prim Care Companion CNS Disord 18(5), September 8, 2016

Kuzminski AM, Del Giacco EJ, Allen RH, et al: Effective treatment of cobalamin deficiency with oral cobalamin. Blood 92:1191–1198, 1998

Kwon JS, Choi JS, Bahk WM, et al: Weight management program for treatment-emergent weight gain in olanzapine-treated patients with schizophrenia or schizoaffective disorder: a 12-week randomized controlled clinical trial. J Clin Psychiatry 67:547–553, 2006

Laje G, Allen AS, Akula N, et al: Genome-wide association study of suicidal ideation emerging during citalopram treatment of depressed outpatients. Pharmacogenet Genomics 19:666–674, 2009

Lam SP, Fong SY, Ho CK, et al: Parasomnia among psychiatric outpatients: a clinical, epidemiologic, cross-sectional study. J Clin Psychiatry 69:1374–1382, 2008

Lamberti JS, Bellnier T, Schwarzkopf SB: Weight gain among schizophrenic patients treated with clozapine. Am J Psychiatry 149:689–690, 1992

Landén M, Eriksson E, Agren H, et al: Effect of buspirone on sexual dysfunction in depressed patients treated with selective serotonin reuptake inhibitors. J Clin Psychopharmacol 19:268–271, 1999

Landry P, Dimitri E, Tessler S, et al: Efficacy of lipid-lowering medications in patients treated with clozapine: a naturalistic study. J Clin Psychopharmacol 28:348–349, 2008

Larsen JR, Vedtofte L, Jakobsen MSL, et al: Effect of luraglutide treatment on prediabetes and overweight or obesity in clozapine- or olanzapine-treated patients with schizophrenia spectrum disorder: a randomized clinical trial. JAMA Psychiatry 74:719–728, 2017

Lauriello J, Lambert T, Anderson S, et al: An 8-week, double-blind, randomized, placebo-controlled study of olanzapine long-acting injection in acutely ill patients with schizophrenia. J Clin Psychiatry 69:790–799, 2008

Lazarus JH: Lithium and thyroid. Best Pract Res Clin Endocrinol Metab 23:723–733, 2009

Lebret T, Hervé J-M, Gorny P, et al: Efficacy and safety of a novel combination of L-arginine glutamate and yohimbine hydrochloride: a new oral therapy for erectile dysfunction. Eur Urol 41:608–613, 2002

Lepkifiker E, Sverdlik A, Iancu I, et al: Renal insufficiency in long-term lithium treatment. J Clin Psychiatry 65:850–856, 2004

Lerer B, Segman RH, Fangerau H, et al: Pharmacogenetics of tardive dyskinesia. Combined analysis of 780 patients supports association with dopamine D3 receptor gene Ser9Gly polymorphism. Neuropsychopharmacology 27:105–119, 2002

Lerner V, Bergman J, Statsenko N, et al: Vitamin B6 treatment in acute neuroleptic-induced akathisia: a randomized, double-blind, placebo-controlled study. J Clin Psychiatry 65:1550–1554, 2004

Lerner V, Miodownik C, Kaptsan A, et al: Vitamin B6 treatment for tardive dyskinesia: a randomized, double-blind, placebo-controlled, cross-over study. J Clin Psychiatry 68:1648–1654, 2007

Leucht S, Cipriani A, Spinelli L, et al: Comparative efficacy and tolerability of 15 antipsychotic drugs in schizophrenia: a multiple-treatments meta-analysis. Lancet 382(9896):951–962, 2013

Levenson JL: Neuroleptic malignant syndrome. Am J Psychiatry 142:1137–1145, 1985

Levinson-Castiel R, Merlob P, Linder N, et al: Neonatal abstinence syndrome after in utero exposure to selective serotonin reuptake inhibitors in term infants. Arch Pediatr Adolesc Med 160:173–176, 2006

Li Z, Maglione M, Tu W, et al: Meta-analysis: pharmacologic treatment of obesity. Ann Intern Med 142:532–546, 2005

Liang CS, Ho PS, Shen LJ, et al: Comparison of the efficacy and impact on cognition of glycopyrrolate and biperiden for clozapine-induced sialorrhea in schizophrenic patients: a randomized, double-blind, crossover study. Schizophr Res 119:138–144, 2010

Libov I, Miodownik C, Bersudsky Y, et al: Efficacy of piracetam in the treatment of tardive dyskinesia in schizophrenia patients: a randomized, double-blind, placebo-controlled crossover study. J Clin Psychiatry 68:1031–1037, 2007

Lieberman JA, Stroup TS, McEvoy JP, et al: Effectiveness of antipsychotic drugs in patients with chronic schizophrenia. N Engl J Med 353:1209–1223, 2005

Linnebank M, Moskau S, Semmler A, et al: Antiepileptic drugs interact with folate and vitamin B12 serum levels. Ann Neurol 69:352–359, 2011

Lipkovich I, Citrome L, Perlis R, et al: Early predictors of substantial weight gain in bipolar patients treated with olanzapine. J Clin Psychopharmacol 26:316–320, 2006

Lobbezoo F, Lavigne GJ, Tanguay R, et al: The effect of the catecholamine precursor l-dopa on sleep bruxism: a controlled clinical trial. Mov Disord 12:73–78, 1997

Loebel A, Cucchiaro J, Silva R, et al: Lurasidone monotherapy in the treatment of bipolar I depression: a randomized, double-blind, placebo-controlled study. Am J Psychiatry 171:160–168, 2014a

Loebel A, Cucchiaro J, Silva R, et al: Lurasidone as adjunctive therapy with lithium or valproate for the treatment of bipolar I depression: a randomized, double-blind, placebo-controlled study. Am J Psychiatry 171:169–177, 2014b

Lohr JB, Liu L, Caligiuri MP, et al: Modafinil improves antipsychotic-induced parkinsonism but not excessive daytime sleepiness, psychiatric symptoms or cognition in schizophrenia and schizoaffective disorder: a randomized, double-blind, placebo-controlled study. Schizophr Res 150:289–296, 2013

Londborg PD, Smith WT, Glaudin V: Short-term cotherapy with clonazepam and fluoxetine: anxiety, sleep disturbance and core symptoms of depression. J Affect Disord 61:73–79, 2000

Lorberg B, Youssef NA, Bhagwagar Z: Lamotrigine-associated rash: to rechallenge or not to rechallenge? Int J Neuropsychopharmacol 12:257–265, 2009

Lu BY, Cullen CE, Eide CE, et al: Antidepressant-induced sweating alleviated by aripiprazole. J Clin Psychopharmacol 28:710–711, 2008

Lu ML, Lane HY, Lin SK, et al: Adjunctive fluvoxamine inhibits clozapine-related weight gain and metabolic disturbances. J Clin Psychiatry 65:766–771, 2004

Maayan L, Vakhrusheva J, Correll CU: Effectiveness of medications used to attenuate antipsychotic-related weight gain and metabolic abnormalities: a systematic review and meta-analysis. Neuropsychopharmacology 35:1520–1530, 2010

Maina G, Albert U, Salvi V, et al: Weight gain during long-term treatment of obsessive-compulsive disorder: a prospective comparison between serotonin reuptake inhibitors. J Clin Psychiatry 65:1365–1371, 2004

Mallikaarjun S, Shoaf SE, Boulton DW, et al: Effects of hepatic or renal impairment on the pharmacokinetics of aripiprazole. Clin Pharmacokinet 47:533–542, 2008

Mansur RB, Ahmed J, Cha DS, et al: Luraglutide promotes improvement in objective measures of cognitive dysfunction in individuals with mood disorders. J Affect Disord 207:114–120, 2017

Manu P, Sarpal D, Muir O, et al: When can patients with potentially life-threatening adverse effects be rechallenged with clozapine? A systematic review of the published literature. Schizophr Res 134:180–186, 2012

Marangell LB, Johnson CR, Kertz B, et al: Olanzapine in the treatment of apathy in previously depressed participants maintained with selective serotonin reuptake inhibitors: an open-label, flexible-dose study. J Clin Psychiatry 63:391–395, 2002

Marder SR, McQuade RD, Stock E, et al: Aripiprazole in the treatment of schizophrenia: safety and tolerability in short-term, placebo-controlled trials. Schizophr Res 61:123–136, 2003

Markowitz GS, Radhakrishnan J, Kambham N, et al: Lithium nephrotoxicity: a progressive combined glomerular and tuberinterstitial nephropathy. J Am Soc Nephrology 11:1439–1448, 2000

Markowitz JS, DeVane CL, Malcolm RJ, et al: Pharmacokinetics of olanzapine after single-dose oral administration of standard tablets versus normal and sublingual administration of an orally disintegrating tablet in healthy volunteers. J Clin Psychopharmacol 46:164–171, 2006

Masand PS, Ashton AK, Gupta S, et al: Sustained-release bupropion for selective serotonin reuptake inhibitor-induced sexual dysfunction: a randomized, double-blind, placebo-controlled, parallel-group study. Am J Psychiatry 158:805–807, 2001

Masters KJ: Pilocarpine treatment of xerostomia induced by psychoactive medications. Am J Psychiatry 162:1023, 2005

Mattson RH, Cramer JA, Collins JF, et al: Comparison of carbamazepine, phenobarbital, phenytoin, and primidone in partial and secondarily generalized tonic-clonic seizures. N Engl J Med 313:145–151, 1985

McBride PE: Triglycerides and risk for coronary heart disease. JAMA 298:336–338, 2007

McElroy SL, Frye MA, Altshuler LL, et al: A 24-week, randomized, controlled trial of adjunctive sibutramine versus topiramate in the treatment of weight gain in overweight or obese patients with bipolar disorders. Bipolar Disord 9:426–434, 2007

McElroy SL, Winstanley E, Mori N, et al: A randomized, placbo-controlled study of zonisamide to prevent olanzapine-associated weight gain. J Clin Psychopharmacol 32:165–172, 2012

McElroy SL, Martens BE, Mori N, et al: Adjunctive lisdexamfetamine in bipolar depression: a preliminary randomized, placebo-controlled trial. Int Clin Psychopharmacol 30:6–13, 2015

McGahuey CA, Gelenberg AJ, Laukes CA, et al: The Arizona Sexual Experience Scale (ASEX): reliability and validity. J Sex Marital Ther 26:25–40, 2000

McGrath PJ, Blood DK, Stewart JW, et al: A comparative study of the electrocardiographic effects of phenelzine, tricyclic antidepressants, mianserin, and placebo. J Clin Psychopharmacol 7:335–339, 1987

McIntyre RS: Aripiprazole for the maintenance treatment of bipolar I disorder: a review. Clin Ther 32 (suppl 1):S32–S38, 2010

McIntyre RS, Lophaven S, Olsen CK: A randomized, double-blind, placebo-controlled study of vortioxetine on cognitive function in depressed adults. Int J Neuropsychopharmacol 17:1557–1567, 2014

McKinney PA, Finkenbine RD, DeVane CL: Alopecia and mood stabilizer therapy. Ann Clin Psychiatry 8:183–185, 1996

McLean JD, Forsythe RG, Kapkin IA: Unusual side effects of clomipramine associated with yawning. Can J Psychiatry 28:569–570, 1983

Meador KJ, Baker GA, Browning N, et al: Cognitive function at 3 years of age after fetal exposure to antiepileptic drugs. N Engl J Med 360:1597–1605, 2009

Meco G, Fabrizio E, Epifanio A, et al: Levetiracetam in tardive dyskinesia. Clin Neuropharmacol 29:265–268, 2006

Meehan AD, Humble MB, Yazarloo P, et al: The prevalence of lithium-associated hyperparathyroidism in a large Swedish population attending psychiatric outpatient units. J Clin Psychopharmacol 35:279–285, 2015

Megna JL, Kunwar AR, Mahlotra K, et al: A study of polypharmacy with second generation antipsychotics in patients with severe and persistent mental illness. J Psychiatr Pract 13:129–137, 2007

Melmed S, Casanueva FF, Hoffman AR, et al: Diagnosis and treatment of hyperprolactinemia: an Endocrine Society Clinical Practice Guideline. J Clin Endocrinol Metab 96:273–288, 2011

Meltzer HY, Bobo WV, Nuamah IF, et al: Efficacy and tolerability of oral paliperidone extended-release tablets in the treatment of acute schizophrenia: pooled data from three 6-week, placebo-controlled studies. J Clin Psychiatry 69:817–829, 2008

Meltzer HY, Cucchiaro J, Silva R, et al: Lurasidone in the treatment of schizophrenia: a randomized, double-blind, placebo- and olanzapine-controlled study. Am J Psychiatry 168:957–967, 2011

Meltzer HY, Elkis H, Vanover K, et al: Pimavanserin, a selective serotonin (5HT)2A-inverse agonist, enhances the efficacy and safety of risperidone, 2 mg/day, but does not enhance efficacy of haloperidol, 2 mg/day: comparison with reference dose risperidone, 6 mg/day. Schizophr Res 141:144–152, 2012

Menkes DB, Larson PM: Sodium valproate for tinnitus. J Neurol Neurosurg Psychiatry 65:803, 1998

Menza M, Vreeland B, Minsky S, et al: Managing atypical antipsychotic-associated weight gain:12-month data on a multimodal weight control program. J Clin Psychiatry 65:471–477, 2004

Merideth CH: A single-center, double-blind, placebo-controlled evaluation of lamotrigine in the treatment of obesity in adults. J Clin Psychiatry 67:258–262, 2006

Merrill DB, Ahmari SE, Bradford JM, et al: Myocarditis during clozapine treatment. Am J Psychiatry 163:204–208, 2006

Meston CM, Worcel M: The effects of yohimbine plus L-arginine glutamate on sexual arousal in postmenopausal women with sexual arousal disorder. Arch Sex Behav 31:323–332, 2002

Meyer JM, Rosenblatt LC, Kim E, et al: The moderating impact of ethnicity on metabolic outcomes during treatment with olanzapine and aripiprazole in patients with schizophrenia. J Clin Psychiatry 70:318–325, 2009

Michelson D, Amsterdam JD, Quitkin FM, et al: Changes in weight during a 1-year trial of fluoxetine. Am J Psychiatry 156:1170–1176, 1999

Michelson D, Bancroft J, Targum S, et al: Female sexual dysfunction associated with antidepressant administration: a randomized, placebo-controlled study of pharmacologic intervention. Am J Psychiatry 157:239–243, 2000

Michelson D, Kociban K, Tamura R, et al: Mirtazapine, yohimbine or olanzapine augmentation therapy for seroton reuptake-associated female sexual dysfunction: a randomized, placebo controlled trial. J Psychiatr Pract 36:147–152, 2002

Mir A, Shivakumar K, Williamson RJ, et al: Changes in sexual dysfunction with aripiprazole: a switching or add-on study. J Psychopharmacol 22:244–253, 2008

Mizoguchi Y, Monji A, Yamada S: Dysgeusia successfully treated with sertraline. J Neuropsychiatry Clin Neurosci 24:E42, 2012

Montague DK, Jarow J, Broderick GA, et al: American Urological Association guideline on the management of priapism. J Urol 170:1318–1324, 2003

Montejo AL, Rico-Villademoros F: Psychometric properties of the Psychotropic-Related Sexual Dysfunction Questionnaire (PRSexDQ-SAL-SEX) in patients with schizophrenia and other psychotic disorders. J Sex Marital Ther 34:227–239, 2008

Montejo-González AL, Llorca G, Izquierdo JA, et al: SSRI-induced sexual dysfunction: fluoxetine, paroxetine, sertraline, and fluvoxamine in a prospective, multi-center, and descriptive clinical study of 344 patients. J Sex Marital Ther 23:176–194, 1997

Monti JM, Torterolo P, Pandi Perumal SR: The effects of second generation antipsychotic drugs on sleep variables in healthy subjects and patients with schizophrenia. Sleep Med Rev 33:51–57, 2017

Moore TJ, Glenmullen J, Mattison DR: Reports of pathological gambling, hypersexuality, and compulsive shopping associated with dopamine receptor agonist drugs. JAMA Intern Med 174:1930–1933, 2014

Morgan JC, Sethi KD: Drug-induced tremors. Lancet Neurol 4:866–876, 2005

Morrell MJ: Folic acid and epilepsy. Epilepsy Curr 2:31–34, 2002

Moss LE, Neppe VM, Drevets WC: Buspirone in the treatment of tardive dyskinesia. J Clin Psychopharmacology 13:204–209, 1993

Movig KL, Leufkens HG, Lenderink AW, et al: Association between antidepressant drug use and hyponatremia: a case-control study. Br J Clin Pharmacol 53:363–369, 2002

Mundo E, Walker M, Cate T, et al: The role of serotonin transporter protein gene in antidepressant-induced mania in bipolar disorder. Arch Gen Psychiatry 58:539–544, 2001

Munetz MR, Benjamin S: How to examine patients using the abnormal involuntary movement scale. Hosp Community Psychiatry 39:1172–1177, 1988

Murphy GM, Kremer C, Rodrigues HE, et al: Pharmacogenetics of antidepressant medication intolerance. Am J Psychiatry 160:1830–1835, 2003

Nagler EV, Webster AC, Vanholder R, et al: Antidepressants for depression in stage 3-5 chronic kidney disease: a systematic review of pharmacokinetics, efficacy and safety with recommendations by European Renal Best Practice. Nephrol Dial Transplant 27:3736–3745, 2012

Naranjo CA, Busto U, Sellers EM, et al: A method for estimating the probability of adverse drug reactions. Clin Pharmacol Ther 30:239–245, 1981

Narula PK, Rehan HS, Unni KE, et al: Topiramate for prevention of olanzapine associated weight gain and metabolic dysfunction in schizophrenia: a double-blind, placebo-controlled trial. Schizophr Res 118:218–223, 2010

Nasrallah HA, Earley W, Cutler AJ, et al: The safety and tolerability of cariprazine in long-term treatment of schizophrenia: a post hoc pooled analysis. BMC Psychiatry 17:305, 2017

National Kidney Foundation: KDOQI Clinical Practice Guidelines for Chronic Kidney Disease: evaluation, classification, and stratification. Am J Kidney Dis 39 (suppl 1):S1–S266, 2002

Newcomer JW, Campos JA, Marcus RN, et al: A multicenter, randomized, double-blind study of the effects of aripiprazole in overweight subjects with schizophrenia or schizoaffective disorder switched from olanzapine. J Clin Psychiatry 69:1046–1056, 2008

Newcomer JW, Ratner RE, Eriksson JW, et al: A 24-week, multi-center, open-label, randomized study to compare changes in glucose metabolism in patients with schizophrenia receiving treatment with olanzapine, quetiapine, or risperidone. J Clin Psychiatry 70:487–499, 2009

Nurnberg HG, Hensley PL, Gelenberg AJ, et al: Treatment of antidepressant-associated sexual dysfunction with sildenafil: a randomized controlled trial. JAMA 289:56–64, 2003

Nurnberg HG, Hensley PL, Heiman JR, et al: Sildenafil treatment of women with antidepressant-associated sexual dysfunction: a randomized controlled trial. JAMA 300:395–404, 2008

Oben JE, Ngondi JL, Momo CN, et al: The use of a Cissus quadrangularis/Irvingia gabonesis combination in the management of weight loss: a double-blind, placebo-controlled study. Lipids Health Dis 7:12, 2008

Oinonen KA, Mazmanian D: To what extent do oral contraceptives influence mood and affect. J Affect Disord 70:229–240, 2002

Olfson M, Shaffer D, Marcus SC, et al: Relationship between antidepressant medication treatment and suicide in adolescents. Arch Gen Psychiatry 60:978–982, 2003

Olfson M, Marcus SC, Shaffer D: Antidepressant drug therapy and suicide in severely depressed children and adults. A case-control study. Arch Gen Psychiatry 63:865–872, 2006

Onakpoya I, Hung SK, Perry R, et al: The use of Garcinia extract (hydroxycitric acid) as a weight loss supplement: a systematic review and meta-analysis of randomised clinical trials. J Obes 2011:509038, 2011

Ormerod S, McDowell SE, Coleman JJ, et al: Ethnic differences in the risks of adverse reactions to drugs used in the treatment of psychoses and depression: a systematic review and meta-analysis. Drug Saf 31:597–607, 2008

Oskarsson B: Myopathy: five new things. Neurology 76 (7, suppl 2):S14–S19, 2011

Oskooilar N: A case of premature ventricular contractions with modafinil. Am J Psychiatry 162:1983–1984, 2005

Ozmenler NK, Karlidere T, Bozkurt A, et al: Mirtazapine augmentation in depressed patients with sexual dysfunction due to selective serotonin reuptake inhibitors. Hum Psychopharmacol 23:321–326, 2008

Pae CU, Marks DM, Masand PS, et al: Methylphenidate extended release (OROS MPH) for the treatment of antidepressant-related sexual dysfunction in patients with treatment-resistant depression: results from a 4-week, double-blind, placebo-controlled trial. Clin Neuropharmacol 32:85–88, 2009

Paul E, Conant KD, Dunne IE, et al: Urolithiasis on the ketogenic diet with concurrent topiramate or zonisamide therapy. Epilepsy Res 90:151–156, 2010

Pavan C, Vindigni V, Michelotto L, et al: Weight gain related to treatment with atypical antipsychotics is due to activation of PKC-beta. Pharmacogenomics J 10:408–417, 2010

Paykel ES, Fleminger R, Watson JP: Psychiatric side effects of antihypertensive drugs other than reserpine. J Clin Psychopharmacol 2:14–39, 1982

Pellock JM, Willmore LJ: A rational guide to routine blood monitoring in patients receiving antiepileptic drugs. Neurology 41:961–964, 1991

Penzer JB, Dudas M, Saito E, et al: Lack of effect of stimulant combination with second-generation antipsychotics on weight gain, metabolic changes, prolactin levels, and sedation in youth with clinically relevant aggression or oppositionality. J Child Adolesc Psychopharmacol 19:563–573, 2009

Perez-Iglesias R, Crespo-Facorro B, Martinez-Garcia O, et al: Weight gain induced by haloperidol, risperidone and olanzapine after 1 year: findings of a randomized clinical trial in a drug-naïve population. Schizophr Res 99:13–22, 2008

Perlis RH, Mischoulon D, Smoller JW, et al: Serotonin transporter polymorphisms and adverse effects with fluoxetine treatment. Biol Psychiatry 54:879–883, 2003

Perry PJ, Lund BC, Sanger T, et al: Olanzapine plasma concentrations and clinical response: acute phase results of the North American Olanzapine Trial. J Clin Psychopharmacol 21:14–20, 2001

Phung OJ, Baker WL, Matthews LJ, et al: Effect of green tea catechins with or without caffeine on anthropometric measures: a systematic review and meta-analysis. Am J Clin Nutr 91:73–81, 2010

Pigott TA, Carson WH, Saha AR, et al: Aripiprazole for the prevention of relapse in stabilized patients with chronic schizophrenia: a placebo-controlled 26-week study. J Clin Psychiatry 64:1048–1056, 2003

Plenge P, Mellerup ET, Bolwig TG, et al: Lithium treatment: does the kidney prefer one daily dose or two? Acta Psychiatr Scand 66:121–128, 1982

Podewils LJ, Lyketsos CG: Tricyclic antidepressants and cognitive decline. Psychosomatics 43:31–35, 2002

Pompili M, Baldessarini RJ: Epilepsy: risk of suicidal behavior with antiepileptic drugs. Nat Rev Neurol 6:651–653, 2010

Pope HG Jr, Kouri EM, Hudson JI: Effects of supraphysiologic doses of testosterone on mood and aggression in normal men: a randomized controlled trial. Arch Gen Psychiatry 57:133–140, 2000

Poulin MJ, Chaput JP, Simard V, et al: Management of antipsychotic-induced weight gain: prospective naturalistic study of the effectiveness of a supervised exercise program. Aus N Z J Psychiatry 41:980–989, 2007

Preskorn SH: Imipramine, mirtazapine, and nefazodone: multiple targets. J Psychiatr Pract 6:97–102, 2000

Preskorn S, Flockhart D: 2010 guide to psychiatric drug interactions. Primary Psychiatry 16:45–74, 2009

Preskorn SH, Kane CP, Lobello K, et al: Cytochrome P450 2D6 phenoconversion is common in patients being treated for depression: implications for personalized medicine. J Clin Psychiatry 74:614–621, 2013

Presne C, Fakhouri F, Noël LH, et al: Lithium-induced nephropathy: rate of progression and prognostic factors. Kidney Int 64(2):585–592, 2003

Pugh RN, Murray-Lyon IM, Dawson JL, et al: Transection of the oesophagus for bleeding oesophageal varices. Br J Surg 60:646–649, 1973

Raeder MB, Bjelland I, Emil Vollset S, et al: Obesity, dyslipidemia, and diabetes with selective serotonin reuptake inhibitors: the Hordaland Health Study. J Clin Psychiatry 67:1974–1982, 2006

Raja M, Azzoni A: Valproate-induced hyperammonemia. J Clin Psychopharmacol 22:631–633, 2002

Rajagopal V, Sundaresan L, Rajkumar AP, et al: Genetic association between the DRD4 promoter polymorphism and clozapine-induced sialorrhea. Psychiatr Genet 24:273–276, 2014

Rasch B, Pommer J, Diekelmann S, et al: Pharmacological REM sleep suppression paradoxically improves rather than impairs skill memory. Nature Neurosci 12:396–397, 2008

Raskin J, Goldstein DJ, Mallinckrodt CH, et al: Duloxetine in the long-term treatment of major depressive disorder. J Clin Psychiatry 64:1237–1244, 2003

Raskind MA, Peskind ER, Kanter ED, et al: Reduction of nightmares and other PTSD symptoms in combat veterans by prazosin: a placebo-controlled study. Am J Psychiatry 160:371–373, 2003

Rasmussen SA, Rosenbush PI, Mazurek MF: The relationship between early haloperidol response and associated extrapyramidal side effects. J Clin Psychopharmacol 37:8–12, 2017

Rathbone J, Soares-Weiser K: Anticholinergics for neuroleptic-induced acute akathisia. Cochrane Database of Systematic Reviews 2006, Issue 4. Art. No.: CD003727. DOI: 10.1002/14651858.CD003727.pub3.

Rau T, Wohlleben G, Wuttke H, et al: CYP2D6 genotype: impact on adverse effects and nonresponse during treatment with antidepressants—a pilot study. Clin Pharmacol Ther 75:386–393, 2004

Ray WA, Chung CP, Murray KT, et al: Atypical antipsychotic drugs and the risk of sudden cardiac death. N Engl J Med 360:225–235, 2009

Reaven GM, Lieberman JA, Sethuraman G, et al: In search of moderators and mediators of hyperglycemia with atypical antipsychotic treatment. J Psychiatr Res 43:997–1002, 2009

Reeves RR, Mustain DW, Pendarvis JE: Valproate-induced tinnitus misinterpreted as psychotic symptoms. South Med J 93:1030–1031, 2000

Reilly JG, Ayis SA, Ferrier IN, et al: QTc-interval abnormalities and psychotropic drug therapy in psychiatric patients. Lancet 355:1048–1052, 2000

Repetto MJ, Petitto JM: Psychopharmacology in HIV-infected patients. Psychosom Med 70:585–592, 2008

Resende Lima A, Soares-Weiser K, Bacaltchuk J, et al: Benzodiazepines for neuroleptic-induced acute akathisia. Cochrane Database of Systematic Reviews 1999, Issue 4. Art. No.: CD001950. DOI: 10.1002/14651858.CD001950.

Reuben A: Hy's law. Hepatology 39:574–578, 2004

Reynolds GP, Zhang ZJ, Zhang XB: Association of antipsychotic drug-induced weight gain with a 5-HT2C receptor gene polymorphism. Lancet 359:2086–2087, 2002

Reynolds GP, Zhang Z, Zhang X: Polymorphism of the promoter region of the serotonin 5-HT(2C) receptor gene and clozapine-induced weight gain. Am J Psychiatry 160:677–679, 2003

Riba MB, Balon R: Competency in Combining Pharmacotherapy and Psychotherapy. Washington, DC, American Psychiatric Publishing, 2005

Richardson GS, Roehrs TA, Rosenthal L, et al: Tolerance to daytime sedative effects of H1 antihistamines. J Clin Psychopharmacol 22:511–515, 2002

Richardson MA, Bevans ML, Read LL, et al: Efficacy of the branched-chain amino acids in the treatment of tardive dyskinesia in men. Am J Psychiatry 160:1117–1124, 2003

Rinnerthaler M, Luef G, Mueller J, et al: Computerized tremor analysis of valproate-induced tremor: a comparative study of controlled-release versus conventional valproate. Epilepsia 46:320–323, 2005

Roeloffs C, Bartlik B, Kaplan PM, et al: Methylphenidate and SSRI-induced sexual side effects. J Clin Psychiatry 57:548, 1996

Ronaldson KJ, Taylor AJ, Fitzgerald PB, et al: Diagnostic characteristics of clozapine-induced myocarditis identified by an analysis of 38 cases and 47 controls. J Clin Psychiatry 71:976–981, 2010

Rosenbaum JF, Fava M, Hoog SL, et al: Selective serotonin reuptake inhibitor discontinuation syndrome: a randomized clinical trial. Biol Psychiatry 44:77–87, 1998

Rothschild AJ: Selective serotonin reuptake inhibitor-induced sexual dysfunction: efficacy of a drug holiday. Am J Psychiatry 152:1514–1516, 1995

Rothschild AJ, Shindul-Rothschild JA, Viguera A, et al: Comparison of the frequency of behavioral disinhibition on alprazolam, clonazepam, or no benzodiazepine in hospitalized psychiatric patients. J Clin Psychopharmacol 20:7–11, 2000

Rummel-Kluge C, Komossa K, Schwarz S, et al: Head-to-head comparisons of metabolic side effects of second generation antipsychotics in the treatment of schizophrenia: a systematic review and meta-analysis. Schizophr Res 123:225–233, 2010

Sachs GS, Renshaw PF, Lafer B, et al: Variability of brain lithium levels during maintenance treatment: a magnetic resonance spectroscopy study. Biol Psychiatry 38:422–428, 1995

Sachs G, Bowden C, Calabrese JR, et al: Effects of lamotrigine and lithium on body weight during maintenance treatment of bipolar I disorder. Bipolar Disord 8:175–181, 2006a

Sachs GS, Sanchez R, Marcus R, et al: Aripiprazole in the treatment of acute manic or mixed episodes in patients with bipolar I disorder: a 3-week placebo-controlled study. J Psychopharmacol 20:536–546, 2006b

Safarinejad MR: The effects of the adjunctive bupropion on male sexual dysfunction induced by a selective serotonin reuptake inhibitor: a double-blind placebo-controlled and randomized study. BJU Int 106:840–847, 2010

Safarinejad MR: Reversal of SSRI-induced female sexual dysfunction by adjunctive bupropion in menstruating women: a double-blind, placebo-controlled and randomized study. J Psychopharmacol 25:370–378, 2011

Sagud M, Pivac N, Mück-Seler D, et al: Effects of sertraline treatment on plasma cortisol, prolactin and thyroid hormones in female depressed patients. Neuropsychobiology 45:139–143, 2002

Saiz-Ruiz J, Montes JM, Ibanez A, et al: Assessment of sexual functioning in depressed patients treated with mirtazapine: a naturalistic 6-month study. Hum Psychopharmacol 20:435–440, 2005

Saletu A, Parapatics S, Anderer P, et al: Controlled clinical, polysomnographic and psychometric studies on differences between sleep bruxers and controls and acute effects of clonazepam as compared with placebo. Eur Arch Psychiatry Clin Neurosci 260:163–174, 2010

Sander JW, Patsalos PN: An assessment of serum and red blood cell folate concentrations in patients with epilepsy on lamotrigine therapy. Epilepsy Res 13:89–92, 1992

Sarma S, Ward W, O'Brien J, et al: Severe hyponatremia associated with desmopressin nasal spray to treat clozapine-induced nocturnal eneuresis. Aust N Z J Psychiatry 39:949, 2005

Schenck CH, Mahowald MW: REM sleep behavior disorder: clinical, developmental, and neuroscience perspectives 16 years after its formal identification in SLEEP. Sleep 25:120–138, 2002

Schittecatte M, Dumont F, Machowski R, et al: Mirtazapine, but not fluvoxamine, normalizes the blunted REM sleep response to clonidine in depressed patients: implications for subsensitivity to alpha(2)-adrenergic receptors in depression. Psychiatr Res 109:1–8, 2002

Schneeweiss S, Setoguchi S, Brookhart A, et al: Risk of death associated with the use of conventional versus atypical antipsychotic drugs among elderly patients. CMAJ 176:627–632, 2007

Schneider LS, Dagerman KS, Insel P: Risk of death with atypical antipsychotic drug treatment for dementia: meta-analysis of randomized placebo-controlled trials. JAMA 294:1934–1943, 2005

Schou M: Effects of long-term lithium treatment on kidney function: an overview. J Psychiatr Res 22:287–296, 1988

Schou M: Forty years of lithium treatment. Arch Gen Psychiatry 54:9–13, 1997

Schwartz TL, Nasra GS, Ashton AK, et al: An open-label study to evaluate switching from an SSRI or SNRI to tiagabine to alleviate antidepressant-induced sexual dysfunction in generalized anxiety disorder. Ann Clin Psychiatry 19:25–30, 2007

Schweiger U, Weber B, Deuschle M, et al: Lumbar bone mineral density in patients with major depression: evidence of increased bone loss at follow-up. Am J Psychiatry 157:118–120, 2000

Scott J, Pope M: Nonadherence with mood stabilizers: prevalence and predictors. J Clin Psychiatry 63:384–390, 2002

Segraves RT, Lee J, Stevenson R, et al: Tadalafil for treatment of erectile dysfunction in men on antidepressants. J Clin Psychopharmacol 27:62–66, 2007

Seidman SN, Pesce VC, Roose SP: High-dose sildenafil citrate for selective serotonin reuptake inhibitor-associated ejaculatory delay: open clinical trial. J Clin Psychiatry 64:721–725, 2003

Serinken M, Karcioglu O, Korkmaz A: Rarely seen cardiotoxicity of lithium overdose: complete heart block. Int J Cardiol 132:276–278, 2009

Serrano-Dueñas M: Use of primidone in low doses (250 mg/day) versus high doses (750 mg/day) in the management of essential tremor. Double-blind comparative study with one-year follow-up. Parkinsonism Relat Disord 10:29–33, 2003

Serretti A, Chiesa A: A meta-analysis of sexual dysfunction in psychiatric patients taking antipsychotics. Int Clin Psychopharmacol 26:130–140, 2011

Shahzad S, Suleman M-I, Shahab H, et al: Cataract occurrence with antipsychotic drugs. Psychosomatics 43:354–359, 2002

Shamir E, Barak Y, Shalman I, et al: Melatonin treatment for tardive dyskinesia: a double-blind, placebo-controlled, crossover study. Arch Gen Psychiatry 58:1049–1052, 2001

Shapiro HI, Davis KA: Hypercalcemia and "primary" hyperparathyroidism during lithium therapy. Am J Psychiatry 172:12–15, 2015

Shekelle PG, Hardy ML, Morton SC, et al: Efficacy and safety of ephedra and ephedrine for weight loss and athletic performance: a meta-analysis. JAMA 289:1537–1545, 2003

Shen J, Ge W, Zhang J, et al: Leptin-2548 G/A gene polymorphism in association with antipsychotic-induced weight gain: a meta-analysis study. Psychiatr Danub 26:145–151, 2014

Shim J-C, Shin JG, Kelly DL, et al: Adjunctive treatment with a dopamine partial agonist, aripiprazole, for antipsychotic-induced hyperprolactinemia: a placebo-controlled trial. Am J Psychiatry 164:1404–1410, 2007

Shlipak MG, Matsushita K, Ärnlöv J, et al: Cystatin C versus creatinine in determining risk based on kidney function. N Engl J Med 369: 932–943, 2013

Shrivastava RK, Shrivastava S, Overweg N, et al: Amantadine in the treatment of sexual dysfunction associated with selective serotonin reuptake inhibitors. J Clin Psychopharmacol 15:83–84, 1995

Silver H, Geraisy N, Schwartz M: No difference in the effect of biperiden and amantadine on parkinsonian and tardive dyskinesia-type involuntary movements: a double-blind, crossover, placebo-controlled study in medicated chronic schizophrenic patients. J Clin Psychiatry 56:167–170, 1995

Simpson GM, Angus JW: A rating scale for extrapyramidal side effects. Acta Psychiatr Scand 212:11–19, 1970

Smith RC, Jin H, Li C, et al: Effects of pioglitazone on metabolic abnormalities, psychopathology, and cognitive function in schizophrenic patients treated with antipsychotic medication: a randomized double-blind study. Schizophr Res 143(1):18-24, 2013

Soares-Weiser K, Maayan N, McGrath J: Vitamin E for neuroleptic-induced tardive dyskinesia. Cochrane Database of Systematic Reviews 2011, Issue 2. Art. No.: CD000209. DOI: 10.1002/14651858.CD000209.pub2.

Sowell M, Mukhopadhyay N, Cavazzoni P, et al: Evaluation of insulin sensitivity in healthy volunteers treated with olanzapine, risperidone, or placebo: a prospective, randomized study using the two-step hyperinsulinemic, euglycemic clamp. J Clin Endocrinol Metab 88:5875–5880, 2003

Spencer T, Biederman J, Coffey B, et al: A double-blind comparison of desipramine and placebo in children and adolescents with chronic tic disorder and comorbid attention-deficit/hyperactivity disorder. Arch Gen Psychiatry 59:649–656, 2002

Spigset O, Hedenmalm K: Hyponatremia and the syndrome of inappropriate antidiuretic hormone secretion (SIADH) induced by psychotropic drugs. Drug Saf 12:209–225, 1995

Spivak B, Mester R, Abesgaus J, et al: Clozapine treatment for neuroleptic-induced tardive dyskinesia, parkinsonism, and chronic akathisia in schizophrenic patients. J Clin Psychiatry 58:318–322, 1997

Srisawat U, Reynolds GP, Zhang ZJ, et al: Methylenetetrahydrofolate reductase (MTHFR) 677C/T polymorphism is associated with antipsychotic-induced weight gain in first-episode schizophrenia. Int J Neuropsychopharmacol 17:485–490, 2014

Stauffer VL, Sniadecki JL, Piezer KW, et al: Impact of race on efficacy and safety during treatment with olanzapine in schizophrenia, schizophreniform, or schizoaffective disorder. BMC Psychiatry 10:89, 2010

Sternbach H: The serotonin syndrome. Am J Psychiatry 148:705–713, 1991

Stewart JW, Harrison W, Quitkin F, et al: Phenelzine-induced pyridoxine deficiency. J Clin Psychopharmacology 4:225–226, 1984

Stoffer SS, Szpunar WE: Potency of brand name and generic levothyroxine. JAMA 244:1704–1705, 1980

Stone NJ, Robinson J, Lichtenstein AH, et al: 2013 ACC/AHA Guideline on the Treatment of Blood Cholesterol to Reduce Atherosclerotic Cardiovascular Risk in Adults: A Report of the American College of Cardiology/American Heart Association Task Force on Practice Guidelines. J Am Coll Cardiol 63 (25 Pt B):2889–2934, 2014

Strauss M, Heinritz W, Hegerl U, et al: Risperidone intoxication in a patient with a genetic predisposition as a "poor [non]metabolizer." Psychiatr Prax 37:199–201, 2010

Stryjer R, Spivak B, Strous RD, et al: Trazodone for the treatment of sexual dysfunction induced by serotonin reuptake inhibitors: a preliminary open-label study. Clin Neuropharmacol 32:82–84, 2009

Suppes T, Vieta E, Liu S, et al: Maintenance treatment for patients with bipolar I disorder: results from a North American study of quetiapine in combination with lithium or divalproex (Trial 127). Am J Psychiatry 166:476–488, 2009

Sussman N, Ginsberg DL, Bikoff J: Effects of nefazodone on body weight: a pooled analysis of selective serotonin reuptake inhibitor- and imipramine-controlled trials. J Clin Psychiatry 62:256–260, 2001

Szalat A, Mazeh H, Freund HR: Lithium-associated hyperparathyroidism: report of four cases and review of the literature. Eur J Endocrinol 160:317–23, 2009

Taira N, Nishi H, Mano M, et al: Pancreatitis induced by valproic acid: report of a case. Surg Today 31:1027–1031, 2001

Tariot PN, Schneider LS, Mintzer JE: Safety and tolerability of divalproex sodium in the treatment of signs and symptoms of mania in elderly patients with dementia: results of a double-blind, placebo-controlled trial. Current Therapeutic Research 62: 51–67, 2001

Taslimi S, Vahidi H, Pourvaziri A, et al: Ondansetron in patients with tinnitus: randomized double-blind placebo-controlled study. Eur Arch Otorhinolaryngol 270:1635–1641, 2013

Taylor MJ, Rudkin L, Bullemor-Day P, et al: Strategies for managing sexual dysfunction induced by antidepressant medication. Cochrane Database of Systematic Reviews Issue 5, Art No CD003382, 2013

Tchoukhine E, Takala P, Hakko H, et al: Orlistat in clozapine- or olanzapine-treated patients with overweight or obesity: a 16-week open-label extension phase and both phases of a randomized controlled trial. J Clin Psychiatry 72:326–330, 2011

Tek C, Ratliff J, Reutenauer E, et al: A randomized, double-blind, placebo-controlled pilot study of naltrexone to counteract antipsychotic-associated weight gain. J Clin Psychopharmacol 34:608–612, 2014

Tengstrand M, Star K, van Puijenbroek EP, et al: Alopecia in association with lamotrigine use: an analysis of individual case safety reports in a global database. Drug Saf 33:653–658, 2010

Terevnikov V, Stenberg JH, Tiihonen J, et al: Add-on mirtazapine improves orgasmic functioning in patients with schizophrenia treated with first-generation antipsychotics. Nord J Psychiatry 71:77–80, 2017

Thase ME, Fava M, Halbreich U, et al: A placebo-controlled, randomized clinical trial comparing sertraline and imipramine for the treatment of dysthymia. Arch Gen Psychiatry 53:777–784, 1996

Thase ME, Youakim JM, Skuban A, et al: Efficacy and safety of adjunctive brexpiprazole 2 mg in major depressive disorder: a phase 3, randomized, placebo-controlled study in patients with inadequate response to antidepressants. J Clin Psychiatry 76:1224–1231, 2015a

Thase ME, Youakim JM, Skuban A, et al: Adjunctive brexpiprazole 1 and 3 mg for patients with major depressive disorder following inadequate response to antidepressants: a phase 3, randomized, double-blind study. J Clin Psychiatry 76:1232–1240, 2015b

Thrush A, Shai I, Bitzur R, et al: Changes in triglyceride levels over time and risk of type II diabetes in young men. Diabetes Care 31:2032–2037, 2000

Tohen M, Castillo J, Baldessarini RJ, et al: Blood dyscrasias with carbamazepine and valproate: a pharmacoepidemiological study of 2,228 patients at risk. Am J Psychiatry 152:413–418, 1995

Tohen M, Sniadecki J, Sutton VK, et al: Number needed to treat or harm analyses of olanzapine for maintenance treatment of bipolar disorder. J Clin Psychopharmacol 29:520–528, 2009

Tondo L, Vásquez G, Baldessarini RJ: Mania associated with antidepressant treatment: comprehensive meta-analytic review. Acta Psychiatr Scand 121:404–414, 2010

Toth P, Frankenburg FR: Clozapine and seizures: a review. Can J Psychiatry 39:236–238, 1994

Trujillo JM, Goldman J: Lixisenatide, a once-daily prandial glucagon-like peptide-1 receptor agonist for the treatment of adults with type 2 diabetes. Pharmacotherapy 37:927–943, 2017

Uca AU, Uğuz F, Kozac HH, et al: Antidepressant-induced bruxism: prevalence, incidence, and related factors. Clin Neuropharmacol 38:227–230, 2015

Ujike H, Nomura A, Morita Y, et al: Multiple genetic factors in olanzapine-induced weight gain in schizophrenia patients: a cohort study. J Clin Psychiatry 69:1416–1422, 2008

Umpierrez GE, Pantalone KM, Kwan AYM, et al: Relationship between weight change and glycaemic control in patients with type 2 diabetes receiving once-weekly dulaglutide treatment. Diabetes Obes Metab 18:615–622, 2016

U.S. Food and Drug Administration: Guidance for Industry: E14 clinical evaluation of QT/QTc interval prolongation and proarrhythmic potential for non-antiarrhythmic drugs. October 2005. Available at: www.fda.gov/downloads/Drugs/GuidanceComplianceRegulatoryInformation/Guidances/ucm073153.pdf. Accessed June 15, 2011.

Usiskin SI, Nicolson R, Lenane M, et al: Gabapentin prophylaxis of clozapine-induced seizures. Am J Psychiatry 157:482–483, 2000

Van Ameringen M, Manci C, Pipe B, et al: Topiramate treatment for SSRI-induced weight gain in anxiety disorders. J Clin Psychiatry 63:981–984, 2002

Van Ameringen M, Mancini C, Patterson B, et al: Symptom relapse following switch from Celexa to generic citalopram. J Psychopharmacol 21:472–476, 2007

Vandenberghe F, Gholam-Rezaee M, Saigí-Morgui N, et al: Importance of early weight gain to predict long-term weight gain during psychotropic drug treatment. J Clin Psychiatry 76(11):e1417–e1423, 2015

van der Hoeven J, Duyx J, de Langen JJ, et al: Probable psychiatric side effects of azathioprine. Psychosom Med 67:508, 2005

Vanderkooy JD, Kennedy SH, Bagby MR: Antidepressant side effects in depression patients treated in a naturalistic setting: a study of bupropion, moclobemide, paroxetine, sertraline and venlafaxine. Can J Psychiatry 47:174–180, 2002

VanderZwaag C, McGee M, McEvoy JP, et al: Response of patients with treatment-refractory schizophrenia to clozapine within three serum level ranges. Am J Psychiatry 153:1579–1584, 1996

Vanina Y, Podolskaya A, Sedky K, et al: Body weight changes associated with psychopharmacology. Psych Serv 53:842–847, 2002

van Laar MW, van Willigenburg AP, Volkerts ER: Acute and subchronic effects of nefazodone and imipramine on highway driving, cognitive functions, and daytime sleepiness in healthy adult and elderly subjects. J Clin Psychopharmacol 15:30–40, 1995

van Marum RJ, Wegewijs MA, Loonen AJ, et al: Hypothermia following antipsychotic drug use. Eur J Clin Pharmacol 63:627–631, 2007

Verrotti A, Basciani F, Morresi S, et al: Serum leptin changes in epileptic patients who gain weight after therapy with valproic acid. Neurology 53:230–232, 1999

Vetter VL, Elia J, Erickson C, et al: Cardiovascular monitoring of children and adolescents with heart disease receiving stimulant drugs: a scientific statement from the American Heart Association Council on Cardiovascular Disease in the Young Congenital Cardiac Defects Committee and the Council on Cardiovascular Nursing. Circulation 117:2407–2423, 2008

Viana Bde M, Prais HA, Camargos ST, et al: Ziprasidone-related oculogyric crisis in an adult. Clin Neurol Neurosurg 111:883–885, 2009

Vidarsdottir S, de Leeuw van Weenen JE, Frölich M, et al: Effects of olanzapine and haloperidol on the metabolic status of healthy men. J Clin Endocrinol Metab 95:118–125, 2010

Vieta E, Torrent C, Garcia-Ribas G, et al: Use of topiramate in treatment-resistant bipolar spectrum disorders. J Clin Psychopharmacol 22:431–435, 2002

Vieta E, Sánchez-Moreno J, Goikolea JM, et al: Effects on weight and outcome of long-term olanzapine-topiramate combination treatment in bipolar disorder. J Clin Psychopharmacol 24:374–378, 2004

Vieta E, Montgomery S, Sulaiman AH, et al: A randomized, double-blind, placebo-controlled trial to assess prevention of mood episodes with risperidone long-acting injectable in patients with bipolar I disorder. Eur Neuropsychopharmacol 22:825–835, 2012

Viktrup L, Pangallo BA, Detke MJ, et al: Urinary side effects of duloxetine in the treatment of depression and stress urinary incontinence. Prim Care Companion J Clin Psychiatry 6:65–73, 2004

Vreeland B, Minsky S, Menza M, et al: A program for managing weight gain associated with atypical antipsychotics. Psychiatr Serv 54:1155–1157, 2003

Wada K, Yamada N, Sato T, et al: Corticosteroid-induced psychotic and mood disorders. Diagnosis defined by DSM-IV and clinical pictures. Psychosomatics 42:461–466, 2001

Wagner J, Wagner ML: Nonbenzodiazepines for the treatment of insomnia. Sleep Med Rev 4:551–581, 2000

Waldinger MD, Hengeveld MW, Zwinderman AH, et al: Effect of SSRI antidepressants on ejaculation: a double-blind, randomized, placebo-controlled study with fluoxetine, fluvoxamine, paroxetine, and sertraline. J Clin Psychopharmacol 18:274–281, 1998

Waldinger MD, Zwinderman AH, Olivier B: SSRIs and ejaculation: a double-blind, randomized, fixed-dose study with paroxetine and citalopram. J Clin Psychopharmacol 21:556–560, 2001

Waldinger MD, Zwinderman AH, Olivier B: Antidepressants and ejaculation: a double-blind, randomized, fixed-dose study with mirtazapine and paroxetine. J Clin Psychopharmacol 23:467–470, 2003

Waldschmitt C, Vogel F, Pfuhlmann B, et al: Duloxetine serum concentrations and clinical effects. Data from a therapeutic drug monitoring (TDM) survey. Pharmacopsychiatry 42:189–193, 2009

Wang HR, Woo YS, Bahk W-M: The role of melatonin and melatonin agonists in counteracting antipsychotic-induced metabolic side effects: a systematic review. Int Clin Psychopharmacol 31:301–306, 2016

Wang PW, Yang YS, Chandler RA, et al: Adjunctive zonisamide for weight loss in euthymic bipolar disorder patients: a pilot study. J Psychiatr Res 42:451–457, 2008

Warburton W, Hertzman C, Oberlander TF: A register study of the impact of stopping third trimester selective serotonin reuptake inhibitor exposure on neonatal health. Acta Psychiatr Scand 121:471–479, 2010

Watanabe N, Omori IM, Nakagawa A, et al: Safety reporting and adverse-event profile of mirtazapine described in randomized controlled trials in comparison with other classes of antidepressants in the acute-phase treatment of adults with depression: systematic review and meta-analysis. CNS Drugs 24:35–53, 2010

Weich S, Pearce HL, Croft P, et al: Effect of anxiolytic and hypnotic drug prescriptions on mortality hazards: retrospective cohort study. BMJ 348:g1996, 2014

Weiden PJ, Daniel DG, Simpson G, et al: Improvement in indices of health status in outpatients with schizophrenia switched to ziprasidone. J Clin Psychopharmacol 23:595–600, 2003a

Weiden PJ, Simpson GM, Potkin SG, et al: Effectiveness of switching to ziprasidone for stable but symptomatic outpatients with schizophrenia. J Clin Psychiatry 64:580–588, 2003b

Weiden PJ, Cutler AJ, Polymeropoulos MH, et al: Safety profile of iloperidone: a pooled analysis of 6-week acute-phase pivotal trials. J Clin Psychopharmacol 28:S12–S19, 2008

Werneke U, Ott M, Renberg ES, et al: A decision analysis of long-term lithium treatment and the risk of renal failure. Acta Psychiatr Scand 126(3):186–197, 2012

Werner JL, Christopher-Stine L, Ghazarian SR, et al: Antibody levels correlate with creatine kinase levels and strength in anti-3-hydroxy-3-methylglutaryl coenzyme A reductase-associated autoimmune myopathy. Arthritis Rheum 64:4087–4093, 2012

Wheatley D: Triple-blind, placebo-controlled trial of Gingko biloba in sexual dysfunction due to antidepressant drugs. Hum Psychopharmacol 19:545–548, 2004

Wingo AP, Wingo TS, Harvey PD, et al: Effects of lithium on cognitive performance: a meta-analysis. J Clin Psychiatry 70:1588–1597, 2009

Winokur A, Sateia MJ, Haves JB, et al: Acute effects of mirtazapine on sleep continuity and sleep architecture in depressed patients: a pilot study. Biol Psychiatry 48:75–78, 2000

Wisniewski SR, Rush AJ, Balasubramani GK, et al: Self-rated global measure of the frequency, intensity, and burden of side effects. J Psychiatr Pract 12:71–79, 2006

Wohlreich MM, Mallinckrodt CH, Prakash A, et al: Duloxetine for the treatment of major depressive disorder: safety and tolerability associated with dose escalation. Depress Anxiety 24:41–52, 2007

Wooltorton E: Risperidone (Risperdal): increased rate of cerebrovascular events in dementia trials. CMAJ 167:1269–1270, 2002

Woods SW, Saksa JR, Baker CB, et al: Effects of levetiracetam on tardive dyskinesia: a randomized, double-blind, placebo-controlled study. J Clin Psychiatry 69:546–554, 2008

Wroe S: Zonisamide and renal calculi in patients with epilepsy: how big an issue? Curr Med Res Opin 23:1765–1773, 2007

Wu RR, Zhao JP, Jin H, et al: Lifestyle intervention and metformin for treatment of antipsychotic-induced weight gain: a randomized controlled trial. JAMA 299:185–193, 2008

Wulf NR, Matuszewski KA: Sulfonamide cross-reactivity: is there evidence to support broad cross-allergenicity? Am J Health Syst Pharm 70:1483–1494, 2013

Wynn GH, Oesterheld JR, Cozza KL, et al (eds): Clinical Manual of Drug Interaction Principles for Medical Practice. Washington, DC, American Psychiatric Publishing, 2009

Yatham LN, Mackala S, Basivreddy J, et al: Lurasidone versus treatment as usual for cognitive impairment in euthymic patients with bipolar I disorder: a randomised, open-label, pilot study. Lancet Psychiatry 4:208–217, 2017

Yazaki Y, Faridi Z, Ma Y, et al: A pilot study of chromium picolinate for weight loss. J Altern Complement Med 16:291–299, 2010

Young RM, Lawford BR, Barnes M, et al: Prolactin levels in antipsychotic treatment of patients with schizophrenia carrying the DRD2*A1 allele. Br J Psychiatry 185:147–151, 2004

Zawadzki JK, Dunaif A: Diagnostic criteria for polycystic ovary syndrome: towards a rational approach, in Polycystic Ovary Syndrome. Edited by Dunaif A, Givens JR, Haseltine F, et al. Oxford, UK, Blackwell Scientific, 1992, pp 377–384

Zesiewicz TA, Elble R, Louis ED, et al: Practice parameter: therapies for essential tremor: report of the Quality Standards Subcommittee of the American Academy of Neurology. Neurology 64:2008–2020, 2005

Zhang WF, Tan YL, Zhang XY, et al: Extract of Ginkgo biloba treatment for tardive dyskinesia in schizophrenia: a randomized, double-blind, placebo-controlled trial. J Clin Psychiatry 72:615–621, 2011

Zhang XY, Tan YL, Zhou DF, et al: Association of clozapine-induced weight gain with a polymorphism in the leptin promoter region in patients with chronic schizophrenia in a Chinese population. J Clin Psychopharmacol 27:246–251, 2007

Ziere G, Dieleman JP, van der Cammen TJ, et al: Selective serotonin reuptake inhibiting antidepressants are associated with an increased risk of nonvertebral fractures. J Clin Psychopharmacol 28:411–417, 2008

Index

*Page numbers printed in **boldface** type refer to tables or figures.*